THE HANDBO

NURSING ASSOCIATES AND ASSISTANT PRACTITIONERS

Sara Miller McCune founded SAGE Publishing in 1965 to support the dissemination of usable knowledge and educate a global community. SAGE publishes more than 1000 journals and over 800 new books each year, spanning a wide range of subject areas. Our growing selection of library products includes archives, data, case studies and video. SAGE remains majority owned by our founder and after her lifetime will become owned by a charitable trust that secures the company's continued independence.

Los Angeles | London | New Delhi | Singapore | Washington DC | Melbourne

THE HANDBOOK FOR NURSING ASSOCIATES AND ASSISTANT PRACTITIONERS

GILLIAN ROWE, SCOTT ELLIS, DEBORAH GEE,
KEVIN GRAHAM, MICHELLE HENDERSON, JANETTE BARNES,
CHRIS COUNIHAN, AMI JACKSON AND JADE CARTER-BENNETT

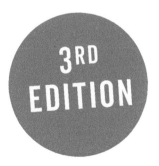

3RD
EDITION

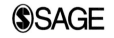

Los Angeles | London | New Delhi
Singapore | Washington DC | Melbourne

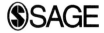

Los Angeles | London | New Delhi
Singapore | Washington DC | Melbourne

SAGE Publications Ltd
1 Oliver's Yard
55 City Road
London EC1Y 1SP

SAGE Publications Inc.
2455 Teller Road
Thousand Oaks, California 91320

SAGE Publications India Pvt Ltd
B 1/I 1 Mohan Cooperative Industrial Area
Mathura Road
New Delhi 110 044

SAGE Publications Asia-Pacific Pte Ltd
3 Church Street
#10-04 Samsung Hub
Singapore 049483

Editorial Arrangement © Gillian Rowe 2023; Chapter 1 © Chris Counihan 2023; Chapters 2, 4, 6, 7, 9, 10 and 13 © Gillian Rowe 2023; Chapter 3 © Michelle Henderson 2023; Chapter 5 © Gillian Rowe and Ami Jackson 2023; Chapter 8 © Deborah Gee 2023; Chapter 11 © Michelle Henderson and Gillian Rowe 2023; Chapter 12 © Scott Ellis 2023; Chapter 14 © Janette Barnes and Jade Carter-Bennett 2023; Chapter 15 © Kevin Graham and Gillian Rowe 2023

Apart from any fair dealing for the purposes of research, private study, or criticism or review, as permitted under the Copyright, Designs and Patents Act, 1988, this publication may not be reproduced, stored or transmitted in any form, or by any means, without the prior permission in writing of the publisher, or in the case of reprographic reproduction, in accordance with the terms of licences issued by the Copyright Licensing Agency. Enquiries concerning reproduction outside those terms should be sent to the publisher.

Editor: Laura Walmsley
Assistant editor: Sahar Jamfar
Production editor: Sarah Sewell
Copyeditor: Jane Fricker
Proofreader: Rosemary Campbell
Indexer: Martin Hargreaves
Marketing manager: Ruslana Khatagova
Cover design: Sheila Tong
Typeset by: C&M Digitals (P) Ltd, Chennai, India
Printed in the UK

Library of Congress Control Number: 2022935610

British Library Cataloguing in Publication data

A catalogue record for this book is available from the British Library

ISBN 978-1-5297-8982-9
ISBN 978-1-5297-8981-2 (pbk)

At SAGE we take sustainability seriously. Most of our products are printed in the UK using responsibly sourced papers and boards. When we print overseas we ensure sustainable papers are used as measured by the PREPS grading system. We undertake an annual audit to monitor our sustainability.

CONTENTS

LIST OF TABLES AND FIGURES

TABLES

FIGURES

ONLINE RESOURCES FOR INSTRUCTORS

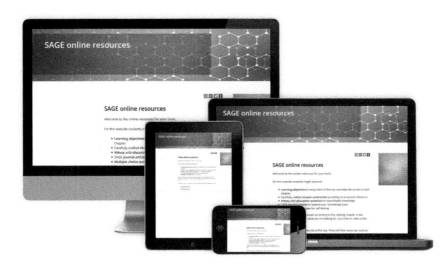

Instructors can visit https://study.sagepub.com/rowehandbook3e to access a **Teaching Guide** featuring chapter overviews and aims, teaching and assessment suggestions and links to additional video content.

ABOUT THE AUTHORS

Gillian Rowe is a full-time writer and researcher working with marginalised groups such as the GRT community. She has edited and authored chapters for this book and has edited and written for the Learning Matters imprint on health promotion and ethics and values for nursing associates. Gillian has extensive experience of the healthcare sector, having been a qualified nurse and then managed a large residential care facility. Gillian completed a PGCE and lectured for Plymouth University; Gillian is an Associate Fellow of the Higher Education Academy (AFHEA).

Janette Barnes completed her Social Work degree in 2009 and worked for Barnardo's supporting children with disabilities and their families. Many of the children were diagnosed with autism – a subject she has continued to research and advise on. Janette has a teaching qualification and delivers training on disability issues and autism. She has also supported and mentored social work students. Janette is currently taking a career break to travel.

Jade Carter-Bennett has been a qualified social worker since 2015, after receiving her BA Hons Social Work Degree from Plymouth University. During this time, Jade has undertaken post-qualification studies with the University of the West of England and obtained her Experienced Social Worker level under the Professional Capabilities Framework in 2021. Jade worked primarily within the Adult Sector but now specialises in Transitions to Adulthood. She has also been involved in working with parents with learning disabilities and has become a Practice Workplace Supervisor, supporting and mentoring social work students.

Chris Counihan completed a PhD in Education at Newcastle University which studied the effects of a peer-mediated literacy intervention with children from rural India. Chris has over 10 years' experience of working and leading on international development and education projects. His primary research interests lie in the field of child development and policy initiatives in education. He is currently developing ideas under the 'Education for All' agenda that targets poverty alleviation and educational empowerment. Chris' research has positively impacted children's learning opportunities in some of the poorest areas of the world, such as India, Ghana, Sierra Leone and Tanzania. Chris is a Lecturer in Education at Northumbria University and a Teaching Fellow of the Higher Education Academy (HEA).

Scott Ellis is a postdoctoral researcher, educator and public health specialist working across multi-disciplinary projects in suicide prevention and social inequalities. He has a wealth of experience in the public health and social care sectors and specialises in research in sexual health and marginalised groups. He works across public and private healthcare; he is an Acute Healthcare inspector for the Care Quality Commission and contributes to the NHS National Institute of Health Research. Scott is a Fellow of the Higher Education Academy (FHEA), a Fellow of Advanced HE (FAHE) and a Fellow of the Royal Society for Public Health (FRSPH).

Deborah Gee is a Senior Lecturer and course leader for Nursing Associates within the School of Health and Social Care at Teesside University. In 2006 Deborah qualified as a registered nurse and has worked within a variety of settings including Neonatal Intensive Care and Community District Nursing. In 2010 Deborah completed her PGDip SCPHN qualification and has significant experience working with families and young children assessing and identifying their health needs, and that of the wider population in her role as a health visitor. Deborah has an MSc in Education in Professional Practice, in addition to holding recognised teacher status with the Nursing and Midwifery Council. Deborah is a Fellow of the Higher Education Academy.

Kevin Graham has been a Lecturer and Programme Leader in Higher Education for many years. He has lectured on a range of subjects, including Health and Social Care, Children and Young People's Studies, Law, Politics and Sociology in colleges in the Northeast at A-Level, Foundation Degree and Honours Degree level. Kevin is also a published author who has worked in a variety of different roles in addition to teaching: this includes managing an education charity for adults with learning difficulties and being a Local Authority Cabinet Member for Adult Social Care. He is a doctoral candidate and his current research interests are political history and theory.

Michelle Henderson is a qualified adult nurse and Specialist Community Public Health Nurse (SCPHN). She completed her first degree at Northumbria University and has also completed an MSc in Healthcare Leadership and is a registered coach having completed an ILM qualification in coaching and mentoring. She has worked in a range of NHS clinical specialties as well as non-NHS settings. She has specialised in public health settings for a number of years, including working as a Sister in Occupational Health at a large foundation trust where she completed her SCPHN degree. Michelle has also worked at Public Health England (now known as UKHSA) as a health protection nurse and Health Education England as workforce lead for Nursing and Midwifery development across the Northeast and Yorkshire. She has also been a practice tutor supporting Trainee Nursing Associates on Open University programmes. She currently works at NHS England as a senior nurse in the Northeast and Cumbria Nursing and Quality team. In her spare time, she is a mentor for the Social Mobility Foundation and is passionate about health inequalities, social mobility, and education and development of the nursing workforce.

Ami Jackson began her nursing career as a cadet nurse and then completed her pre-registration training at Northumbria University in 2007. She went on to complete a Practice Development degree in 2013. Ami has worked in a variety of areas including stroke rehabilitation, acute older persons' medicine, intensive care and orthopaedic surgery. Ami became a ward sister on an orthopaedic trauma unit and developed significant experience in leadership and management. More recently, Ami was a Practice Placement Facilitator, leading on pre-registration nursing programmes within her local NHS Trust. Ami now tutors Training Nursing Associates at Teesside University and is completing a master's degree in Global Leadership.

ACKNOWLEDGEMENTS

The authors wish to express their very great appreciation to Laura Walmsley, Becky Taylor, Charlène Burin, Alex Clabburn and Jade Grogan at SAGE for their help, advice and guidance.

We would also like to give our love and thanks to our partners, families and friends for their continued support during the writing of this third edition.

Our especial thanks go to Lewis Wade, John Wheatley and Roo Cooper for their amazing drawings. Our thanks also go to Danni Nash, Rebecca Woodman, John Wheatley and Wade Lewis for allowing us to use photographs of their arms for various chapters.

We would particularly like to thank our contributing students and trainee nursing associates: Julie Greenslade, Heather Tilmouth, Heather Saint, Lindsey Shaw, Susan Beany and Gillian Nesbit.

We are also grateful to Dolores Campanario at the World Health Organization for her help with WHO authorised images. Also, many thanks to the following for their amazing support in granting us use of their images: Krishna Stone at GMHC.org, Teri Christenson at Drugfree. org, Marc van Gurp at Osocio.org, Thelma Simmons at communityhealth. ku.edu, Ford Higson at Ishtm.ac.uk, Brian Chittock at aidsvancouver.org, Alan Davidson at the Better Life Chances Unit, Scottish Government, and more thanks to Charlène Burin and Jade Grogan at SAGE for access to designs created in-house.

ABOUT THE BOOK

In choosing to study for the role of Nursing Associate or to enter into a higher level practitioner apprenticeship, you are following a career choice made since the role was officially created by the NHS and Community Care Act 1990 and the *Shape of Caring Review* in 2015. The recorded history of caring goes back to the ancient Greeks and Egyptians, and Ayurvedic practitioners have an equally long history. In Christian countries, caring was provided by monks and nuns, and we still call female ward managers 'Sister' as a result of this. Nursing auxiliaries followed Florence Nightingale to the Crimean War (1854–6) but it took until 1955 for the auxiliary role to be formalised. After the 1990 Act, the auxiliary role within the NHS was renamed 'Healthcare Assistant' (HCA).

The Cavendish Review (2013) explains that the NHS treats HCAs and the registered nurses who supervise them as separate workforces. Cavendish continued, stating that 'A glaring example is the failure to consider how the move to all-degree nursing would affect the career prospects of HCAs. Good hospitals and care homes are now unable to promote some of their best assistants into nursing roles. This is a waste of talent which must be overcome by urgently developing new bridging programmes' (p. 58). Higher level care workers and band 4 healthcare practitioners (HCPs)/healthcare assistants (HCAs) deserve a career progression and some form of recognition for the work they do, and the assistant practitioner (AP) and new nursing associate (NA) roles go some way to meeting that recognition.

Nursing associate and assistant practitioner students enter programmes of study from a variety of routes; many of you were previously either HCAs or care workers and you are transitioning into the role of a regulated healthcare professional. As these roles mature, it will become easier to make the mental transition and accept more responsibility. The first nursing associate cohorts were pioneers in this programme and suffered from role ambiguity and a lack of role clarity. There was a lack of understanding within employing organisations and among mentoring staff who didn't really understand what the role was, or viewed it as a modern version of the old state enrolled nurse (SEN). This led to questions about the longevity of the role, but given the acute shortage of trained staff, this is unlikely to be an issue for a significant period of time. The local apprenticeship route offers an affordable opportunity for career progression without the burden of student debt and the need for geographical relocation.

You will experience an exciting range of opportunities as you progress through placements which will influence your career aspirations, and if you adopt a 'can do' attitude and a positive outlook to each learning opportunity you will achieve your goals. Remember that your lecturers and supervisors want you to succeed and will support you every step on your journey to becoming a qualified Nursing Associate (NA) or Assistant Practitioner (AP). We hope this book facilitates your learning and encourages you to become a knowledgeable and thoughtful health practitioner.

This book has been constructed by considering the Standards of Proficiency for Nursing Associates, the apprenticeship standards, and the Learning Domains for the Nursing Associate training programme, these are highlighted at the beginning of each chapter and the tables of apprenticeship standards and learning domains is at the end of the book. Many aspects of the Foundation Degrees in Associate Practitioner, Health and Social Care and Healthcare Practice are also included within this book, so we hope you find it a useful addition to your library.

LEARNING FEATURES: ENGAGING WITH THE TEXT

The book has pedagogic content for you to use as aids to learning, Go Further readings, links to websites and journal articles and reflective activities. These have been designed to stretch and challenge you and deepen your knowledge. This will also help you to become an active independent learner. For the third edition we have included reflections from trainee nursing associates, and we hope these will support your understanding of theory into practice.

ICONS

Throughout the book you will see icons in the margin for 'Values', 'Communication and Interpersonal Skills', 'Chapter Cross-references' and 'Person-centred Approach'. These flag up places where these skills are highlighted to support you to deliver high quality care.

Values

Communication
& Interpersonal
Skills

Chapter
Cross-
references

Person-
centred
Approach

A NOTE ON TERMINOLOGY: HOW ARE THEY KNOWN?

Throughout this book, those for whom we care are called 'patients'. This is because it is too unwieldy to write 'patient slash client slash service user' each time they are mentioned. So please mentally insert the name you use at your work setting, and we apologise if it gets annoying.

REFERENCE

Cavendish, C. (2013) *Review of Healthcare Assistants and Support Workers in NHS and Social Care*. London: Department of Health. Available at: www.gov.uk/government/publications/review-of-healthcare-assistants-and-support-workers-in-nhs-and-social-care

PART ONE

ACADEMIC, PERSONAL AND PROFESSIONAL DEVELOPMENT

1

DEVELOPING ACADEMIC STUDY SKILLS: TECHNIQUES AND GUIDANCE FOR UNDERGRADUATE STUDENTS

CHRIS COUNIHAN

STANDARDS OF PROFICIENCY FOR NURSING ASSOCIATES (2018)

Relevant Platforms include:

Platform 1:1.7 Describe the principles of research and how research findings are used to inform evidence-based practice.

Platform 1:1.13 Demonstrate the numeracy, literacy, digital and technological skills required to meet the needs of people in their care to ensure safe and effective practice.

Platform 1:1.15 Take responsibility for continuous self-reflection, seeking and responding to support and feedback to develop professional knowledge and skills.

Question everything – identify any assumptions that may have been made including the author's stance and what an opposing argument may be; whether there is enough evidence to justify their conclusions and investigate alternative views.

Julie Greenslade, BA (Hons) Student

This chapter will introduce you to the skill set needed to succeed as a higher level student, through using the internet to engage in research, how to sift through the research to locate the information you need and then how to use the information gained properly and to reference it to Harvard convention.

Glossary

- **HE** Higher education
- **Referencing** Ensuring that you do not commit plagiarism
- **Reflection** The deliberate consideration of troubling thoughts
- **Theory** A hypothesis that has been tested and a theory formulated

INTRODUCTION

This chapter provides a snapshot of various techniques, skills and concepts required for enhancing quality learning outputs in higher education (HE). Each section contains guidance, review and practice examples for transfer into your own study domain. In the first section, we consider how previously acquired skills can be useful in a variety of HE learning situations. Second, we look at how to conduct effective searches online to maximise your time spent analysing, critiquing and producing. Finally, we revisit practical concepts of referencing works in your assignments. Use this chapter as your mini support guide at the beginning or during your course of study.

PREPARING TO LEARN IN HIGHER EDUCATION

It might seem a little odd, but the best way to learn is to revisit skills you already possess. For example, let's say you can speak a second language, but your learning goal is to master how to write it. In this case, you look at what you have already understood about the language and build a plan for learning how to write it. Understanding the tools for the job through problem solving, personal reflection and development are essential to your success in HE. Recognition of prior learning is key for your plans as you take previously acquired skills and implement them into future learning activities.

One of the problems when we think about learning is the relationship it has with schooling, which may lead to the resurfacing of old nightmares and panic-stricken worry. I include myself in this. You might reflect on a disastrous learning journey; moreover, you might feel unrewarded or unchallenged – hence your interest now in studying for a degree. Lots of neurological research has your back here. When threatened, our brains go into shutdown. The amygdala, which is in the centre of our brains, is trained in the art of detecting stressful events and determining whether you turn into a Persian Kitten, like me, or a Spartan Warrior, roar!

Fortunately, learning has changed, and HE offers open forums to include discussion, debate and personal reflection, thus enabling you to make your own mind up. One of its strengths is the desire to recognise skills and use them in a variety of academic contexts. We might consider academic reading, writing and presenting ideas as being too challenging, but we all have skills that we can use for academic study. The truth is, we use most of these unconsciously every day, which makes them perfect to be developed for academic study.

You already possess remarkable abilities for making analytical, creative and practical judgements. Consider when buying an item of clothing: you analyse the price, shape and colour. Perhaps you will compare it with another piece of clothing before making a decision. Furthermore, being creative doesn't necessarily mean you will build a robot that writes essays; instead, you will deploy solutions based on personal and professional experiences. Finally, being practical, here you will draw upon skills that have not been taught to you, things you are able to do naturally without pause for thought. Recognise when you can select one (or more) of your superpowers when approaching learning in the HE environment. You may be pleasantly surprised at how well they will serve you. Learning to use your intellectual faculties, such as asking questions of the texts you are reading, is a skill that you will need to develop. Table 1.1 gives you guidance.

Robert Sternberg (1985) has researched intelligence all around the world. He views intelligence in his 'triarchic model', which includes the three classifications shown in Table 1.1.

Table 1.1   Using your intelligence

Analytical	Creative	Practical
Intellectual capability to problem solve, complete tests and make informed judgements	Intellectual capability to tackle unusual problems drawing on pre-existing skills and experiences – the 'thinking outside of the box' approach to problems	Intellectual capability to deploy 'tacit' skills to a unique set of problems. There might not be an exam, course or guidance for such a scenario and it depends on your interaction with the experience first hand

See examples of how you could apply Sternberg's model below to help with your own reflections.

Analytical	George, a second-year degree student is tasked with comparing two academic health diversity journal articles. Using his analytical skills, George reviews each article for underlying themes, messages and emergent discussion points before making a list he will use for critical comparative judgement.
Creative	Noah and James are working together on a project set by their tutor. The task is to produce a digital presentation on evaluating polypharmacy and the risk of adverse health conditions. The digital presentation is open to interpretation and as such, Noah and James must decide how to present their findings. They decide to use their newly acquired digital skills from attending a study skills workshop to develop a Microsoft Sway presentation. They creatively bring together text and media to explain key definitions and current risks associated with polypharmacy.
Practical	Hallie is working on developing her referencing skills. She starts to look at different stylistic ways to reference in-text (e.g. author followed by date and secondary referencing). Hallie realises there are many ways to use and apply references in her academic work. Hallie then writes out several different approaches and highlights them with different colours. Highlighting using various colours has helped Hallie recall and memorise techniques in the past. Hallie uses this skill to help practise her referencing styles, which she intends on using in future written academic assignments.

⚙️ Activity 1.1

Using Sternberg's triarchic model of intelligence, reflect on your own learning and work experiences, then write down one example for each. See the table above for descriptions and examples.

DEVELOPING SKILLS AND TECHNIQUES FOR ONLINE SEARCHES

Let's look at some of the basic skills. When researching a topic, it is vital that you are able to locate the information required to fulfil assessment criteria. The following five tips will demonstrate how to effectively navigate along the information highway:

1. **Control 'F'** – The Time Saver! It operates a mini-search function within any web page, article and/or other word processing software. It works by pressing the 'Control' button (Command button if you are using a Mac) followed by the 'F' button on your keyboard. From here, a box

will appear in the top right of the browser. Typing any word into the box and pressing return will automatically search the entire document for your chosen word. This command can be particularly useful if you are reviewing/searching an article for predetermined keywords.

2. **Boolean** searches can enable a specific focus for a keyword and term searches.Type in the following commands separately to narrow down searches:

   a. OR – you might want to search for two separate terms such as 'NHS OR Private' – the OR function will list the number of sites that relate to the first or second term.
   b. You can combine your searches using phrase and key terms in parentheses, such as 'Obesity treatment (NHS OR Private)' which will list sites that relate to 'Obesity treatment' on sites containing the words 'NHS' and 'Private', separately.
   c. BUT – this allows terms to be specified while limiting other possible connections. For example, 'Skin cancer BUT NOT melanoma'. Searches will eliminate sites containing 'melanoma' skin cancers and concentrate on listings of non-melanoma hits.
   d. ADJ – this command will look for a term that is positioned within a specified distance (number of words). For example, say you search for 'Public Health obesity ADJ 4'. The search will retrieve all records of 'public' 'health' 'obesity' within four words of each other.
   e. Google Advanced Search provides a variety of variables (language, date, region, etc.) for searches and can be found at: www.google.com/advanced_search

3. **Authority** – Published work and material found online comes in a variety of forms, such as traditional academic articles found in journals, newspapers, magazines, blogs and the like. When considering authority in your searches, you must make a judgement on information presented to you. You should ask yourself the following questions:

   a. Who is the author and how are they the expert?
   b. Has it been verified by academic peers (known as peer review)?
   c. How do I know that it isn't made up?

4. **Evidence** – It's all about the evidence. It is vital to question everything, unleashing your analytical and evaluative reasoning skills. This means that you must analyse a number of sources before using information in your assignments. Ask the following questions:

   a. Is the information from opinion or based on studied research material?
   b. Is there similar evidence that verifies the original claim(s)? Are there other studies, ideas or information that say the same thing?
   c. Does the article offer a balanced view, that is, the inclusion of counter-evidence?

5. **Time** – As with most things, there is a shelf life. Fortunately, web pages don't smell bad when they go off. The truth is that web pages don't really go off at all, instead, they go into hiding and then reappear when something triggers an associated interest. Fans and users of Twitter will be familiar with trending media; this is essentially the same process. A web page might trend again and accelerate to a higher ranking along the information highway. As Google ranked it highly, you assume that the information is current and decide to use it in your assignment. WARNING! You must investigate the publication date as the web page might have resurfaced from years past and be outdated. You will need to check the date of the original source before employing sentences like these in your work:

    a. Recent evidence suggests …
    b. The latest statistics show …

    How far back should one go? There's no consensus on this, but as with the terms above – recent and latest – there is an assumption that information is current or is the leading frame of thought at that time. Of course, if your assignment asks that you include historical accounts then you have the licence to trace longer developments but keep these focused. Seminal theories, famous debates/arguments and other historical content should form the basis of your enquiry.

ASSESSMENTS AND THE APPLICATION OF ANALYTICAL, CRITICAL AND EVALUATIVE REASONING

UNDERSTANDING ASSESSMENTS

When developing degree level programmes within HE, course leaders have a wealth of assessment methods in their arsenal to choose from. Course leaders will select assessments based on overall module objectives and the interdisciplinary skills students are required to demonstrate. What is important to understand is that your degree programme is designed specially to accelerate your personal, professional and academic skills and knowledge. Well-planned modules include a broad range of skills and relative assessment methods for subsequent demonstration.

Nightingale et al. (1996) originally suggested eight learning outcomes demonstrable while studying in HE. They include the following:

*   Thinking critically and making judgements
*   Problem solving and developing plans
*   Performing procedures and demonstrating techniques
*   Managing and developing oneself

- Accessing and managing information
- Demonstrating knowledge and understanding
- Designing, creating and performing
- Communicating

⚙ **Activity 1.2**

Write down one example for each of the eight learning outcomes that you have demonstrated in the work or school environment. Include a short description of what you did and how you did it.

As you can see from Nightingale et al. (1996), there are broad learning outcomes with some interconnections (i.e. communicating and performing) while others are diverse (critical thinking vs creative outputs). The point is your degree will encompass each one through a range of skill/vocational assessment methods. But which methods are suitable against each competency? Figure 1.1 provides a synthesis of Nightingale et al.'s (1996) taxonomy and provides details on the types of assessments used against grouped skills.

Figure 1.1 is by no means an exhaustive list of core competencies or definite assessments. Instead, it provides a snapshot of the skills/vocational competencies allied to assessment methods that you are likely to face. Course leaders will consider the broader spectrum, so immediate tasks relate to module assessment tasks, tracking your development across the degree programme.

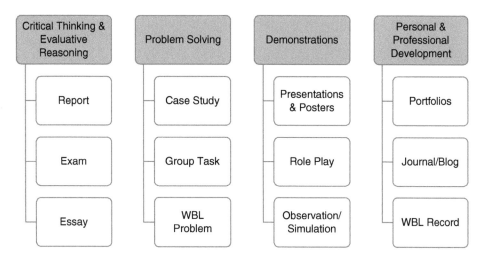

Figure 1.1   Grouped skills and assessment methods

ESSAYS

Essays are perhaps the most common assessment type in HE. They can vary in length and require time for researching themes, sorting notes, creating arguments and summarising main points. Essays are intended to inform your lecturers as to how well you have understood salient theories, arguments and themes about a studied topic. Let's consider the following essay question from a Healthcare Practice course:

> Justify what is meant by quality of care? Critically appraise the theoretical dimensions of organisational cultures in a chosen UK healthcare provider.

To approach the question, it is easier to break down what it is asking us to present for assessment. We can do this in a variety of ways. Firstly, we recognise the keywords, which are usually the verbs as they ask us to do something. In the question above, we note the following verbs and their meaning as:

- Justify – to provide evidence for a claim in knowledge
- Appraise – to evaluate the quality of something through assessing its worth

We use the terminology to help navigate our research about the topic and start to plan the structure of our essay. Remember that an essay is like a story, with a beginning, a middle and an end, you use the essay title to guide how the story (the narrative) goes. Always consult your college's style guide and ask to see samples of previous students' work so you have a clear idea of what is expected of you. Some colleges do not allow the use of Google; although Google Scholar is a good place to search for journal articles or books, you should learn to use your internal platform (Moodle, Blackboard, NHS database/digital services). Ask for help in the library, someone there will support you to use the system.

For the question above, we might adopt the following structure:

Introduction

- To outline how the essay is structured – signposting to core themes such as key policy care documents and legislation. We might consider introducing specific theories that will be referred to, and the organisation chosen as our case study. Essay introductions should offer a sequence to improve the transitions between themes, concepts and major ideas.

Middle paragraphs

- Definitions and legal representations of quality of care from a UK perspective
- Salient arguments and key academic debates on future directions of quality of care

- Description of chosen healthcare provider and how they implement/ challenge the above (using your placement as a physical reference)
- Examine chosen provider by linking theory to practice in relation to organisational culture

Conclusion

- A summary of the main findings and themes throughout the essay. This will include a brief recap of how you answered the essay question followed by concluding remarks. No new ideas or theories should be introduced here, only a summary of what was investigated and interpreted through your careful analysis.

Essay questions and learning outcomes/objectives arrive in various formats. Module guides illustrate what is required for assessment and these will be indispensable when you start to plan your essay. Below are some of the common directive terms, as adapted from Lewis' (1999: 42) comprehensive list of words (and associated meanings) used in essay questioning:

- Analyse – look at multiple parts of something (theme, argument, idea) and examine each in detail
- Describe – provide a detailed account of your subject/topic – usually, answers the what of something
- Discuss – investigate various accounts of something – multiple views or using various arguments giving reasons for each angle
- Compare – look for the similarities and differences of something
- Explain – an interpretation followed by an accurate account of something
- Evaluate – supported by valid evidence, an appraisal of something which might include your own reflections (if related to work placement or learning journeys)
- Identify – recognise an important part of something and include brief descriptions
- Interpret – understanding the reality of something, making clear and informed judgements
- Justify – make a clear argument for something supported by valid and justifiable evidence

⚙️ Activity 1.3

Look at the following passages and detect the descriptive, critical and explanation voices. Choose only one for each passage and note down the differences for each.

(Continued)

1. Cystic fibrosis is a condition that is inherited that affects the performance in the lungs and kidneys due to the presence of thick and sticky mucus (NHS, 2016). In the UK, statistics show that one in every 2500 babies are born with the disease. It is suggested that improvements that relate to newborn screening tests have a better clinical condition when compared to patients diagnosed clinically within the first 10 years of life (Dankert-Roelse and Vernooij-van Langen, 2011).

2. Cystic fibrosis is a condition that is inherited that affects the performance in the lungs and kidneys due to the presence of thick and sticky mucus (NHS, 2016). In the UK, statistics show that one in every 2500 babies are born with the disease.

3. Cystic fibrosis is a condition that is inherited that affects the performance in the lungs and kidneys due to the presence of thick and sticky mucus (NHS, 2016). In the UK, statistics indicate that one in every 2500 babies are born with the disease. It is suggested that improvements that relate to newborn screening tests have a better clinical condition when compared to patients diagnosed clinically within the first 10 years of life (Dankert-Roelse and Vernooij-van Langen, 2011). However, this is not universally agreed due to complications, following screening, leading to a course of treatment when there are no physical signs of respiratory problems (Dankert-Roelse and Vernooij-van Langen, 2011). The arguments are multifaceted, but studies have identified parental factors in screening decisions. One study found parental preference for early diagnosis even if it led to untreatable outcomes (Plass et al., 2010). However, other studies report increased anxiety levels when waiting for additional diagnostic testing (Dankert-Roelse and Vernooij-van Langen, 2011). In summary, parental factors alone cannot sway this argument; further clinical evidence is required and discussed as a major theme of this report.

Answers are at the end of the chapter.

REPORTS

Often confused with essays and vice versa, reports might contain various different ideas within specific sections. This is the distinction between the traditional essay and a report. Table 1.2 details a typical report structure with supporting explanations of each section.

It is important to check your module guide, as specific guidance will be presented on stylistic measures for assessment. Reports come in all shapes and include different elements. You should always refer to the guidance as set by your HE provider.

Table 1.2　Report structure

Structure	Explanation
Introduction	• Includes an abstract or executive summary situated at the beginning and provides a descriptive account of the main findings
Main body	• Presents the main ideas and arguments in different sections (these might be numbered) • Multiple sections can be used to bring together a variety of ideas that interlink with the main topic, for example: 1.2　Malaria 　　1.2.1　Malaria Prevention 　　1.2.2　Malaria Diagnosis • The above example showcases the topic of malaria followed by its constituent sections. Each relates to the overarching topic (malaria) but provides further details on prevention followed by diagnosis
Conclusions	• A comprehensive conclusion drawing upon each section of the report • May include a personal reflection section or recommendations
References	• Inclusion of all source types – academic/non-academic
Graphical	• May include diagrams, charts, tables and other graphical illustrations

BLOGS/REFLECTIVE DIARY

Throughout your academic and vocational learning journeys, you will be required to reflect on particular tasks that you undertake. These might be assessed through a diary/blog or as part of classroom exercises such as role-playing. Reflection is a key part of your ability to understand your previous and new experiences. Jasper (2003: 2) describes the process of being reflective as 'the way that we learn from an experience in order to understand and develop practice'. In this regard, you will learn from an experience before redesigning it for practice based on newly acquired skills. The process is continuous and spirals, as new experiences will arrive, and the process is repeated. Documenting this in your studies can be tricky as you are developing skills, knowledge and vocation concurrently throughout a lifelong learning process. Therefore, it is more about taking a snapshot of skill acquisition rather than a description of polished mastery. Fortunately, there are various models and cycles that can help you to capture your development. The two you might come across in your programme are Kolb's (1984) Experiential Learning Cycle and Gibbs' Reflective Cycle (1988) (see Figure 1.2), which improved on Kolb's work in educational reflection theory. Both provide a conceptual framework that you can use in reflective tasks you undertake.

> ## Go Further 1.1
>
> See Chapter 2, Personal and Professional Development, for in-depth detail on how to engage in reflection. You can find more about Kolb's Experiential Learning as it relates to public health practitioners by following this link to a free article which demonstrates the use of the cycle as an aid to research: 'Reflection as part of continuous professional development for public health professionals: a literature review' at: http://jpubhealth.oxfordjournals.org/content/early/2012/10/16/pubmed. fds083.full. It is typically presented to students in a cyclic format to help construct deeper, more meaningful reflections.

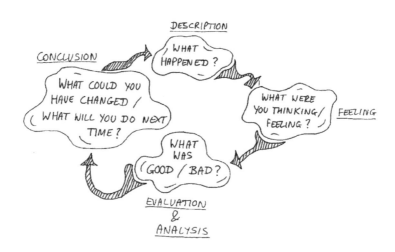

Figure 1.2   Gibbs' Reflective Cycle (1988)

It is not uncommon for students to receive feedback stating the need to be more critical and to bring counterarguments or differing perspectives into their work. Perhaps the reason behind this is to do with the negative connotations of taking a critical approach. You might think of criticality as the protagonist in provoking or upsetting someone. It is a falsism to criticise personally and act without justification or evidence in any domain, not least academic study. The other factor is to do with learning new material. It is impossible to write critically if we do not have all of the information to hand. This requires an analytical approach because we need to locate, appraise and evaluate material before including it in our work. For example, you might be writing about health and wellbeing – which is a broad area covering many categories, perspectives and actors. Taking the analytical approach requires careful synthesis of all associated parts, identifying crossover relationships and trends when researching material. One way to achieve this is through a concept map. This is a visual method for connecting themes and investigating trends and relationships. Not to be confused with mind maps, they are more structured – looking in detail at how (and why in some cases) themes are connected. Figure 1.3 illustrates a basic concept map that investigates health and wellbeing.

The connected arrows indicate the relationship between different parts and the theme. The theme lifestyle has links to exercise, diet and sleep. The visual aspect of creating a concept map helps us to arrange complex information. Our brains are very good at deciphering complex visual material and arranging them into meaningful categories. There are a number of good references online for creating a concept map, but the process usually considers the gathering of themes (brainstorming) and organisation – you might use sticky notes to write out themes. Then, a drafting process of laying out material, exploring connections. Finally, these are written to show which themes connect to main and sub-themes. Going through this process enables us to understand important components and their relationship to the topic we are researching. It is a useful starting point for consolidating ideas and preparing for the next step of critical and evaluative writing.

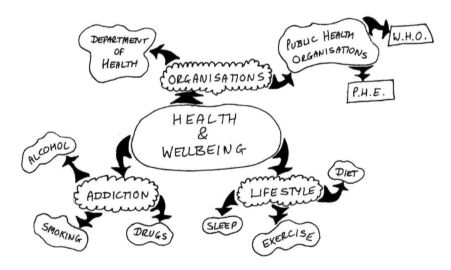

Figure 1.3   Health and wellbeing concept map

After completing a concept map and subsequent investigation into relationships and trends, the next stage will be to write about them, thus moving from the descriptive to the critical and evaluative stages of your assignment. Using the search tips we discussed earlier, you will locate a bank of pertinent scholarly evidence in preparation for writing your assignment. It might be useful to extend your concept map to bridge between the positive and negative arguments about something. A good critical analysis will be balanced and reflective before leading to an overall summation of a topic. In this way, you should remain independent and impartial to what is being said. Your focus is bringing attention to the key arguments and perspectives on said phenomena. Only when a reasoned and justifiable conclusion has been made can it be considered critically approved.

ANNOTATING ACADEMIC ARTICLES

After conducting initial searches, you will have selected one or two academic articles you think are appropriate to your topic. One useful technique to use when narrowing down articles is skim reading. Fortunately, academic articles include an abstract – which is a summary of what the article contains. You will be able to do keyword searches and apply techniques as discussed earlier to highlight anything of importance and focus on the details required.

Think of academic articles as a sales pitch. Recall a time when someone was trying to sell you something. Think about their approach and the language they used. Academic articles won't sell you a car, or anything tangible for that matter, but they will offer you an idea. Authors will use convincing language to grab your attention and get you on their side – so to speak. This isn't a trick or a mind control attempt; instead, articles go through a process of falsification, where other academics review and question the scientific rigour of what is presented and discussed. Personal beliefs will always need support from evidence of studied phenomena. Keep this in mind when developing your own critical concepts.

Thinking critically can springboard you to write critically. Sounds simple, but you need to know what you are looking for. Critical annotation can help, so let's start with the following article by Fujii (2021), who researched the sleep quality and personality traits of patients with Parkinson's disease pre- and post-diagnosis to determine how these factors affected patients' quality of life. Like all good science, the article explains the problem area, introduces us to methods and procedures of how they collected their data, presented results and discussed their findings. Generally speaking, this is how all academic articles are presented. We start to analyse the present article by understanding its main headlines. Let's consider asking the following questions:

- What is the main problem area(s) the article specifically addresses?
- Who were the participants in the study?
- How did the author(s) go about collecting their data?
- What were the final results and were these positive/negative?

The above will help to shape a descriptive overview, which we include in our final essay. It might be written like this:

> Fujii (2021) researched the subjective sleep traits and personality pre- and post-Parkinson's disease (PD) diagnosis to determine the implications of these traits for multiple home care strategies. Using a cross-sectional survey research design, results suggest patients with PD reported a post-diagnosis decrease in sleep time but this increases during nap time. Other findings included the study subjects reporting becoming tense easily but they did not report feeling irritated or angry. The subjective assessment suggested a post-diagnosis worsening of sleep quality in patients with PD.

Following the description part, we then move into the critical stage. To help us, let's consider asking the following questions:

- What types of methods did the author(s) use? Were they appropriately performed?
- Was each method viable for each of the results presented? Could there be another way? Provide details on improvements, if any.
- Did the author(s) interpret results accurately through an informed discussion?
- Was there mention of the limitations of the study? What were they? How does this affect the overall results?
- What other evidence is out there to contest/agree with these findings?

The above are some questions that we may ask ourselves when applying criticality. It is useful to make notes in the margin of the paper or use digital markers if preferred. Annotating each section will no doubt throw up further questions, thus it is important to keep the focus on what it was that originally drew your attention to the paper. Always ask yourself – 'how will this article feature in my final assignment?'

Once we have analysed the article we come to add in our critical points. All academic articles will have a limitation section or some reference to how they would either do the study again or some justification on the issues surrounding data collection/analysis. If we run a Control-F search for limitations in our article we locate a section dedicated to the study's limitations. Staying with our example, we note the study reports several limitations that we could use for the basis of a critique. One example is where it is suggested the 'data obtained from the questionnaire could be limited by poor memory of experiences prior to PD diagnosis' (Fujii, 2021: 152). This is rightfully a limitation, as the survey is self-reporting, which means people who present as having PD may find it challenging to recall pre-diagnosis memories. Building in our critical element from the descriptive could read like this:

Fujii (2021) researched subjective sleep traits and personality pre- and post-Parkinson's disease (PD) diagnosis to determine the implications of these traits for multiple home care strategies. Using a cross-sectional survey research design, results suggest patients with PD reported a post-diagnosis decrease in sleep time but increases during nap time. Other findings included the study subjects reporting becoming tense easily but they did not report feeling irritated or angry. The subjective assessment suggested a post-diagnosis worsening of sleep quality in patients with PD. However, there are several limitations to the study. One of them linking to the study design – a self-reporting survey. Patients reporting on survey item questions prior to PD diagnosis might be considered unreliable as participants may have poor recollections prior to PD diagnosis. This threatens the validity and reliability of the inferences and conclusions drawn.

The critical element uses information in the article to draw attention to the limitations of this type of research. Indeed, all articles will have their limitations, and this enables us to explore critically what exactly is going on. To take this one step further is to review similar studies and compare findings. Here you will build up a better picture of analysis, patterns and trends before offering a well-informed critical appraisal.

INVESTIGATING REFERENCING: STUDENTS' ANATHEMA

Before we start, consider the following syllogism (deductive reasoning in which a conclusion is derived from two premises – Definitions.net, 2016):

I provide references in my work,

References in my work lead to better quality,

Better quality equals better grades, all because I provided references.

To get to its core, referencing deals with the proof and acknowledgement of others' work used in a specific context within your own. When searching for anything, you will select appropriate material to help build an answer against your assignment goals. This takes time, as you will need to search, read and select appropriate literature or other media. Indeed, referencing others' works serves a dual purpose and in its literal sense requires you to show support of a claim by providing a reference from an appropriate source. Consider the following claims and note the differences before selecting the one you think is more trustworthy:

1. Cystic fibrosis has improved over the years mainly due to early diagnosis, targeted therapies and specialised units.

2. There has been an improvement in the diagnosis, treatment and specialised care for cystic fibrosis patients in recent years (O'Sullivan and Freedman, 2009).

Although written differently, both put out the same idea and seem genuine, both make bold claims about something but only one can be classed as being credible. You should have selected the second claim, as it is supported by an in-text reference. Adding academic references will significantly improve the quality of your work and showcases your knowledge. Again, option two starts this process by including a credible source from a peer-reviewed journal – in this case, *The Lancet*. It will need improving, bringing in alternative views (using and extending upon additional sources) and summarising before moving on. Let's investigate the styles of referencing you will need to master.

REFERENCING: THE BASICS

Most HE courses will follow the Harvard referencing system to stylise your citations and lists. There are other systems, and it is best to read your course handbook or speak to your lecturer should your institution follow a different system. The internet and bookstores are ablaze with guidance on how to develop your referencing skills. One thing to note here is the layout of different media sources (e.g. book, blog, video, audio) that have different reference layouts. This goes beyond this chapter, but there is further guidance in the Further reading section at the end of this chapter.

There are two important steps to remember when using references. Firstly, references that include the author's name, date of publication, title and publisher are located at the back of your work. This is known as your reference list. Secondly, references that are used within your work (known as in-text references or citations) include only the author(s) name(s), the date of publication and a page number if you use a direct quote. These simple rules are the basics of using and applying references in your work. It's a good idea to practise stylistically to get used to different ways to integrate citations into your own work.

IN-TEXT REFERENCES

Let's look at this more closely with examples of how in-text references can be shaped to fit your style of writing and improve its flow. As we have seen previously, writing essays and reports requires various techniques to enable the transition between descriptive, critical and explanatory voices. The following are different in-text styles, the first one suggests a descriptive approach:

- Counihan (2015) suggests that universal peer learning originated in India as a pedagogical package before being shipped worldwide.

The descriptive style might be useful when introducing a new theme or perspective. Alternatively, it can be written with the author's name at the end, but notice the different arrangement with the brackets:

- Universal peer teaching was a pedagogical package that was developed in India before being sent worldwide (Counihan, 2015).

Lastly, we might reference a direct quote. A quotation is used to emphasise a specific point or show support for one of our arguments and it looks like this:

- As Counihan (2015: 291) suggests, 'At the height of its popularity, the method garnered interest from kings, tsars and early educational reformers who were keen to raise standards, particularly access to education for the poor.'

As before, the reference can go at the end of the paragraph or sentence. It depends on the flow of your work and whether the quote is long enough to break away from the main body of text, or short enough to remain as part of the same sentence. There is no universal agreement here so do check course handbooks; but generally, anything longer than three sentences requires indenting and separating from the main body of text. When referencing a direct quote, that is, when you have used exactly the same words as the author(s), you must provide a page number, as can be seen in the parentheses above.

SECONDARY REFERENCES

Some colleges do not allow secondary referencing and expect you to find the original research, and where possible, you should do this to ensure accuracy. Secondary sources mean that the original authors' work may be misinterpreted or misquoted – you will only find out if you read their words yourself. In some cases, the original work may be in another language, and you have to read it in translation, or the original is out of print (this is especially true of sociology or psychology books and journal articles). Also, sadly, some works are behind paywalls, and you cannot freely access all of the article or research. Always ask the librarian if they can access or obtain work for you; they have mystical skills in getting hold of original work. In the event of using secondary referencing, ensure you acknowledge who you are citing; examples are given below.

As with in-text references, the same process of including a source and placing it near content you have written remains the same, the only difference being the style it is presented in. Sometimes when researching material, we might come across sources we are unable to access, or that information is missing. Let's assume we have come across interesting material in a book and want to use it. However, we cannot gain access to the citation, thus, we think about discarding it. Don't do it! We can still use it by following the basic rules of secondary sourcing.

Let's now look at this in more detail with a worked example. Starting with an extract from an essay we are developing on cystic fibrosis, a secondary reference will be styled like the following:

- In 1959, Gibson and Cooke pioneered a method that revolutionised the diagnosis of cystic fibrosis (cited in Filbrun et al., 2016).

Notice the similarity of providing an author's name and date, the same as we did for our in-text reference in the previous section. However, let's dissect the above into two sentences to master secondary referencing styles.

The first sentence refers to a study completed in 1959 by Gibson and Cooke, and this is what we want to use in our essay. Usually, we would cite it following the *in-text* rules, as before – (Gibson and Cooke, 1959). However, we are unable to find the complete source for our reference list but still want to include it. Therefore, if we consult the second sentence from our example above, we will notice the *(cited in)* reference style. This is because Filbrun and her colleagues (the *et al.* part, note that the first time you use a reference, you should include the names of all the authors, and use *et al.* each time thereafter) have written about the method pioneered by Gibson and Cooke in their own publication. Thus, we are able to acknowledge (and use in our essay/report) the material we want (i.e. Gibson and Cooke) by citing Filbrun and colleagues' book. Finally, you will not need to include the Gibson and Cooke citation in your reference list. Instead, you only include information related to the Filbrun publication. The Further reading section of this chapter has helpful interactive links and information on how to create a reference list incorporating both in-text and secondary referencing styles.

Referencing will take some time getting used to. Remember to paraphrase sentences into your own words, unless you use a direct quote. Some students consider using multiple quotes to eat up word counts. This won't do, because assessors will want to know what you have understood and whether you can synthesise major arguments, themes and perspectives required at this level of study.

Paraphrasing (also précising, or summarising) is an important skill to learn if you want to avoid charges of plagiarism (stealing someone else's work). In its most basic form, plagiarism is passing off ideas or content developed by others as your own and without direct reference or permission to do so. Plagiarism can take many forms and it's useful to know how to avoid common pitfalls. A useful educational tool developed for nursing students is provided by Goodwin and McCarthy (2020), who explain plagiarism for nurses, and this article provides an overview with workable examples. Full reference for this article is in the reference section.

If you go back and look at the Counihan quotes, you see the first two are paraphrases and the last is a direct quote; if you are quoting you must use 'quotation' marks. HE assignments are usually submitted through a plagiarism checker such as Turnitin: this system recognises quotation marks and disregards the words between. Thus, if you do not use quotation marks, the system will flag the words up as plagiarised, and this will have implications for your grading.

DOING EVIDENCE-BASED RESEARCH

Evidence-based practice helps to fill the theory-to-practice gap in nursing. Undergraduate nurses engage in research as part of developing their professional practice; it is part of what makes the nursing profession current and up-to-date. Nurses contribute to and access evidence-based research which informs practice. For instance, Mulhall (1998) considers that nurses caring for patients with cannulas would want to understand why infection and thrombophlebitis occurs, therefore they would research randomised controlled trials showing the various ways in which cannula sites are cleansed and dressed to ensure best safe, effective practice. According to Nieswiadomy and Bailey (2018: 2), nursing research is a 'systematic objective process of analysing phenomena of importance to nursing' designed to develop new knowledge and skills that ultimately lead to better practice.

Research nearly always begins with a question or an idea (this is called a hypothesis): you want to find something out. Evidence-based practice finds out what works and, equally importantly, what doesn't work. The main medical research database is hosted by the Cochrane Library, where researchers conduct meta-analysis: this looks at the grouping of previous research in specific areas and draws conclusions using statistical methods of analysis. Whilst conducting a meta-analysis during your undergraduate programme of study is unrealistic, nurses will need good levels of numeracy skills to retrieve meaning from meta-analytical review findings. Meta-analytical reviews follow a rigorous methodological structure and studies present their findings quantitatively, e.g. using descriptive and inferential statistics. More generally, nurses must make effective use of their numeracy skills in sometimes challenging and fast-paced situations. For example, understanding conversion between decimals and fractions, calculating dosages for use in prescribing medication and working with time calculations are all part of the job in the practical sense.

Back to research. Nurses ask many questions, and there are many ways of engaging in research; the type of questions will guide the types of research paradigm used to explore answers. Nurses use the scientific method, ethnography, grounded theory, cohort studies and randomised controlled trials and all other spectrums of options suitable for research. Nurses who are research orientated are more likely to implement the findings within their practice and to disseminate them through their workplace, leading to improved evidence-based praxis.

Research is always conducted to a specific formula. The first step is ensuring your project is legal and ethical, especially when researching with children and vulnerable adults. You must demonstrate how you will protect your participants from harm. All universities and trusts have an ethics committee, and you should submit your proposal for review before conducting any research. Next you must recruit your research participants; they will have to give you written permission and you have obligations of confidentiality and safeguarding under medical research rules. Your participants also have the right to withdraw at any time during the life of the research, if they choose to do so, you must remove and destroy all their data. Your participants also have the right to see the data you hold and to read the completed research documents.

You must then consider your method of doing the research. This will be driven by the knowledge you are looking for and the participants; so, for instance, if you wanted to know how effective a particular day surgery is, you might consider examining readmission rates. Your participants will initially be selected from medical records, and you might then want to interview a representative sample of patients drawing on the knowledge gained from the records. You would also engage in a literature review, reading what previous researchers have found; this then would give some comparisons with your own setting. Your methodology states why you have chosen a particular research method and why it is the most suitable for your research; your findings or results are the data you have generated during your enquiry, and you would then discuss what these mean for future practice. Dissemination is sharing your work with a wider audience, try to get your work published by a reputable journal such as the *British Journal of Nursing* or *The Nursing Times*; you could also attend conferences and give seminars to nurses working in the same field, or seminars to your ward staff if it is something that purely relates to your setting; and finally you could use social media and blogging to get your message out.

There are many good textbooks which offer full guidance for engaging in research, some more specialist than others; look for one that most meets your research needs. Most university libraries have a good selection to choose from.

⚙ Activity 1.4

When nurses critically reflect on their own practice it will lead them to think about questions. To help construct evidence-based practice research, clarifying key aspects as part of a systematic/critical review of studies is necessary if the outcomes are to be of any reliable and valid use in practice. The PICO (population, intervention, comparator and outcome) model provides a useful strategy to bring together key aspects to help answer the research question:

- Population – researchers will identify relevant participants (e.g. patients) who are included in the study. This may include patient characteristics linked to the primary problem or specific research question.
- Intervention – what are the details of the intervention and what is being considered? Researchers will locate different types of interventions (e.g. testing a specific drug) and provide information about included interventions relevant to the problem area.
- Comparator – what will researchers compare the intervention to? Researchers will offer details on the comparator (e.g. drug A vs drug B – which is more effective?).
- Outcome – the results are important but what do we think the outcome will be? How will it affect the patient positively? Researchers will provide further details.

The study by Louie et al. (2021) takes an evidence-based practice approach to identify programmes that were effective in providing care in drug and alcohol settings. They followed systematic review research principles and suggested outcomes of programme effectiveness using the PICO model. The study is available here via open access link: www.ncbi.nlm.nih.gov/pmc/articles/PMC7931583/
Read the study and then answer the following questions:

Q1: In the Population and Intervention sections – identify what is meant by 'inclusion' and 'exclusion' criteria. Write a few sentences on why these are important at the early stages of the research enquiry.
Q2: Write down a few sentences on how you think Louie et al.'s (2021) study contributed to the development of future practice.

CHAPTER SUMMARY

- You have recognised the transparency in personal skills and how they can be utilised in academic contexts.
- You have investigated, developed and applied techniques for conducting contextualised searches for online material.
- You have understood the assessment processes involved in HE and developed an awareness of descriptive, explanatory and critical voices to be used in academic writing and relative assignments.

- You have taken an in-depth practical look at referencing, its various styles and how it can be applied to academic assignments.

⚙ Answers to Activity 1.3

1   = Explanation
2   = Descriptive
3   = Critical

⚙ Answers to Activity 1.4

Q1: Stating the inclusion and exclusion criteria in a systematic or critical review used in evidence-based practice is extremely important. Inclusion criteria helps to identify the specific characteristics/traits of a study population that must be fulfilled for their 'inclusion' into the review. Similarly, identifying specific characteristics/traits that are not required for the review should also be explained. For example, if you wanted to review evidence of a specific drug used to treat a specific age group this would need to be justified through the inclusion and exclusion criteria.

Q2: Any answers relating to the key findings of the review that offered the following to advance practice:

- Clinician beliefs and attitudes
- Modes of learning – possibly modified to levels of education
- Awareness of the influence of patient and clinician gender on the implementation outcome

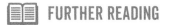 FURTHER READING

WEBSITES

These websites will help you with your research skill development:

- The *British Medical Journal* has an excellent resource for reading and researching different types of academic articles and how to read them. It is available at: www.bmj.com/about-bmj/resources-readers/publications/how-read-paper
- See Julian Treasure detail how to give an excellent presentation in his TED talk, which can be found at: www.ted.com/talks/julian_treasure_how_to_speak_so_that_people_want_to_listen?language=en

- Review your referencing skills with *Cite Them Right: The Basics of Referencing*, available at: www.citethemrightonline.com/Basics
- Academic phrasebank found at www.phrasebank.manchester.ac.uk/

VIDEOS

- See how to create an end-of-text reference list by viewing this useful YouTube video: www.youtube.com/watch?v=QtfXN8QYJik
- How to write a nursing essay: www.youtube.com/watch?v=aScAV3C_F3w
- How to write a reflective essay: www.youtube.com/watch?v=whKS AKSMFs8

BOOKS

These texts will all support your study skills development:

- Burns, T. and Sinfield, S. (2016) *Essential Study Skills: The Complete Guide to Success at University* (4th edn). London: Sage.
- Jasper, M. (2003) *Beginning Reflective Practice*. Cheltenham: Nelson Thornes.
- Kolb, D.A. (1984) *Experiential Learning: Experience as the Source of Learning and Development*. Englewood Cliffs, NJ: Prentice-Hall.
- Lewis, D. (1999) *The Written Assignment: A Guide to the Writing and Presentation of Assignments*. Kelvin Grove: Queensland University of Technology.

REFERENCES

Counihan, C. (2015) Endogenous education in India and the implications of universal peer teaching in the 19th century. In P. Dixon, S. Humble and C. Counihan (eds), *Handbook of International Development and Education*. London: Edward Elgar.

Dankert-Roelse, J.E. and Vernooij-van Langen, A. (2011) Newborn screening for cystic fibrosis: pros and cons. *Breathe, 8*: 24–30.

Definitions.net (2016) Syllogism. Available at: www.definitions.net/definition/syllogism

Filbrun, A.G., Lahiri, T.R. and Ren, C.L. (2016) *Handbook of Cystic Fibrosis*. Cham: Adis Publishing.

Fujii, C. (2021) The post-diagnosis sleep quality of patients with Parkinson's disease. *British Journal of Neuroscience Nursing, 17*(4): 148–54.

Gibbs, G. (1988) *Learning by Doing: A Guide to Teaching and Learning Methods*. Oxford: Oxford Further Education Unit.

Goodwin, J. and McCarthy, J. (2020) Explaining plagiarism for nursing students: an educational tool. *Teaching and Learning in Nursing, 15*(3): 198–203.

Jasper, M. (2003) *Beginning Reflective Practice*. Cheltenham: Nelson Thornes.

Kolb, D.A. (1984) *Experiential Learning: Experience as the Source of Learning and Development*. Englewood Cliffs, NJ: Prentice-Hall.

Lewis, D. (1999) *The Written Assignment: A Guide to the Writing and Presentation of Assignments*. Kelvin Grove: Queensland University of Technology.

Louie, E., Barrett, E.L., Baillie, A., Haber, P. and Morley, K.C. (2021) A systematic review of evidence-based practice implementation in drug and alcohol settings: applying the consolidated framework for implementation research framework. *Implementation Science*, *16*, 22 (2021). https://doi.org/10.1186/s13012-021-01090-7

Mulhall, A. (1998) Nursing, research, and the evidence. *Evidence-Based Nursing*, *1*: 4–6.

NHS (2016) Cystic fibrosis. Available at: www.nhs.uk/Conditions/cystic-fibrosis/Pages/Introduction.aspx

Nieswiadomy, R. and Bailey, C. (2018) *Foundations of Nursing Research* (7th edn). New York: Pearson Education.

Nightingale, P., Te Wiata, I.T., Toohey, S., Ryan, G., Hughes, C. and Magin, D. (1996) *Assessing Learning in Universities*. Sydney: Professional Development Centre, University of New South Wales.

O'Sullivan, P.B. and Freedman, D.S. (2009) Cystic fibrosis. *The Lancet*, *373*(9678): 1891–904.

Plass, A.M., Van El, C.G., Pieters, T., et al. (2010) Neonatal screening for treatable and untreatable disorders: prospective parents' opinions. *Pediatrics*, *125*: 99–106.

Sternberg, R.J. (1985) *Beyond IQ: A Triarchic Theory of Intelligence*. Cambridge: Cambridge University Press.

2

PERSONAL AND PROFESSIONAL DEVELOPMENT

GILLIAN ROWE

STANDARDS OF PROFICIENCY FOR NURSING ASSOCIATES (2018)

Relevant Platforms include:

Platform 1:1.6 Understand the professional responsibility to adopt a healthy lifestyle to maintain the level of personal fitness and wellbeing required to meet people's needs for mental and physical care.

Platform 1:1.7 Describe the principles of research and how research findings are used to inform evidence-based practice.

Platform 1:1.10 Demonstrate the skills and abilities required to develop, manage and maintain appropriate relationships with people, their families, carers and colleagues.

Platform 1:1.13 Demonstrate numeracy, literacy, digital and technological skills required to meet the needs of people in their care to ensure safe and effective practice.

Platform 1:1.15 Take responsibility for continuous self-reflection, seeking and responding to support and feedback to develop professional knowledge and skills.

Platform 1:1.16 Act as an ambassador to their profession and promote public confidence in health and care systems.

Platform 4:4.1 Demonstrate an awareness of the roles, responsibilities and scope of practice of different members of the nursing and interdisciplinary team, and their own role within it.

Personal development begins with self-awareness. You get to know who you really are; your values, beliefs and the dreams you wish to pursue. True fulfilment can never come from chasing other people's dreams.

Abraham Maslow (1954)

This chapter is aimed at helping you become an independent learner and to become an effective student. It will also support you to become a reflective learner and develop the skill of reflective writing and journal keeping. Furthermore, it will introduce you to evidence-based practice and team working. As part of your Nursing and Midwifery Council (NMC) registration you are required to:

… keep your knowledge and skills up to date, taking part in appropriate and regular learning and professional development activities that aim to maintain and develop your competence and improve your performance.

(22.3, NMC Code, 2018)

Glossary

- **Personal development** Improves your self-identity and self-awareness
- **Professional development** Earning or maintaining your professional credibility
- **Reflection** Giving serious thought or consideration to something
- **Reflective guide** Using a guide to help you clarify your thinking
- **IT** Information technology

INTRODUCTION

Personal and professional development is a lifelong process, and as Abraham Maslow so nicely puts it, it begins with self-awareness, getting to know who you are and what your strengths and challenges are. The world of health and social care changes rapidly; new ideas, changing legislation, improving standards and different ways of working all add to the changing landscape. Continuous development comes about by reading journals, taking courses, and attending seminars or conferences and deepening your understanding of how change affects what you do and how you do it. A good example of this is in Chapter 4 on values and ethical frameworks, which discusses the changes brought about by the Francis Report and the introduction of the six Cs into your day-to-day work. Recall that the NMC Code of Practice requires you to 'gather and reflect on feedback from a variety of sources, using it to improve your practice and performance' (9.2, NMC Code, 2018) to ensure that your practice reflects your professional development.

Becoming a student and adopting an enquiry-based outlook is a big change in your life; it is hard work and demands that you put aside time to engage in study. It also asks that you question what you do and how you do it, and this learning process is formularised by using reflective practices such as journal keeping. This chapter will guide you through the process and sits alongside Chapter 1 on academic study skills, which will support you in your academic work.

GETTING STARTED

Independent learning requires commitment and discipline. To make it easier for yourself, try to organise a study space. The family dining table is not suitable as you will need to move your stuff continually (and things will get lost). You will need somewhere to put all the books you buy and borrow, and your folders. This could be a big box (at least it is all together), a filing cabinet and desk, or your own study room. Your study space needs to be free of distractions, so keep clutter to a minimum.

You will need a laptop or large tablet and an internet connection, and a software package such as MS Student, as you will need a range of office software (e.g. Word, PowerPoint, Publisher and Excel in MS Office). Ask your college if they offer a free MS suite, many do. Apple Mac for students requires an institutional log in but they also offer deals. Linux offer their office suite equivalent free but there may be compatibility issues. Some larger universities will offer a free tablet such as an iPad.

LEARNING RESOURCES

Books are another big budget item. You will need various key texts for each module you study, and although there will be a few copies of each book on the reading list in your college library, usually they are restricted to 7- or 14-day loans. Buying your books secondhand from a previous student or by checking out deals on eBay or Amazon is a good way to get reasonably priced textbooks. Sage Catalyst is a subscription access to a range of Sage textbooks; your HEI may subscribe to this service.

Your college may well subscribe to an e-journal account such as Athens, which will allow you free access to health journal articles; however, these subscriptions are remarkably expensive and smaller colleges without university partnerships may not be able to afford them. In which case, most journal publishers have 'open access' articles which are free to view. Colleges may also have institutional subscriptions to relevant monthly publications (such as *Nursing Times*) which should be in the library. Always remember that the librarian is your friend and will help you obtain books and articles through the college book exchange system.

Go Further 2.1

You can freely access NHS digital, evidence.nhs.uk and learning resources on the Royal College of Nursing (RCN) website. Other sites are MEDLINE databases, PubMed, Cochrane Library, PsycINFO, Web of Science (open Athens log in), SCOPUS, PROSPERO and many others.

BECOMING A STUDENT

When you are a beginning student, it is easy to feel intimidated by how much you must learn – it seems endless. There is a new language to learn, long complicated words that you need to spell, understand and use. You may feel that you do not bring anything to the table in the classroom, or that your views are not of value. However, everyone has knowledge and experience of value, and you will develop confidence as you read and learn more, and this will help you find your voice. Do not feel scared to put your hand up and ask if you do not understand something; you will not be the only one and you will probably be doing your shyer class-mates a favour. It is important that during your protected hours, that you behave as a student, ask questions and treat each activity as a learning opportunity.

Look for independent learning opportunities by watching YouTube channels such as Khan Academy and Bosman Science and read your module textbooks to support your learning. Textbook publishers often have online learning materials too to support the textbook content. Sage has an amazing website and most of Sage's textbooks offer online learning materials. Go to Sage Publishing, and click the resources button, look for 'students' in the drop-down list, then select the discipline you are looking for, search at the bottom on the textbooks for online resources.

You can join online forums dedicated to the knowledge you seek, watch TED talks, and take free online courses such as edX or FutureLearn. All the information you need is available but ensure you use reputable sites (there is a lot of misinformation, fake news, and downright rubbish out there too).

LEARNING ABOUT HOW YOU LEARN

To complete a higher education degree or higher apprenticeship you need to think about how you learn. Everyone has a learning style; you may well have completed an assessment of your learning style when you were younger, but our learning styles change as we get older. Figure 2.1 refers to four learning styles which we use in training and practice.

Think about the differences in the way you learnt at school or FE college (where you may have done A-Levels, BTEC or NVQs). Look at Table 2.1 to see how you will learn on university-level programmes.

In order to take responsibility for your own learning, you need to understand how you learn. You may be familiar with VARK, which means Visual, Audio, Reading and Kinetic. Table 2.2 shows how each term relates to practical learning skills.

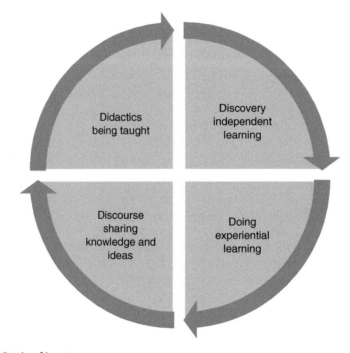

Figure 2.1   Circle of learning

Table 2.1   Types of learning

Learning at lower level	Learning at higher level
Information given by teachers	Self-directed learning
Listening	Active participation
Shared responsibility for learning	Personal responsibility for learning

Table 2.2   VARK

Visual: Watching YouTube, TV, observing others	Reading: textbooks, articles, online materials
Audio: listening to podcasts or the radio, listening to explanations	Kinetic: learning by doing

So what is learning? It is concerned with the acquisition of knowledge that can be retained and applied. Learning is said to take place when you can make sense of something and reinterpret it into your own words and can apply something into a skill or action. However, the act of acquiring new knowledge and skills is the start of your learning journey; as a nursing associate, it is not enough to understand concepts, you need to apply them to a variety of patients and situations. Kong Qui (better known as Confucius) was a Chinese philosopher in the fourth century BCE and he said, 'By three methods we may learn wisdom: first, by reflection, which is the noblest; second by imitation, which is the easiest; and third by experience, which is the bitterest' (Confucius). Experience can be gained from poor decision making which is then used to make good decisions (bitter experience), but David Kolb (1984) designed the Experiential Learning Cycle as a way of learning and practising (Figure 2.2).

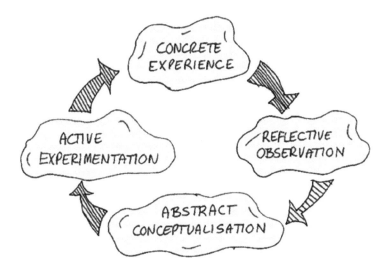

Figure 2.2   Kolb's Experiential Learning Cycle

1. Concrete experience might be trying something new or looking at a known thing in a new light, or a new way of doing things, adapting to change.
2. Reflective observation is about thinking about what happened, how you did, what went well, what didn't work.
3. Abstract conceptualisation can prompt you to make changes.
4. Active experimentation means doing it again, but a different way.

And this takes you back to the beginning of the cycle. Kolb (1984) says effective learning takes place when all four parts of the cycle have been visited. The cognitive psychologist Jean Piaget (1964) said that children learn through a process of assimilation and accommodation, that they build on knowledge (called scaffolding). They start out with a schema (an idea) which may be used in different situations (assimilation) or changed (accommodation) when the schema doesn't work. He considers that equilibration drives children's search for understanding, and balance comes from mastery. Piaget only applies his theory to children, not adult learners, and focuses on development not just learning, but you can see a relationship between this model and the Kolb model.

Generally, the students most likely to succeed are students who attend lectures. There is a direct correlation between attendance and achievement. It is not always the brightest student who achieves the highest degree classification but the one who has a willing attitude and an enquiring mind. This is what the psychologist Carol Dweck (2006) calls 'a growth mindset', which is a belief that talent will only get you so far, whereas hard work and dedication makes for great accomplishment. No one achieves great things without years of effort and practice. Once you know how you learn, you can consider the barriers to your learning. Table 2.3 is based on a survey I conducted with students to identify their barriers. Do any of these apply to you?

Table 2.3   Thinking about the things that can get in the way of your studies

I'm terrible at time management – always have been!
I know what I need to do – I just can't make myself do it
I can't work unless I'm under pressure
I'm just lazy – no other explanation!
I always leave everything to the last minute – it's just the way I am!
I never have enough time to do what I want

GOOD TIME MANAGEMENT

We have all been here, even your lecturers! However, unless you really are the kind of person who can sit up all night and hand in a first-class paper, it will help if you can plan your time management for the next 15 or 30 weeks of study. Go Further 2.2 explains that poor time management can result in students leaving their course. There are many apps to help you with time management such as Remember the Milk, Focus Keeper, Evernote and Trello. MindNode is great for mind mapping. Focus@will is good for those with ADHD. One of the more fun ones is Forest. Gantt charts are easy to create and use too; you can find out more about Gantt charts here: www.mindtools.com/pages/article/newPPM_03.htm

---

Go Further 2.2

Students often report that their inability to manage their time is the biggest problem they face when trying to fit in everything that has to happen in the home, at work and study. A study by Adams and Blair (2019) found that 'effective time management is associated with greater academic performance and lower levels of anxiety in students'. On their website, the National Union of Students (NUS) have an advice page to help you with time management.

NON-STUDY OBLIGATIONS

Keeping a weekly record is critical to staying on track. Some weeks will be the same, but others may need to accommodate trips to medical facilities either for yourself or another family member, children's sports day, parents' evening, creating a birthday party or going to a wedding (try not to arrange your own wedding in term time) and learning to drive. Do not forget to programme in household chores such as shopping, cooking, washing and cleaning.

Moving to a new house or finding a new home is something that happens a lot for students. It is better to move in the term breaks if possible. Moving is stressful enough without the added burden of study, and universities generally do not accept moving (other than in emergency) as a reason for an extension on your hand-in dates.

Organising childcare and planning how to cope when it falls apart, or when the children are sick, is important. If you are a nursing associate apprentice, you will have a job and work shifts and these needs should be programmed in. You might also work irregular hours or night shifts or be on call; somehow these must be accommodated. Students are noted for having a hectic social life and therefore you should be no different and this needs to be considered when planning your study time. Also, try to give yourself some 'me' time to unwind. Look at Activity 2.1 and consider if this activity would help you with time management.

⚙ Activity 2.1   Make a time planner

Download Google 'printable weekly planner' and print some copies off, filling them in at the beginning of each week. This activity will add evidence for your portfolio as well as keeping you up-to-date on your studying.

If you are keeping a weekly diary, use backward planning. When you write a due date in your diary/planner, go back a week, and give yourself a reminder that the due date is approaching.

(Continued)

It really is essential that you keep track of 'hand-in dates'. Here sticky notes are your friend.

Use a colour-coding system. Keep some coloured sticky notes on hand and use those for reminders that a due date or other important event is approaching. For instance, use a yellow (amber) sticker to serve as a warning 7 days before your assignment is due in, and a red one for 2 days before hand-in. You can do all of these things on your phone or laptop if you prefer.

Think about the things that soak up your time, called time sponges. Look at Table 2.4 and see how many you waste time on.

What can you do?

Deactivate social media or use it as reward for 2 hours spent studying. Do Activity 2.2 to decide what would work for you.

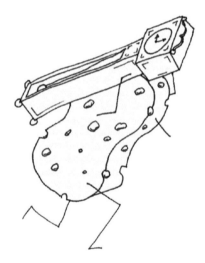

Figure 2.3   Time sponge

Table 2.4   Time sponges: How many of these do you waste time on?

Friends' Instagram/TikTok/Twitter posts

Netflix/YouTube

Checking out Vinted /Amazon/eBay

WhatsApp chat group

Pinterest/Bustle

Making brownies

Instagramming a picture of your brownies

Television/iPlayer/YouTube/Soccer Rally Arena

Opening a new tab ... Facebook/Instagram/TikTok again

⚙ Activity 2.2   Make a chart of your time sponges

Your personal time sponges	What may work for you

When we perceive tasks as difficult, inconvenient, or scary, we may shift into pro-crastination mode with self-sabotaging statements.

- I'll wait until I'm in the mood to do it.
- There's plenty of time to get it done.
- I work better under pressure, so I don't need to do it right now.

GETTING STARTED AND STAYING ON TRACK

- Complete small tasks straight away rather than putting them off. This will encourage you to begin tackling larger tasks needing attention.
- Break difficult or 'boring' work into sections. This allows you to approach a large task as a series of manageable parts.
- Don't try to write a whole assignment in one sitting. Write it section by section.
- If you have 'writer's block', try writing something – anything – down. Even if you change it completely later, at least you have made a start. The alternative is having nothing at all.
- Make a mind map of your assignment title. This should give you the main keywords. Look at the example in Figure 2.4 to see how it can guide your research and structure your essay.

If you find yourself losing direction, sit back and think of why you are doing this course, remembering your goals can put everything into perspective.

SUMMARY OF KEY STAGES IN MANAGING YOUR TIME

- Organising your study time – give yourself treats and rewards, take frequent short breaks away from your books or computer. Run around the block or to the park and back to get your circulation flowing.
- Planning ahead – be organised and aware of both college and work and social commitments.
- Prioritisation – discover what needs to be done by when, expect to study at home for at least 2 hours for each hour spent in class.

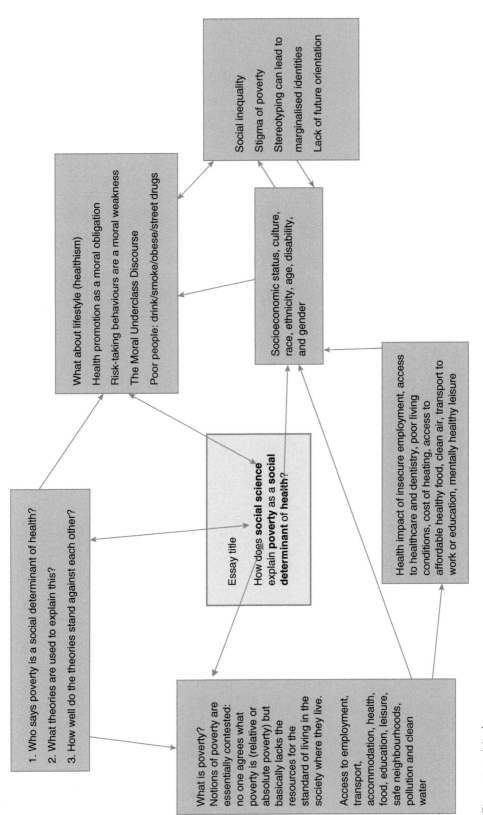

1. Who says poverty is a social determinant of health?
2. What theories are used to explain this?
3. How well do the theories stand against each other?

What about lifestyle (healthism)

Health promotion as a moral obligation
Risk-taking behaviours are a moral weakness
The Moral Underclass Discourse
Poor people: drink/smoke/obese/street drugs

Social inequality
Stigma of poverty
Stereotyping can lead to marginalised identities
Lack of future orientation

Socioeconomic status, culture, race, ethnicity, age, disability, and gender

Essay title

How does **social science** explain **poverty** as a **social determinant** of **health?**

Health impact of insecure employment, access to healthcare and dentistry, poor living conditions, cost of heating, access to affordable healthy food, clean air, transport to work or education, mentally healthy leisure

What is poverty?
Notions of poverty are essentially contested: no one agrees what poverty is (relative or absolute poverty) but basically lacks the resources for the standard of living in the society where they live.

Access to employment, transport, accommodation, health, food, education, leisure, safe neighbourhoods, pollution and clean water

Figure 2.4   Mind map

- Action planning – how will you complete tasks and stay motivated?
- Evaluating your progress on a regular basis – how are you getting on and are you on schedule?

TECHNICAL AND PRACTICAL ASSESSMENT

In Chapter 1, you learned about academic assessment and how to write academically. However, you will also perform assessments online: you might have taken a Self-Directed Learning Readiness Assessment (SDLRA) or an Online Learning Readiness Assessment, which assess your ability to engage in self-directed or problem-based learning. You will also be expected to complete some distance learning using online packages such as SafeMedicate.

You will also undertake practical assessments called Objective Structured Clinical Examination (OSCE) or OSCA depending on setting: both mean that you will have an objective, structured clinical assessment of your skills. Depending on your employing organisation and training facility, you may have a practice assessment document which identifies any skills and knowledge that require further work and records the competencies and skills you have attained. The NMC explains that assessment should be evidence-based and that (standard 7.3) 'practice assessors make and record objective, evidenced-based assessments on conduct, proficiency and achievement, drawing on student records, direct observations, student self-reflection, and other resources'. Further details of the assessment standard are given in Box 2.1

Box 2.1   Standards framework for nursing education

5.10   Students are assessed across practice settings and learning environments as required by their programme

5.12   Practice assessment is facilitated and evidenced by observations and other appropriate methods

5.13   Students' self-reflections contribute to, and are evidenced in, assessments

5.14   A range of people including service users contribute to student assessment

---

You will be given a scenario and a patient (real, actor or manikin) and you will be observed in your interactions according to the task given. The OSCE is designed to test clinical skill performance and competence in a real-world situation. Most OSCEs will be a selection of stations, each with a specific task, and each station will have a different examiner, usually a lecturer but they might also be a clinical practitioner. Each candidate is asked the same questions or asked to perform the same procedure or asked for an interpretation of given data. The OSCE is a demonstration of praxis, the combination of theoretical knowledge and practical clinical skills.

You are likely to be assessed on your communication skills (with both staff and patients and their families), your knowledge and application of infection control and health and safety, your theoretical and technical knowledge of the task you are to perform, your skill in undertaking the task, and finally, your documentation of the process.

UNDERTAKING A SWOT ASSESSMENT

SWOT is an acronym for Strengths, Weaknesses, Opportunities and Threats. You can identify things in each area that either support your learning or are barriers to your learning. Use Table 2.5 for some ideas to help you to write this. Once you have identified your barriers (weakness and threats) consider how you might overcome them and what changes you may need to make.

Table 2.5   Ideas for a SWOT assessment

Some ideas for Strengths or Weaknesses	Some ideas for Opportunities or Threats
Time management Work ethic Confidence	Available time for study
Communication skills Empathy	Student finance
Ability to follow instructions Showing initiative	Job availability Pay/salary
Can work in a team Independent	Family Current employment
Understand confidentiality Tactful Patient Reliable	Government policies
IT literate Flexible Numeracy skills	Skill set Travel time
Relevant work experience Social skills	Educational support/study
Working under pressure Organised Multi-tasking	support Relationships

ASSESSMENT INTERVIEWS

You will have an initial, mid point and end point placement interview where you will evidence your learning in that placement. You will engage in self-assessment and reflection on the progression of your learning needs. The next section offers you details on how to become reflective and examines reflective guides.

BECOMING REFLECTIVE

Reflective practice (RP) is a crucial component of health professionals' practice. For students, RP is a way to increase their professional competence and improve patient care (McLeod et al., 2019).

What is reflection, and why do we do it? Reflection is something of an art and a skill; it is the process of mulling over our day and thinking about events that may have puzzled us. The purpose of reflection is to facilitate learning from experience and develop critical thinking; it can also enhance your problem-solving skills. Engaging in higher education and higher vocational training teaches you to learn to think as effectively as you learn to write. Academic life gives you the opportunity to reflect on your college learning, such as a thought-provoking lecture or practical, or reflecting on feedback which might give you advice on how to improve your work.

You must learn to have an open mind, to not be judgemental, and to examine your thought processes. Your reflective journal is more than a simple account of your working day – it is an examination of your working day. Reflection can allow you to experience the wonder of your learning, being totally amazed or shocked by new knowledge. A part of the reflective process is the willingness to self-criticise, to change or challenge beliefs, actions, assumptions and practice. As McLeod at al. (2019: 50) considered, 'Students perceived RP as an important catalyst for personal and professional development. They reported using reflection to reconsider clinical decisions, identify gaps in their knowledge and skills, and enhance patient-centred care.'

Professor Jenny Moon (2006: 162) says that 'we reflect on things that are relatively complicated. We do not reflect on a simple addition sum – or the route to the corner shop. We reflect on things for which there is not an obvious or immediate solution.' John Dewey (1933: 12) said, 'Reflection has two interconnected qualities, that of being troubled by some phenomenon and doubting the evidence, and of searching for answers which will remove the problem and doubt.' Reflection is about self-learning and seeking answers; it is also about being self-aware as it involves your beliefs, values, qualities, strengths and limitations. When engaging in reflection you are considering your role, actions and inactions in any given situation. Do Activity 2.3 and see how engaging in reflection supports your learning about your practice.

⚙ Activity 2.3

Think about an event that has occurred, something that made you stop and think. Reflection is a conscious action and gives you the opportunity to evaluate the experience. Learning journals are not usually written in 'the third person', you can say 'I think' or 'I feel' and this gives you an authentic voice in your work.

What happened? (Describe)	What was my role in this? (Analyse)
How did I feel about this? (Evaluate)	What did I learn? (Self-awareness)

REFLECTIVE GUIDES

We often use a reflective guide to aid reflection. This is because sometimes it is hard to look at something from other perspectives or take on board other people's views. By using a guide, we can examine an experience from 360 degrees. The most commonly used guide is Gibbs' Reflective Cycle (1988) (see Box 2.2), which lends itself particularly well to repeated experiences, allowing you to learn and plan from things that either went well or did not go well. There is another image of Gibbs' cycle in Chapter 1.

Box 2.2   Gibbs' Reflective Cycle

- Description of the experience
- Feelings and thoughts about the experience
- Evaluation of the experience, assess both the good and bad
- Analysis to make sense of the situation
- Conclusion as to what you learned and what you could have done differently
- Action plan for how you would deal with similar situations in the future

---

All reflective cycles have similar components (see Figure 2.5). More recently the REFLECT model has been created specifically for nurses by Barksby et al. (2015), as it was felt that Gibbs' cycle was overly complex, difficult to recall in a practice setting and somewhat repetitive, whereas REFLECT is also a handy acronym and easy to remember. Table 2.6 show the seven stages of REFLECT, standing for Recall, Examine, Feelings, Learning, Exploring, Creating and Timescale.

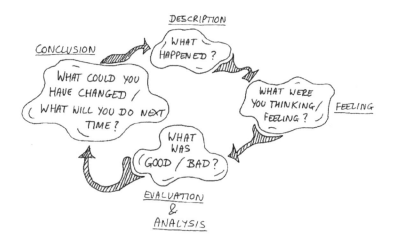

Figure 2.5   Reflective cycle

Table 2.6   REFLECT

R	Recall the events (**stage 1**) Describe the event you wish to reflect on
E	Examine your responses (**stage 2**) Consider what you were thinking and doing at the time
F	Acknowledge feelings (**stage 3**) How did you feel at the time of the event; how did you feel after?
L	Learn from the experience (**stage 4**) Explain what you learned
E	Explore options (**stage 5**) Explain what you would do next time there is a similar event
C	Create a plan of action (**stage 6**) Create a plan for the future, what you will do next time
T	Set timescale (**stage 7**) Set a time for when you will create your plan

Donald Schön (1984) wrote extensively on the value of reflection (mainly in education) but his work considered two types of reflection: reflection on action and reflection in action (Table 2.7).

Table 2.7   Schön's two types of reflection

Reflection on action	**Reflection in action**
Reviewing that occurs after an event	Continually assessing while actually acting

Schön considers the ability to reflect in action as 'professional artistry'; this means that if a situation develops while participating in an activity, you are able to intervene, respond and make changes. He states:

> The practitioner allows himself [*sic*] to experience surprise, puzzlement, or confusion in a situation which he finds uncertain or unique. He reflects on the phenomenon before him, and on the prior understandings which have been implicit in his behaviour. He carries out an experiment which serves to generate both a new understanding of the phenomenon and a change in the situation. (Schön, 1984: 68)

Quite often in healthcare we are presented with an 'accepted picture', which may be based on preconceived ideas, received wisdom or unconscious bias; we become reflective when presented with information that does not fit this accepted pattern and engage in 'retrospective' reflection. To become reflexive thinkers and engage in conscious processing, we need to attend to our intuitive thoughts (Rolfe, 2001). Read Scenario 2.1 and think about how reflection has helped Anya to support her client.

📋 Scenario 2.1   Mr Smith

Mr Smith suffers from dementia and lives in a dementia care unit. His behaviour at meal times is puzzling. He happily eats breakfast and supper but will not eat his lunch. At lunch time he pushes his chair back, leaves the table and sits in an armchair. Anya (apprentice TNA) found that if she brought him a biscuit and a cup of tea, he would accept these. At a team meeting Anya discussed his behaviour with her manager and she asked if she could organise a family meeting to find out how to resolve this situation and support his nutritional needs.

Anya met with Mrs Smith, who told Anya about Mr Smith's life. She said he was a proud man, who had worked as a miner in the coal industry. They worked hard to buy a house and raise their children, and there was little spare money. Mr Smith insisted that they saved up if they wanted something new as he was afraid of getting into debt. They had had family holidays, usually staying in 'Bed and Breakfast' guest houses near the coast.

After Mrs Smith had left, Anya wondered about where Mr Smith thought he was now; she knew from conversations she had with him that he was not orientated to time and location, but he knew he was not at home. Anya mulled over Mrs Smith's comment about Mr Smith being a proud man and his attitude to money. The next day at lunch time, when Mr Smith was assisted to the table, he again pushed his chair away. Anya said to him that lunch had already been paid for but Mr Smith still went to the armchair. Anya rang Mrs Smith and related the day's events. Mrs Smith said that Mr Smith usually paid cash when they were out for lunch. The following day, when Anya was supporting Mr Smith with getting dressed, she put some money in his pocket and told him it was to pay for his lunch. At lunch time, she assisted him to the table and reminded him to pay for his food with the money in his pocket. Mr Smith put the money on the table and ate his lunch.

1.   Apply the Gibbs' or REFLECT cycle to this case study. How many times did Anya go through the cycle?

By applying reflective practice, Anya was able to support Mr Smith with his nutrition in a way that he was comfortable with.

Some journal/practice assessment document (PAD) work will be based on your clinical experiences; these will be structured around the patient's care. Your structure might be:

1. Objective (or goal) of an intervention
2. Outcome (good, neutral, poor)
3. Evaluation (did the intervention work)
4. Plan (amend the care plan).

Each of these headings will require links to theoretical models of care and reflective thinking.

KEEPING A REFLECTIVE JOURNAL

Those of you who have completed NVQs will be familiar with the concept of 'naturally occurring evidence'; this is learning that takes place as you go about your day-to-day work. Keeping a reflective journal is a way to capture this evidence and gives you an opportunity to see how your knowledge and skill grow over time.

A reflective journal is different from a personal diary, as it examines your professional practice; it also does not need daily recording but should be used regularly. Your placement supervisor may ask to see your journal, so ensure that you respect confidentiality and do not identify patients/clients/staff or settings by name or places.

Which format you use for your journal is up to you – it could be a paper portfolio, an e-journal or a personal blog or vlog, or your training organisation's e-portfolio system. Either way, it must be kept securely, and password protected.

It is also a way of keeping things in perspective when you are feeling overwhelmed in placement. Sometimes traumatic things occur which you need to make sense of, or you have experienced a difficult or challenging situation, or maybe you have worked in a team that has achieved success (good things need to be thought about too).

Your journal is also a good place to make links between theory and practice as well as making notes on research you have undertaken (or need to undertake) to support your learning. By keeping a journal in practice and placement, you have something to look back on to support your report or essay writing or your observed structured clinical examination (OSCEs). Remember that you will have to evidence journal keeping in your continuous professional development portfolio for your registration revalidation. Your revalidation reflections will centre on your learning experience (CPD activity, reflecting on feedback and experience in practice) and how this relates to themes in the code of practice. As part of revalidation, you will need to provide five reflective accounts for your mandatory reflective discussion.

Journal work must be honest. Try to faithfully capture the experience so that you can analyse and evaluate the situation; you need to question your actions and consider if you would do the same thing again in the same situation or if you would change your action and consider how this would affect an outcome. It might be useful to write your experience down or record it on your phone and revisit it a few days later when you have had time to assimilate events or calm down if something has upset you. Your views might change, or you may have deepened your learning by research or talking to your mentor.

HOW SHOULD A JOURNAL BE WRITTEN?

Each entry of the journal will have its own agenda and requirements. As you develop your skill in reflection, Moon (2008) says you should move from basic description to profound evaluation. Therefore, you should travel along a continuum:

Action > Understanding > Reflection > Critical reflection

Table 2.8 shows you the different reasons for keeping a journal.

Table 2.8   Reasons to keep a journal

Reflect on doing something for the first time

Challenge received wisdom

Think about how this experience connects with previous experiences

Record key events and experiences

Clarify or provide solutions to problematical issues

Provide a means to extend knowledge and skills

A place to experiment with and develop writing styles

Increase your self-awareness

Evaluate your personal and professional growth

Store ideas or material that could be used in an assignment

YOUR LEARNING JOURNAL

When you write your journal, you are engaging in independent learning, and you are writing about things that are meaningful to you. It is an opportunity to make links with disparate information from different sources such as class notes, handouts, conversations you have with your supervisor/patients/ward staff. Your writing can also identify gaps in your knowledge and guide your research.

EVIDENCE-BASED PRACTICE

Your journal can also contribute to your knowledge of evidence-based practice (EBP). This practice marries together the principles of clinical expertise, best-evidence research and the patients' values and feedback. The integration of these things can help support the patient care process, and help you develop and understand your practice, why decisions are made, lessons you have learnt and the implications of these for your future practice. David Sackett (1996: 71) said that evidence-based practice is 'the conscientious, explicit and judicious use of current best evidence in making decisions about the care of the individual patient. This means integrating clinical expertise with the best available clinical evidence from systematic research.' Adopting the principles of EBP into your thinking and reflection shows that you are willing to learn from experience and to change things, and that you are open to new ideas and new ways of supporting your patients.

You will want to consider:

- What internal/external factors were influencing you?
- What knowledge/values did or should have informed you?
- How did your actions match your beliefs and knowledge?
- What factors made you act in incongruent ways?
- What are you going to do the same or differently in this type of situation next time it happens?

Watch the recommended YouTube videos in Go Further 2.3 to gain a better understanding of critical thinking and how to apply it to EBP. Chapter 10 has a reflection on evidence-based practice written by TNA Heather; if you read that, it might act as a guide for your own reflections.

Go Further 2.3

Watch this YouTube video to support your development of critical thinking: Critical Thinking Part 1: Definition, Connection to the Nursing Process, Benefits and Levels: www.youtube.com/watch?v=GnrPz1AlnW0 and this video about EBP in Gateshead: www.youtube.com/watch?v=5Gkc8gg8CPU

TEAM WORKING

Healthcare practitioners will always be part of a team, whether you are in a care setting, clinic, domiciliary working or on a ward, therefore team working skills are essential. Teams come together for different purposes and small teams will be part of a larger grouping. Look at Table 2.9 to get an idea of who is in a multi-disciplinary team (MDT) and a multi-agency team (MAT). Multi-disciplinary teams consist of the staff within a setting, while multi-agency teams are part of the wider health and social care community.

The King's Fund states that:

Where multi-professional teams work together, patient satisfaction is higher, healthcare delivery is more effective, there are higher levels of innovation in ways of caring for patients, lower levels of stress, absenteeism and turnover, and more consistent communication with patients. (The King's Fund, 2017)

Teams that work well are clear in their roles and goals and support each other in achieving them; effective teams therefore experience less stress. The value of interdisciplinary and multi-disciplinary teams is that alternative and competing perspectives are carefully discussed, leading to better quality patient care. Teams who meet regularly with a clear shared purpose and are a mix of the organisation's hierarchy and are seated in the premise of person-centred care, can provide effective service to the patient. Cultivate your skills as a team player and understand your role within the team – no matter how junior, your input will be valued.

Table 2.9   Multi-disciplinary teams and multi-agency teams

Multi-disciplinary teams	Multi-agency teams
Matrons/Nurses (RGNs/RMNs/Midwives)	Health visitors (could also work in MDT too)
Healthcare Assistants	Community matrons/Nurses (RGNs/RMNs/Midwives)
Healthcare Practitioners/Nursing Associates	Domiciliary support workers/residential care staff
Doctors/Surgeons/Anaesthetists/Consultants	Social workers
Therapists	Police/Probation officers/Youth Offender Teams
Diagnosticians	Youth workers
Dieticians	Therapists
Paramedics	Housing support workers

WORKING IN A TEAM

While you are at college, you will probably experience working in a team. You will certainly be in a team on placement or in your working environment. The team members may have chosen themselves or you may be allocated a team. Good teams, however, don't just happen, you need a common purpose, and everyone needs to contribute using their skills, talents and knowledge.

Tuckman (1965) first described the mechanisms involved in creating teams and named them 'Forming, Storming, Norming, and Performing' (Figure 2.6). The first role of the team is to appoint a leader or organiser who has the responsibility of ensuring the team achieves its objectives. The forming stage involves the team getting to know each other and becoming familiar with the goals; this can be an anxious time and the team leader needs to take a dominant role to get the ball rolling. Quite often the team has meetings about setting realistic and achievable objectives and will use such aids as a Gantt chart or Prince2 so that the objectives are planned and agreed in a timely manner.

The storming stage is the trickiest, as this is when the purpose of the goals and the leadership role are challenged. Quite often conflict arises as people have different ways of working or disagree with approaches to problem solving. Members may withhold their cooperation or leave the

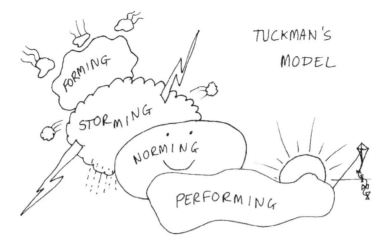

Figure 2.6   Tuckman's model

team at this stage. If the team survives this then they move on to norming, which is when the team accepts their role, starts to socialise together and works collegially. It then achieves the performing stage and works effectively without friction and the leader can step back or delegate part of the role as the team functions well.

A fifth stage, 'adjourning', is sometimes included: this is when the team has completed the task it was formed for, and the members move on to other things. It is important to achieve closure for the group on a positive note, as this stage has sometimes been called the 'mourning' stage. Therefore, the sadness felt at the break up of the team should be managed by transition or some sort of ceremony to celebrate the team's success.

Teams are dynamic: personnel change, goals change, healthcare teams work across disciplines and each member brings a different skill set; communication is the key that promotes good relationships within the team. Everyone should have a clear idea of both their roles and boundaries, who delegates to them and who they delegate to, so no one individual is asked to perform tasks beyond their remit or skill set. Clear lines of management and reporting structures should be established, so if things need to be escalated, each individual knows the chain of responsibility. Everyone in the team has a duty of care and is accountable for their actions (and inactions); therefore, if you are asked to perform a task for which you have not had adequate training, it is your duty to refuse the task and seek supervision.

CONFLICT AND COMPLAINT IN TEAM WORKING

Managing conflict within a team depends on the ability of the team to put the patient front and centre and to deal with personality problems in a mature adult manner. This does not always happen, especially when working and personal relationships are involved.

Conflict can arise if the dispute is a professional criticism of patient care. Nobody likes to be criticised, but poor practice needs to be challenged. Done tactfully and without animosity, it can be a learning process; done badly, resentment can seriously affect the team's ability to function collaboratively. However, not challenging poor practice puts the patient at risk; nursing teams are overstretched and cannot carry someone who is lazy or indifferent in their attitude.

The Thomas–Kilmann Conflict Instrument (TKI) was devised by doctors Ralph Kilmann and Kenneth Thomas in 1974. Designed for resolving conflict between co-workers; these conflicts may be due to individual differences or task-related differences. Resolution is predicated on two modes: Assertiveness and Cooperation (see Figure 2.7). Competitors tend to high assertiveness and low cooperation, this mode is most effective in situations where a fast resolution is needed, usually given by someone in a position of power. Avoiders tend to have less power or less investment in the conflict, although sometimes a conflict has to be faced, at other times it may not be worth the bother. Accommodators try to see both sides of an argument and will look for points of cooperation, and collaborators will seek an equitable resolution or compromise where everyone gets something of what they wanted.

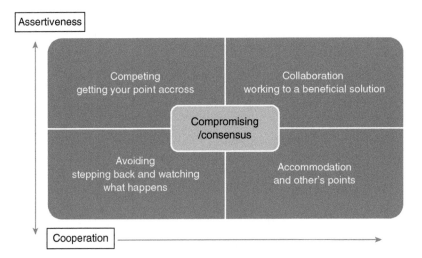

Figure 2.7   The Thomas-Kilmann Conflict Model (1974)

Complaints about poor practice that come from patients or their families need to be dealt with promptly, quite often they want to raise concerns and feel that no one is listening to them. To prevent escalation, listen to what they have to say and respond appropriately, if they are angry or distressed, keep calm, it is probably not you they are angry about. If it is something not easily remedied, escalate to the senior staff and document what has happened, how you tried to resolve it and where it was escalated to.

You can signpost patients and their families to the Patient Advice and Liaison Service (PALS), who will try to resolve their issue internally; or patients and families can contact the NHS Complaints Advocacy Service, who are an independent service, and most local trusts have a branch of Healthwatch, who can also offer support.

KEEPING FIT TO PRACTISE

You need to maintain a healthy lifestyle and a level of personal fitness in order to do a very physically and mentally challenging job. This is part of your professional values and is contained within the NMC Code of Practice: 'maintain the level of health you need to carry out your professional role' (20.9) (NMC, 2018). Chapter 13, Introduction to Mental Health and Wellbeing, will help you to develop mental resilience; keeping physically fit asks you to think about your lifestyle.

Drinking alcohol socially is fun, a night out with good friends in the pub is a great way to relax or sharing pizza and beers while Netflixing. However, when one or two drinks becomes five or six, you are not going to be fit to drive or to be on duty the following morning. You cannot perform at your best with a hangover; if this leads to poor decision making, you might put someone's life at risk. Alcohol should be treated with respect and should not be part of your daily routine; if it becomes your go to coping strategy, you need to engage in reflection and consider a healthier option. After a 12-hour shift, the last thing you need is someone telling you to get some exercise but getting out into the fresh air and walking in nature is a proven way to wind down. Join a team or a choir. If they are too competitive or expensive, start a singing club with your friends or fellow college students.

Try to eat healthily; junk food is accessible and cheap, but the toll it takes on your body is the price you pay later. Nurses are known to live on coffee and chocolate, hospital cafes seldom provide reasonably priced healthy options, and food queues often mean your break involves eating your meal as quickly as you can, neither tasting nor enjoying it. This is especially true when you are on night duty, when the cafe or canteen is usually closed and all that is available are stale snacks in a vending machine. Plan ahead: make up a couple of healthy packed lunches on your day off and keep them in the fridge ready to grab when you go off to work or college. Your body will thank you for it.

CHAPTER SUMMARY

- You have been introduced to the skills of being a successful student, including preparing to study, learning how to study, and learning how to identify your barriers to study.
- You have also learned how to become reflective and keep a reflective journal.
- It has introduced you to notions of evidence-based practice and given you some theoretical underpinning of team working for health and social care both at placement and in college.

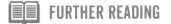 **FURTHER READING**

BOOKS

Reading these texts will deepen your understanding of study skills and reflection:

- Dweck, C. (2006) *Mindset: How You Can Fulfil Your Potential.* New York: Ballantine Books.
- Gibbs, G. (1988) *Learning by Doing: A Guide to Teaching and Learning Methods.* Oxford: Oxford Polytechnic, Further Education Unit.
- Kolb, D.A. (1984) *Experiential Learning: Experience as the Source of Learning and Development.* Englewood Cliffs, NJ: Prentice-Hall.
- Moon, J. (2006) *Learning Journals: A Handbook for Reflective Practice and Professional Development* (2nd edn). London: Routledge.
- Moon, J. (2008) *Reflective Writing: Some Initial Guidance for Students.* Available at: http://services.exeter.ac.uk/cas/employability/students/reflective.htm
- Price, B. and Harrington, A. (2016) *Critical Thinking and Writing for Nursing Students* (3rd edn). London: Sage.
- Schön, D. (1984) *The Reflective Practitioner: How Professionals Think in Action.* New York: Basic Books.
- Thompson, S. and Thompson, N. (2008) *The Critically Reflective Practitioner.* Basingstoke: Palgrave Macmillan.

VIDEOS

- Being reflective and keeping a reflective diary: www.youtube.com/watch?v=kAslHSKelkM
- Gibbs' Cycle tutorial for nursing and midwifery students: www.youtube.com/watch?v=BLfCp7KTCBU

REFERENCES

Adams, R. and Blair, E. (2019) Impact of time management behaviors on undergraduate engineering students' performance. *SAGE Open*. https://journals.sage pub.com/doi/full/10.1177/2158244018824506

Barksby, J., Butcher, N. and Whysall, A. (2015) A new model of reflection for clinical practice. *Nursing Times*, *111*(34/35): 34–5.

Dewey, J. (1933) *How We Think*. Boston: Heath and Co.

Dweck, C. (2006) *Mindset: How You Can Fulfil Your Potential*. New York: Ballantine Books.

Gibbs, G. (1988) *Learning by Doing: A Guide to Teaching and Learning Methods*. Oxford: Further Education Unit, Oxford Polytechnic.

Kolb, D.A. (1984) *Experiential Learning: Experience as the Source of Learning and Development*. Englewood Cliffs, NJ: Prentice-Hall.

Maslow, A. (1954) *Motivation and Personality*. New York: Harper.

McLeod, G.A., Vaughan, B., Carey, I., Shannon, T. and Winn, E. (2019) Pre-professional reflective practice: strategies, perspectives and experiences. *International Journal of Osteopathic Medicine*, *35*: 50–56. https://doi.org/10.1016/j.ijosm.2019.11.005

Moon, J. (2006) *Learning Journals: A Handbook for Reflective Practice and Professional Development* (2nd edn). London: Routledge.

Moon, J. (2008) *Reflective Writing – Some Initial Guidance for Students*. Available at: http://services.exeter.ac.uk/cas/employability/students/reflective.htm

NMC (Nursing and Midwifery Council) (2018) Code of Practice. Available at: www. nmc.org.uk/standards/code/read-the-code-online/#fourth

Piaget, J. (1964) *The Psychology of the Child*. New York: Basic Books.

Rolfe, G. (2001) *Critical Reflection for Nursing and the Helping Professions: A User's Guide*. Basingstoke: Palgrave Macmillan.

Sackett, D. (1996) Evidence based medicine: what it is and what it isn't. *British Medical Journal*, *312*: 71–72.

Schön, D. (1984) *The Reflective Practitioner: How Professionals Think in Action*. New York: Basic Books.

The King's Fund (2017) Improving NHS culture. Teamworking. Available at: www. kingsfund.org.uk/projects/culture/effective-team-working

Tuckman, B. (1965) Developmental sequence in small groups. *Psychological Bulletin*, *63*: 384–99.

3

LEADERSHIP AND TEAMWORK IN HEALTH AND SOCIAL CARE

MICHELLE HENDERSON

STANDARDS OF PROFICIENCY FOR NURSING ASSOCIATES (2018)

Relevant Platforms include:

Platform 1:1.3 Understand the importance of courage and transparency and apply the duty of candour, recognising and reporting any situations, behaviours and errors that could result in poor health outcomes.

Platform 1:1.5 Understand the demands of professional practice and demonstrate how to recognise the signs of vulnerability in themselves or their colleagues and the actions required to minimise risks to health.

Platform 1:1.8 Understand and explain the meaning of resilience and emotional intelligence, and their influence on an individual's ability to provide care.

Platform 1:1.12 Recognise and report any factors that may adversely impact safe and effective care.

Platform 1:1.15 Take responsibility for continuous self-reflection, seeking and responding to support and feedback to develop professional knowledge and skills.

Platform 4:4.2 Demonstrate an ability to support and motivate other members of the care team and interact confidentially with them.

Platform 4:4.6 Demonstrate the ability to monitor and review the quality of care delivered, providing challenge and constructive feedback when an aspect of care is delegated to others.

Platform 4:4.7 Support, supervise and act as a role model to nursing associate students, healthcare support workers and those new to care roles. Review the quality of the care they provide, promoting reflection and providing constructive feedback.

Platform 4:4.8 Contribute to team reflection activities, to promote improvements in practice and services.

Platform 5:5.2 Participate in data collection to support audit activity and contribute to the implementation of quality improvement strategies.

Platform 5:5.5 Recognise when inadequate staffing levels impact on the ability to provide safe care and escalate concerns appropriately.

Platform 5:5.7 Understand what constitutes a near miss, a serious adverse event, a critical incident and a major incident.

Platform 5:5.8 Understand when to seek appropriate advice to manage risk and avoid compromising quality of care and health outcomes.

Platform 5:5.9 Recognise uncertainty and demonstrate an awareness of strategies to develop resilience in themselves. Know how to seek support to help deal with uncertain situations.

Annex A Skills 4.1–4.5, 5.1–5.4.

The NHS needs people to think of themselves as leaders not because they are personally exceptional, senior or inspirational to others, but because they can see what needs doing and can work with others to do it.

Turnbull-James (2011: 18)

This chapter will develop your awareness of the background to leadership, management and team working in current health and social care sector contexts. As you work through the chapter, you will understand the background to some of the key milestones in leadership and management in the NHS, the development of leadership skills and qualities and how the use of reflection contributes to your professional development, and how you can seek leadership opportunities irrespective of your grade or position within your workplace and beyond.

Glossary

- **Care Quality Commission (CQC)** The regulatory and inspection body for health and social care
- **Emotional intelligence** Defined as self-awareness, self-regulation and a level of empathy and understanding of others' perspectives
- **Healthwatch** Healthwatch England, established as an effective, independent consumer champion for health and social care
- **The Berwick Review (2013)** This report is about patient safety, which includes the importance of leadership
- **The Francis Report (2013)** The findings following investigation into the failings at Mid Staffordshire NHS Trust
- **The Shape of Caring Review (Raising the Bar) (2015)** This document looks at the overarching value of high quality education for the caring professions with a focus on HCAs and nurse associate roles

INTRODUCTION

It is never too early to start thinking about leadership skills in health and social care regardless of the stage you are at in your health and social care career. Leadership has never been more important. Changes to the way health and care is commissioned, increasing use of technology and the financial challenges faced require those working in health and social care to utilise skills of leadership regardless of position or grade. Cross-boundary working between statutory, private and voluntary providers and the changing landscape of how services are provided mean leadership skills are crucial. Change is constant but quality remains paramount.

It is therefore recognised that those embarking on careers in health and social care and studying professional programmes need to understand the importance of leadership and team working in current contexts.

Leadership can no longer be seen as position-related, exclusive to those at the top or at certain stages of their careers or training – leadership skills are required at all levels. Literature supports a move away from traditional hierarchical approaches (The King's Fund, 2011); leadership is about working with, and inspiring others. Leadership skills are required when you are supervising, involved in project work or carrying out your day-to-day duties, and therefore it is important to start to think about your views of leadership, and how you can develop leadership skills within your role and beyond. The aim of this chapter is to introduce you to leadership within health and social care practice and to enable you to start thinking about the concept and the skills development you will need early in your learning journey. The first part of the chapter will look at what leadership is, examining the current debates between leadership and management. The second part will look at why leadership is important and how it impacts on quality of care. The final part will explore skills for leadership development, including the value of self-assessment and reflection, looking after your own wellbeing and identifying learning opportunities. The NMC Code asks you to 'Act as an advocate for the vulnerable, challenging poor practice and discriminatory attitudes and behaviour relating to their care' (3.4, NMC Code, 2018) and 'Provide leadership to make sure people's wellbeing is protected and to improve their experiences of the health and care system' (25.0, NMC Code, 2018). This chapter will support your learning development as a leader.

LEADERSHIP VS MANAGEMENT – WHAT'S THE DIFFERENCE?

There are many debates about the differences between leadership and management.

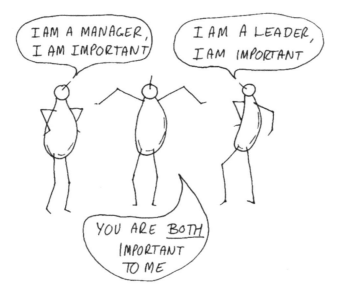

Figure 3.1   Leaders and managers are both important

John Kotter provides a definition:

Management is a set of processes that keep an organisation functioning. They make it work today – they make it hit this quarter's numbers. The processes are about planning, budgeting, staffing, clarifying jobs, measuring performance, and problem-solving when results did not go to plan. Leadership is very different. It is about aligning people to the vision that means buy-in and communication, motivation and inspiration. (Kotter, 1996: 25)

However, the difference is not as clear-cut as Kotter's definition, written over 20 years ago, implies. A report in the *Health Service Journal* argues we focus too much on definitions and identifies that we should look more towards action for practice to reduce bureaucracy and maximise leadership resources in the NHS (HSJ, 2015).

Whilst leadership may be seen as the skills to sell vision, or motivate individuals towards a vision, how this is achieved may be dependent on someone's leadership style or how they utilise power (which will be covered later on in this chapter). Therefore, to suggest that all leaders are capable of selling a vision and motivating others may be inaccurate, as not all leaders achieve such goals – in fact some fail spectacularly. We therefore may need to start to think about the title we give to people as leaders and what is actually meant by leadership and management. This might not always mean those traditionally seen as being in charge or at the top.

Whilst some authors may argue the differences between leadership and management and attempt to make them distinct in their roles, it is key to remember that both have a valued role within healthcare. Management ensures the day-to-day workings run smoothly, managing resources, people and budgets for example. Without these sets of skills many key functions in healthcare would not occur. If we think of leadership as setting direction and inspiring vision, it is clear to see how such skills are important to ensure change is moved forward as an example.

It is important to remember that managers can be leaders and leaders can be managers, or these can be very separate individual roles. Instead of comparing leadership vs management, it is therefore suggested that perhaps such roles should be seen as a circle; a continuum of interaction dependent on circumstance and situation, neither one more important than the other, and how leadership skills should be developed by all involved in healthcare regardless of formal job title.

Figure 3.2 highlights some of the differences and similarities of leadership and management.

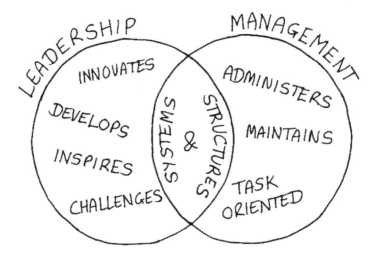

Figure 3.2   Similarities of leadership and management

Scenario 3.1   Reflection on scenarios where you may have used leadership skills

1. Think of a time when you may have advocated or spoke up for a patient OR
2. Mentored or supervised a student or new member of staff OR
3. Voiced your concerns to colleagues about an area of practice.

What skills did you use?

Why were they important?

How did you feel?

Would you have done anything differently?

All of the above are examples where you will have used leadership skills – you just may not have realised this at the time

WHERE ARE WE NOW? A SNAPSHOT OF MANAGEMENT AND LEADERSHIP

If Florence Nightingale was carrying her lamp through the corridors of the NHS today, she would almost certainly be searching for the people in charge.

The Griffiths Report (1983)

Over 30 years ago, the Griffiths Report (1983) looked at management within the NHS. The report author, Sir Roy Griffiths, made this statement as he was concerned at the lack of management in the NHS. The report remarked on the absence of management or leaders who held responsibility, and attempted to encourage a role for clinicians more closely involved in management decisions and created the vision of the general manager. Fast forward to 2011, and the King's Fund still identified that those in clinical roles need to be engaged more in managerial decisions. There had been comments or statements that there were 'too many managers' and 'too many chiefs and not enough Indians'. The King's Fund report (2011) argued that both leaders and managers should be of equal value and that the disregard for the value of managers needed to be addressed as it is damaging to patient care and the morale of the workforce. Furthermore, the report noted there was no evidence that there were too many managers. The NHS Plan (2001) brought back the (modern) matron. This came off the back of a public consultation that showed people wanted strong visible leadership. The plan also identified that leadership was about drive and innovation, not just seniority, and called for a move towards all those involved in healthcare thinking about leadership, and their role within this.

MID STAFFORDSHIRE FAILINGS

In 2008, Mid Staffordshire NHS Trust was investigated due to its high mortality rate. What was uncovered identified one of the most significant failings the NHS had seen since its inception. Key factors identified from the initial investigations were the lack of management and leadership. In 2010, a full public inquiry was launched, chaired by Sir Robert Francis QC. The final report identified reasons why things went so wrong, and the report made many recommendations. The main themes suggested a need to encourage a culture of openness and transparency; a system of accountability for all; a system promoting clinical leadership that put patients first as a priority in achieving this.

Following on from the Francis Inquiry, in 2013 Sir Bruce Keogh was asked to lead a review of 14 hospital trusts which had persistently high mortality rates. Eleven of the 14 trusts inspected were put into special measures and scheduled for re-inspection, and the review report set out key areas for improvement of care. Again, the importance of leadership and management featured within this report. Professor Berwick was asked to look at how 'zero harm' could be made a reality in the NHS. The Berwick Review (2013) made in total 10 recommendations with core themes around transparency, continual learning, regulation and seeking patient and carer opinions. At the heart of all the themes that emerged was the need for leadership, and those willing to promote high standards and speak up when things are going wrong.

Since the inquiries following the Mid Staffordshire failings, there have been many published documents attempting to address the key issues of ensuring that such failings do not occur again and stressing that developing leadership skills can help to achieve this goal.

LEADERSHIP DURING THE COVID-19 PANDEMIC

On 11 March 2020, the World Health Organization declared a global pandemic caused by a novel emerging coronavirus named SARS-CoV-2 causing coronavirus disease 19 (or Covid-19 as it is commonly known). This followed an emerging situation of increased respiratory illness and deaths starting in China in December 2020.

The first case in the UK was reported on 31 January 2021 and there have been over 22 million samples reported as positive and nearly 200,000 deaths (as of July 2022) (data.gov, 2022). On a global scale there have been over 5 billion cases and over 6 million deaths reported to WHO as of July 2022 (WHO, 2022), but figures are likely to be lot higher than this due to reporting mechanisms in some parts of the world.

This has changed how we all work in health and social care. Some areas of practice saw increasing demand on resources such as critical care, medical wards and care homes. Staff working in organisations were sometimes asked to support areas where demand was high for health and social care. This involved some individuals coming out of their usual area of practice and learning new skills and supporting in different areas than they were accustomed to.

Partnership working was vitally important between the NHS, social care, the local authority, and communities.

Scenario 3.2   Reflection on scenarios where you may have used leadership skills

If you were working in a health and social care setting during 2020 and 2021, reflect on your role during the pandemic and after.

1.   Has your role changed? Were you required to take on new tasks or learn new skills?
2.   Did you work with different people or teams?

If so, reflect upon what skills you think you required during this period. Do you think you used skills of leadership?

LEADERSHIP AND QUALITY OF CARE

NHS England (2016) suggests that quality care is:

1.   Care that is clinically effective
2.   Care that is safe
3.   Care that provides a positive experience for patients

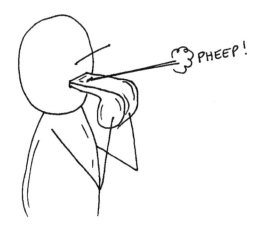

Figure 3.3   Whistleblowing

Leadership behaviours are one of the key factors in quality of care. Ensuring care is clinically effective may mean that care is evidence-based and utilises the latest and most up-to-date methods/technology or treatment. It may mean identifying when practices need to change or identifying new ways of working for service improvement and helping to trial and lead change. Service improvement requires leadership skills in communication, negotiation and getting people on board to support and manage change. Skills for Care (2021) found that over 90% of social care services rated good or outstanding for being well-led by the Care Quality Commission (CQC) were also rated good or outstanding overall.

Care that is safe requires those who deliver it to have integrity and to hold high standards and support others to do the same. In his report *Freedom to Speak Up*, Sir Robert Francis aimed to create conditions for NHS staff to speak out, share good practice and get care providers to make improvements when things go wrong (Francis, 2015). This links very much with transparency and the move towards organisations being assessed by the CQC on how transparent and open they are. As healthcare workers, we all have a duty, morally and ethically, to speak up and voice concerns if things go wrong. Whistleblowing or reporting concerns is essential for safe care and working environments. This requires not just an awareness that we should speak up when things are going wrong, but who to speak up to. Finally, care that provides a positive experience for clients or patients involves auditing the service provided or monitoring patient satisfaction outcomes through patient feedback or complaints. Both practical and personal skills are essential for improving client/patient experience and outcomes.

⚙ Activity 3.1

Think about your current workplace or placement. Are you aware of any policies about raising concerns or whistleblowing? You need to understand your organisation's whistleblowing policies.

- How does the thought of needing to use such policies make you feel?
- What skills and personal qualities do you think would be required when you need to use such policies?

Go Further 3.1

Read this independent review:

Francis, R. (2015) *Freedom to Speak Up: An Independent Review into Creating an Open and Honest Reporting Culture in the NHS*. Available at: www.gov.uk/government/publications/report-of-the-mid-staffordshire-nhs-foundation-trust-public-inquiry

---

Go Further 3.2

To find out more about this, read the full report:

Francis, R. (2013) *Report of the Mid Staffordshire NHS Foundation Trust Public Inquiry: Executive Summary*. London: The Stationery Office.

⚙ Activity 3.2

The King's Fund, an independent charity, has undertaken much research into leadership in healthcare. Read the following documents commissioned by the King's Fund:

The King's Fund (2014a) *Culture and Leadership in the NHS*. Available at: www.kingsfund.org.uk/publications/culture-and-leadership-nhs

The King's Fund (2014b) *Developing Collective Leadership for Health Care*. Available at: www.kingsfund.org.uk/sites/files/kf/field/field_publication_file/developing-collective-leadership-kingsfund-may14.pdf

The King's Fund (2015) *The Practice of System Leadership: Being Comfortable with Chaos*. Available at: www.kingsfund.org.uk/publications/practice-system-leadership

What are the themes throughout the three publications on the position and view of leadership in healthcare today?

How does this fit with your experiences of practice? Consider writing a short reflection on the differing aspects of leadership.

POLICY AND FRAMEWORKS FOR LEADERSHIP

The *Five Year Forward View* (NHS England, 2014) talks about strong leadership and supports the value of the NHS Leadership Academy – a national organisation responsible for leadership training and development in the NHS. The review by Lord Rose (2015), *Better Leadership for Tomorrow*, recognised that change was full scale in the NHS, but perhaps people in the frontline of services were not fully skilled or prepared to participate in this change. It emphasised the importance of seeking out talent and developing staff and considered the importance of equipping them with the right skills and direction to meet the challenges.

Working across boundaries and organisations is an example of such current challenges. West et al. (2015) argue there is urgent need for leadership across boundaries within and across organisations. This means working collectively and cooperatively, which is in effect collective leadership. Financial challenges and the way the NHS is changing in terms of how it delivers services require those working in it to have different sets of skills, as services can no longer run in isolation. West et al. (2015) consider that collective leadership is more crucial due to the changing nature of service provision. Czabanowska et al. (2014) state that a horizontal approach to leadership and working with others rather than a top-down approach is required, meaning leadership skills and behaviours that foster inclusion, collaboration and engagement in sharing leadership roles regardless of position or grade should be encouraged.

The *Shape of Caring Review (Raising the Bar)*, published by Health Education England in March 2015, focused on the role of the care assistant and the development of the associate practitioner and nursing associate role, firmly putting value on such roles within healthcare and their importance to frontline care. Establishing such roles also requires a focus on leadership development in staff who may not previously have had any formal leadership development opportunities.

Leading Change, Adding Value (NHS England, 2016) is a national framework that recognises the value nurses have in leadership, and strongly promotes leadership to achieve the 'triple aims of: better patient outcomes, better patient experiences and better use of resources'. The report suggests that as the face of healthcare changes, healthcare workers will need to have coaching and mentoring skills to be able to support patients and work with others and be confident practitioners who will in turn require leadership skills.

A national framework acknowledges the importance of leadership development which demonstrates the current value and drive that is being placed on leadership. NHS Improvement (2016) launched *Developing People – Improving Care*, a multi-agency effort. It aims to address four key themes:

- Developing systems leadership skills
- Improvement skills for staff at all levels
- Compassionate inclusive leadership skills
- Talent management, developing people and investing in leaders of the future

Skills for Care is the strategic body for workforce development in adult social care in England and is a delivery partner with the Department of Health and Social Care. Together they developed a framework for leadership qualities. The framework is styled as a tool for describing the attitudes and behaviours needed for high quality leadership at all levels across the social care workforce (Skills for Care, 2021).

The NHS Leadership Academy developed a healthcare leadership model that looked at nine dimensions that were deemed as important for those leading in healthcare:

- Inspiring shared purpose
- Leading with care
- Evaluating information
- Connecting our service
- Sharing the vision
- Engaging the team
- Holding to account
- Developing capability
- Influencing for results

Go Further 3.3

Review the Health and Social Care Leadership frameworks by visiting these websites then consider your critical reflection by answering the questions below.

NHS Healthcare Leadership Model: www.leadershipacademy.nhs.uk/resources/healthcare-leadership-model/

Skills for Care Leadership Qualities Framework for Social Care (2013): www.skillsforcare.org.uk/Support-for-leaders-and-managers/Developing-leaders-and-managers/Leadership-Qualities-Framework.aspx

Are there similarities between the health and social care models?

Are there any differences between the health and social care models?

Do you think there is anything missing in the models?

THE NHS LONG-TERM PLAN

NHS England published its long-term plan in 2019, revealing how the health service will develop over the next 10 years. NHS England has stated in the long-term plan that, together with NHS Improvement, they will introduce a new NHS leadership code. Compassion, collaboration and inclusion are key themes going forward in how leaders work within the service.

So what does all this mean for those embarking on a career in health and social care? Current demands on the health service require those working in it to be aware that change is constant, that they should have an understanding of the importance currently being placed on leadership skills, and that we need to stop thinking of leadership as being someone else's role. Utilising and developing confidence in leadership skills can have benefits for patient care, and for personal and professional development.

THE INTRODUCTION OF INTEGRATED CARE SYSTEMS (ICS)

On 11 February 2021, the Department of Health and Social Care released the White Paper: Integration and Innovation: Working Together to Improve Health and Social Care for All.

One of the big changes set out in the paper is around the establishment of Integrated Care Systems (ICS) as statutory bodies in all parts of England. Clinical Commissioning Groups (CCG) were dissolved on 1 April 2022. ICS intend to work closely together across health and social care to address the needs of local populations and work towards the goals contained in the long-term plan. The ICS board has strategic oversight across a geographical region. The ICS health and care partnerships are responsible for planning and developing health, public health and social care needs within their region. The ICS partnerships are made up of representatives from health and social care, local authorities and third parties such as the private and voluntary sectors. The aim is that closer and more integrated ways of working will mean organisations can tackle local issues utilising the best resources available for their population.

This means our roles may change in health and social care as the ICS evolve in the regions where we work. Partnership work will evolve therefore: building and developing leadership and team working skills, not just in your own organisation but with others across the health and social care systems, are important for future working.

WHY IS LEADERSHIP ESSENTIAL FOR TEAM WORKING?

> Teamwork is essential in the provision of healthcare. The division of labour among medical, nursing and allied health practitioners means that no single professional can deliver a complete episode of healthcare.
>
> Leggat (2007: 11)

Evidence is clear that where teams work well staff feel more engaged and deliver better care. Leadership is central to this, and the development of leadership skills is the starting point to contributing to a positive team working culture. Collaboration is required in a healthcare system that now crosses boundaries between statutory, non-statutory and voluntary services.

The importance of human factors such as how teams work together is crucial in terms of impact on patient safety (WHO, 2009). Teams bring together a range of skills both technical and personal; they bring diversity and different perspectives. Learning to work with others is essential. Part of the journey is beginning to understand how your own leadership skills can influence your position in team working. The influence of respected team members can be as powerful as those with positional power, and therefore we can all contribute and play a valuable role within team working.

<hr>

📖 Case Study 3.1   Emmie

Emmie is brought to the A&E in an ambulance after being found collapsed at home by her neighbour. The initial impression by the clinical team is that Emmie looks like she may have had a stroke.

- Which members of the MDT (multi-disciplinary team) will have inputted into Emmie's care so far from the moment her neighbour dialled 999?

Emmie is moved to a medical ward for further care. She is starting to improve but her neighbour confides to a nurse that she has been struggling for a while and finds it difficult to climb the stairs. Emmie's only son lives in Australia. Medically, Emmie is well enough to build towards going home but still has some weakness from her stroke.

- Which members of the MDT may be involved at this stage?

Assessment finds Emmie is not safe to return to her own home alone; a social worker will now liaise with social services and care providers to get Emmie back to her own home with support.

- As the named person looking after Emmie so far, why is it important to be working with all the MDT members to build towards discharging her home?
- What skills may you need to manage all the different assessments and updates occurring in Emmie's care between the MDT members involved?

<hr>

SUPERVISION

The supervising and support of health and social care trainees and students is vital to their education and development, and indeed forms an important part of a trainee nursing associate's competency assessment (NMC, 2018). It is essential for quality of care and requires many leadership skills. Many organisations now have practice facilitators and associated specialists who can offer additional support to learners. Supervision brings responsibility, ensuring that the learner is offered support and has access to a wide range of learning experiences. This will require skills in planning and communication when delivering complex learning information; it also considers the need to assess and identify when individual healthcare workers are meeting competencies or identifying where fitness to practise issues may arise. As you progress through your training and post-qualifying, you too will become a supervisor to others who are training.

Supervisors should ensure that any instructions given are clearly understood; this is especially relevant when delegating duties. The supervisor should ensure the person who has been delegated a duty understands the task and is competent to perform it. The supervisor should also offer constructive feedback and act in the role of critical friend by supporting learning and practical skills development. The process of supervision facilitates the individual to reflect on their learning, knowledge acquisition and competence and link theory to practice (praxis).

Supervisors should be mindful of the code of conduct, and you should stand as a role model. Feedback is essential in helping learners to identify their strengths and tackle areas that need improvement. Understanding what to do when things go wrong is also important in supervision. Standards for your supervision and assessment (NMC, 2018) can be accessed so you understand the expectation of those who will be registered professionals. Supervision should ultimately support independent learning that is safe, and you will be supervised as a learner, but you will be expected in future to supervise others. Nursing associates and some healthcare practitioners will supervise and delegate work to others, so it is important that the skills of supervision include giving clear instructions and explanations and offering constructive feedback that facilitates reflection.

📖 Case study 3.2   Josie

Josie is a qualified nursing associate, and she is helping to support a first-year trainee nursing associate on a 6-week placement. The student is being supervised by one of the qualified nurses on her unit.

Josie has concerns that she has repeatedly gone over how to take a blood pressure reading and what the readings mean with the student. Other staff members have reported that the student keeps asking the same questions too, but it is not obvious that these concerns are being tackled.

1.   How might Josie approach the situation to help support the student?

2.   Who can Josie speak to/make aware about her concerns?

3.   What skills might Josie have used in dealing with the situation?

LEADERSHIP QUALITIES AND DEVELOPMENT

Having discussed the current situation in leadership, and why it's important to work towards developing skills in leading, we will now consider what skills or personal qualities may be beneficial in leadership and how these can be developed or promoted.

WHAT LEADERSHIP SKILLS ARE REQUIRED?

Much debate exists on what are the most beneficial and influential skills needed for leadership. These skills are part of a toolbox that you will need, and which ones you use are situation dependent. This chapter has hopefully allowed you to start thinking about the kind of skills you may require. The next section will look at some key areas for consideration.

Activity 3.3

Download a copy of the Healthcare Leadership Model from the Leadership Academy at: www.leadershipacademy.nhs.uk/wp-content/uploads/dlm_uploads/2014/10/NHSLeadership-LeadershipModel-colour.pdf
In turn, take one of the nine NHS Leadership Academy behaviours:

- In each behaviour, there is a 'What it is not' section
  - How do you think the 'what it is not' behaviours described occur in practice?
  - What can be done to prevent such behaviours occurring?
- Now look at the 'What it is' section associated with each behaviour
  - How can these behaviours be promoted?

Roebuck (2011) suggests that influencing, decision-making skills, briefing a team, running a task, giving feedback and learning how to build networks are all key to leadership development. But if we strip away these practical skills, what are the actual skills and tools which some people may inherently have or need to focus on developing?

COMMUNICATION SKILLS

Developing enhanced verbal communication skills is the backbone to any leadership task. No matter what stage we are at in our careers, we can always remind ourselves to review and reflect on how we verbally communicate with others. Communicating accurately and with an awareness of paralinguistics (tone, pitch, volume) are essential building blocks in verbal communication. Also, you may need to develop your skill at questioning and presenting information to others.

Nonverbal skills are essential. Being able to listen effectively is just as important as being able to convey information. Working on the nonverbal aspects of listening such as eye contact, taking time and using silence is important. Boynton (2009) suggests this can demonstrate physically that you have listened. Active listening is important as it shows respect, and that people are valued; it is also a means of building trust (Battle, 2006). Boynton (2009) suggests this can be demonstrated through not interrupting and allowing others to finish their sentences. Listening may help you to invest in someone's emotional bank account, which is invaluable in collective and transformational leadership styles (Covey, 2004).

Go Further 3.4

The following link is to an RCN article on communication skills www.rcn.org. uk/clinical-topics/Patient-safety-and-human-factors/Professional-Resources/ Communication

---

EMOTIONAL INTELLIGENCE

Goleman et al. (2013) argue that leadership qualities such as developing vision and generating ideas are important, but equally important is the emotional intelligence of leadership. What is emotional intelligence? It can be defined as self-awareness, self-regulation and a level of empathy and understanding of others' perspectives. Having such skills can help to increase positivity and motivation in others and improve our interactions. Frankle (2008) suggests it is the ability to understand and read people's viewpoints and perspectives and put aside glory hunting and ego. Frankle also suggests that personal emotional intelligence is about self-awareness of your own needs and emotions, and the ability to motivate yourself. Controlling your own emotions in situations helps to overcome difficulties in working with others who have different styles and approaches to your own. Covey (2004) argues that self-awareness and looking after one's own emotional wellbeing is essential in leadership.

RESILIENCE

Resilience can be defined as the ability to recover and bounce back from difficulties or adversities. Much has been written about resilience in childhood studies and in such areas as recovery from trauma and abuse, examining what makes certain people recover from difficult life situations. NHS professionals (2020) identifies that resilience is about engaging with and utilising others for your own support and development. This can help to support and manage your emotions, and aids learning from past experience and to seek and use protective factors.

The personal qualities that add to an individual's resilience are being reflective and self-aware. Being more mindful and self-aware may enable individuals to have better capacity to address complex situations. A key factor in resilience is support mechanisms, such as building good relationships in your team and knowing where to go when advice is needed or when things are difficult.

However, the topic of resilience is a complex one. How much should we expect people to be resilient and when perhaps is it cultural or organisational factors that may be impacting on a person's workplace? The concept in health and social care is a difficult one, and resilience is not about taking on too much or not speaking up when you are struggling for fear of being judged as not coping. Therefore, think of resilience as more about building support mechanisms and networks to deal with work issues and complexities, but not to the extent where the underlying causes and cultures are not tackled.

INTERNAL LOCUS OF CONTROL

Rotter (1990: 492) describes the internal locus of control as 'the degree to which persons expect that reinforcement or an outcome of their behaviour is contingent on their own behaviour or personal characteristics'. People with a high internal locus of control believe in their own ability to control themselves and influence the world around them. They see their future as being in their own hands, and that their own choices can lead to success or failure. West et al. (2015) consider that when what happens around you is under your control, you are motivated to take action to influence events; this is associated with a tendency to be proactive rather than passive. Therefore, developing a focus on situations you have control over can help to eliminate stress and manage the situation more effectively.

POWER

As we move towards a landscape in healthcare where leadership will be more shared and encouraged, you need to understand the role power has in leadership.

The online Oxford Dictionary (2016) defines power as: 'The capacity or the ability to direct or influence the behaviour of others or the course of events'. French and Raven (1959) identified five types of power in a classification that is still relevant today:

- **Legitimate**: Legitimate power could be seen as the type of power that managers have due to position or hierarchy. This comes from the belief that a person has the right to make demands, and to expect others to follow commands. This type of power may have influence to an extent in that people may follow commands that they feel are expected of them for fear of repercussions, but this power may be lost along with position. This is not to say legitimate power is always a negative. Legitimate power if used productively can have great impact by being influential.
- **Reward**: Reward power can be subjective. This type of power seeks compliance from people by offering rewards. This could be a promotion or

offering preferential treatment. This type of power can run out if reward promises are not kept, and there is a potential that it could be seen as unethical to offer advantages to a person for carrying out a command. It could be also seen as manipulative.

- **Expert**: Expert power is gained when others may admire or value your knowledge or expertise. Yukl (2012) suggests that expert power is one of the most useful in leadership in getting people on board, but expert power does not come overnight and needs to be developed, and trust gained from those who see your expert knowledge as something of value. It is worth noting that expert power can also be lost if those in possession do not maintain their knowledge and trust could be lost along with power if the person seems arrogant or unapproachable with their expert knowledge.
- **Referent**: Referent power is a very different kind of power; it is not commanded by someone's position or title but is gained through an individual's respect for or loyalty to that person, often based on personal characteristics. This type of personal power can have great reach and is not easy to achieve. Referent power in leadership is the ability of a leader to gain the respect of others, which is not affected by position or hierarchy (although can be present in those in positions of authority).
- **Coercive**: Coercive power uses the force of an action by use of fear or repercussions if orders are not followed. This type of power may be used in certain circumstances (i.e. in disciplinary meetings) but its use in day-to-day leadership can have a negative effect by using fear to achieve compliance.

The way in which power is used may be interchangeable based on the situation and therefore different sources of power may be used in different circumstances. How power is used may also come across positively or negatively depending on how it is delivered, and this may be in relation to an individual's leadership style or personality. An autocratic leader can alienate staff; a laissez-faire leader could allow poor care to happen unchallenged. Democratic or participatory leadership is about influencing others to understand and agree about what needs to be done and how to do it – this then becomes transformational leadership. Improvement is more likely as staff have developed organisational relationships and understand the goals and how to achieve them.

It is important, however, to recognise that being over-reliant on certain types of power may not always gain the best outcome. Activity 3.4 asks you to engage in reflective practice. For more information on how to be reflective, look at Chapter 2, Personal and Professional Development.

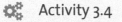

Activity 3.4

Think about some of your current or previous managers or leaders. Thinking about the powers described above, what types of power do you think they used or possessed? What were the good points about that power and how was it used? What were the downsides, or when didn't it work well?

LOOKING AFTER YOUR OWN WELLBEING

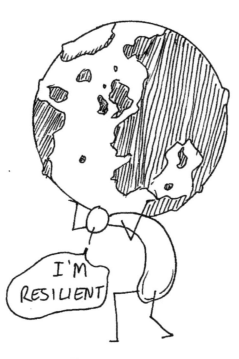

Figure 3.4   Looking after your own wellbeing

Looking after your health and wellbeing is also a very important factor in personal, professional and leadership development (see more in Chapter 13, Introduction to Mental Health and Wellbeing). There is much evidence about the value that healthy and motivated staff bring to the quality outcomes of service users in healthcare (Boorman, 2009). Health and social care is challenging and maintaining a work–life balance is essential. Staff are health and social care's most valuable asset, and whilst much is being done to support staff to stay well and healthy in organisations, there are things you can do and be aware of. It is important to consider your own wellbeing as a building block to strong and effective leadership.

⚙ Activity 3.5   Supporting your health

Have a look online at the RCN 'Healthy Workplace Toolkit' at: www.rcn.org.uk/healthy-workplace/healthy-workplaces
What are your thoughts on the toolkit?

- How useful have you found reading it?
- Do you know how to access support for your health and wellbeing in your organisation? Give examples of where you may seek both physical and mental support inside and outside the workplace.

Useful links:

www.england.nhs.uk/supporting-our-nhs-people/support-now/staff-mental-health-and-wellbeing-hubs/

https://people.nhs.uk/guides/abc-guide-to-being-personally-resilient/

UNDERSTANDING THE IMPORTANCE OF SELF-ASSESSMENT AND REFLECTION IN LEADERSHIP DEVELOPMENT

Self-assessment is a building block to developing into a reflective practitioner, which is an essential skill in leadership, and skills in reflection are required to be able to self-assess.

Rothstein and Burke (2010) stress the importance of self-awareness in leadership. If you want to be effective, especially in healthcare where change is fast paced, you will need to continually learn, grow and adapt. Therefore, self-assessment can be seen as invaluable in personal effectiveness to establish strengths and areas for development in leadership. Identify that those who truly understand themselves and how their behaviours can impact on others are more self-aware, have more sense of emotional control and stability. Sometimes not enough emphasis is put on concentrating on your strengths, and therefore it could be argued that carrying out self-assessment, recognising strengths and how they could be maximised are just as important as identifying any challenges. Sometimes, due to work pressures, you do not often get time to consider what your true strengths are and what you do well.

It is still important to identify areas of challenge, things that require improvements or development. Healthcare professionals have a responsibility bound by their professional body to continue to develop and address areas for improvement, especially in light of the renewed revalidation for nursing associates and the mandatory need to demonstrate personal development in practice (NMC, 2018). Healthcare workers are also expected to assess and develop their skills as stated in their code of ethics. Rothstein and Burke (2010) argue that whilst many theorists discuss those born with natural abilities and qualities to lead, through self-assessment, review and feedback, achieving effective leadership skills is within everyone's reach.

Whilst Rothstein and Burke (2010) argue that self-assessment is a building block to advancing individual personal effectiveness, it is also important to understand and appreciate the psychological factors and ethics and morals an individual has as these can often be seen as factors in leadership styles (Deinert et al., 2015; Judge and Bono, 2000). Therefore, completing an online Myers–Briggs personality test may be beneficial.

Finally, to evaluate only what you see as strengths and weaknesses may fail to uncover how you are perceived by others. Multi-source feedback processes help you not just to be aware of what you believe are your strengths and weaknesses but what others believe are your strengths and weaknesses (which may not be the same at all). Jack and Smith (2007) identified in the Johari Window that there is a blind spot in our self-knowledge, therefore 360-degree feedback is useful for identifying areas you may not have been aware of. The Johari Window is a psychological tool created by Luft and Ingham in 1955 as a model to improve self-awareness and personal development. It is a key tool in skill assessment as it encourages openness and a willingness to understand other people's views of your professional strengths and weaknesses. Taking into account the views of others can be a strong motivator to address behaviours to improve leadership practice. It allows the practitioner to demonstrate ownership of their own development.

⚙ Activity 3.6

Research some of these self-assessment tools and consider the pros and cons of each method.

Type of assessment tool	Pros	Cons
360-degree feedback (such as Leadership Academy tool)		
Johari Window		
Personality self-assessment (such as Myers–Briggs)		
SWOT		

(Continued)

- 360-degree feedback: www.leadershipacademy.nhs.uk/resources/healthcare-leadership-model/supporting-tools-resources/healthcare-leadership-model-360-degree-feedback-tool/
- Personality test: www.16personalities.com/free-personality-test
- Johari Window: www.mindtools.com/CommSkll/JohariWindow.htm

IDENTIFYING OPPORTUNITIES FOR LEADERSHIP DEVELOPMENT

Leadership is about drive and innovation, not about seniority.

NHS Plan (2001)

The final part of this chapter will give ideas for how you could develop your leadership skills both as a health and social care worker and as a student or trainee on placement.

Within our own workplaces and educational establishments, there are a wealth of opportunities that allow us to develop a deeper understanding of how the healthcare system works and how leadership skills are utilised on a daily basis.

SHADOWING SENIOR COLLEAGUES AND IDENTIFYING OPPORTUNITIES ON PLACEMENT

Being able to observe what others do is a good learning opportunity to see how they manage a team or how they may deal with difficult situations or competing demands that all require leadership skills. This observation can be informal or formal. Informally, it may be about taking more notice of how others interact. Formally, it would be asking your manager if you could shadow someone in your organisation or on placement for the day. Write up reflective notes later to help you to break down the leadership activities.

COURSES AND DEVELOPMENT PROGRAMMES

Many organisations will have internal courses or programmes that you may be able to access. Try to make yourself aware of the internal continuing professional development opportunities available. There are a wealth of CPD opportunities through FutureLearn, the NHS, conferences and annual meetings or local societies. You can also take free online courses from the Social Care Institute for Excellence (SCIE), FutureLearn, the Open University or NHS Leadership Academy, and nearly all universities offer free (non-certified) courses.

SOCIAL MEDIA

Social media can be a useful resource in keeping abreast of current debates in healthcare leadership and most large organisations now have their own Twitter account, for example. This can be an easy way of staying up-to-date with the latest documents and policies and can allow you to become involved in debates (being mindful of any comments you make and how they may be perceived). Remember that whatever you post online, you may lose control of, and it may be shared further and wider than you anticipated. There are lots of guides around using social media as a health professional, which offer support with what may or may not be appropriate to share.

APPRAISAL/INDIVIDUAL PERFORMANCE REVIEW (IPR)

Once you are employed, the identification of development doesn't stop there. An appraisal usually happens annually for employees and allows for the individual to reflect and understand their role and the part they play in their team and organisation. It also allows time to set work objectives for the coming year and discuss achievements from the previous year. It then allows a plan for identifying the knowledge and skills you may need to do your job well and achieve the organisation's objectives and your own professional goals. Appraisals are very important for your personal development so utilise them well. Prepare before your appraisal, think about what you might like to be involved in, or work towards. As part of this, think about what you will need to do to get to your goal. Appraisal is a great opportunity to discuss with your manager courses you are interested in or opportunities you want to pursue. You must also revalidate your qualification, so maintaining a reflective diary is essential as you will need to produce evidence of continuous professional development.

OTHER OPPORTUNITIES

At all levels of your healthcare career, you can look for wider opportunities outside of your placement or employment through volunteering, sitting on boards or acting as an advisor. NICE and the CQC are just two examples of national organisations that look for those working in health and social care to contribute to their work through sessional or ad hoc work. Using your students' voices and opinions can be a good opportunity for professional development and leadership skill development.

CHAPTER SUMMARY

- We all have the potential, regardless of grade or position in healthcare, to use leadership skills within our roles to ensure quality of care for our

- clients and patients, whilst also working towards professional and personal development.
- This chapter has introduced the concept of leadership in current healthcare practice.
- Hopefully, the chapter has demystified what leadership is and given practical direction to how leadership opportunities can be utilised and developed.

📖 FURTHER READING

The following websites and texts will support your development, knowledge and understanding of leadership and management.

WEBSITES

- The Foundation of Nursing Leadership: www.nursingleadership.org.uk/resources_free.php
- Florence Nightingale Foundation: https://florence-nightingale-foundation.org.uk/
- The Health Foundation: www.health.org.uk
- The King's Fund: www.kingsfund.org.uk
- NHS Employers: www.nhsemployers.org/resources
- NHS Leadership Academy: www.leadershipacademy.nhs.uk
- NMC Social Media Guide: www.nmc.org.uk/standards/guidance/social-media-guidance/
- Royal College of Nursing: www.rcn.org.uk

TEXTS

- Ellis, P. and Abbott, J. (2014) Leadership and management skills in health care. *British Journal of Cardiac Nursing*, 9(2): 96–9.
- Grant, L. and Kinman, G. (2013) *The Importance of Emotional Resilience for Staff and Students in the Helping Professions*. York: Higher Education Academy.
- National Skills Academy (2015) *The Leadership Qualities Framework for Adult Social Care*. London: Department of Health/The National Skills Academy.
- NHS England (2016) *Leading Change, Adding Value: A Framework for Nursing, Midwifery and Care Staff*. Available at: www.england.nhs.uk/wp-content/uploads/2016/05/nursing-framework.pdf
- NHS Improvement (2016) *Developing People, Improving Care*. Available at: https://improvement.nhs.uk/resources/developing-people-improving-care/.

- Rose, S. (2015) *Better Leadership for Tomorrow.* NHS Leadership Review. London: Department of Health. Available at: www.gov.uk/government/ publications/better-leadership-for-tomorrow-nhs-leadership-review

VIDEOS

- NHS Leadership Academy (various videos): www.youtube.com/channel/ UCRDUK0VYbv64-mMKlXYIH3A
- Professor Michael West: Leadership in today's NHS: www.youtube.com/ watch?v=0RXthT32vcY
- Compassionate Leadership Skills for NHS Frontline Staff, Dr Sarah Watts and Brian Rich: www.youtube.com/watch?v=0J3gsx6o9ts

REFERENCES

Battle, C. (2006) *Effective Listening.* New York: American Society for Training and Development.

Berwick, D. (2013) *A Promise to Learn – A Commitment to Act: Improving the Safety of Patients in England.* London: Department of Health.

Boorman, S. (2009) *NHS Health and Well-Being Review.* London: Department of Health.

Boynton, B. (2009) How to improve your listening skills. *American Nurse Today*, 4(9): 50–1.

Covey, S.R. (2004) *The 7 Habits of Highly Effective People: Restoring the Character Ethic.* New York: Free Press.

Czabanowska, K., Malho, A., Schröder-Bäck, P., Popa, D. and Burazeri, G. (2014) Do we develop public health leaders? Association between public health competencies and emotional intelligence: a cross-sectional study. *BMC Medical Education*, 14: 14–83.

data.gov (2022) Covid-19 virus data. Available at: https://coronavirus.data.gov.uk/

Deinert, A., Homan, A., Boer, D., Voelpel, S. and Gutermanna, D. (2015) Transformational leadership sub-dimensions and their link to leaders' personality and performance. *Leadership Quarterly*, 26(6): 1095–120.

Francis, R. (2013) *Report of the Mid Staffordshire NHS Foundation Trust Public Inquiry: Executive Summary.* London: The Stationery Office.

Francis, R. (2015) *Freedom to Speak Up: An Independent Review into Creating an Open and Honest Reporting Culture in the NHS.* London: The Stationery Office.

Frankle, A. (2008) What leadership styles should senior nurses develop? *Nursing Times*, 104(35): 23–4.

French, J.P.R. and Raven, B.H. (1959) *The Bases of Social Power.* Ann Arbor: University of Michigan, Institute for Social Research.

Goleman, D., Boyatzis, R. and McKee, A. (2013) *Primal Leadership: Unleashing the Power of Emotional Intelligence.* Cambridge, MA: Harvard University Press.

Griffiths, E.R. (1983) *NHS Management Inquiry.* Available at: https://navigator. health.org.uk/theme/griffiths-report-management-nhs

HSJ Future of NHS Leadership (2015) *Ending the Crisis in NHS Leadership: A Plan for Renewal.* Available at: www.hsj.co.uk/Journals/2015/06/12/y/m/e/HSJ-Future-of-NHS-Leadership-inquiry-report-June-2015.pdf

Jack, K. and Smith, A. (2007) Promoting self-awareness in nurses to improve nursing practice. *Nursing Standard*, 21(32): 47–52. doi: 10.7748/ns2007.04.21.32.47.c4497.

Judge, T. and Bono, J. (2000) Five factor model of personality and transformational leadership. *Journal of Applied Psychology*, 85(5): 751–65.

Keogh, B. (2013) *Review into the Quality of Care and Treatment Provided by 14 Hospital Trusts in England: Overview Report.* London: NHS England.

Kotter, J. (1996) *Leading Change.* Boston: Harvard Business School Press.

Leggat, S.G. (2007) Effective healthcare teams require effective team members: defining teamwork competencies. *BMC Health Services Research*, 7: 17.

Luft, J. and Ingham, H. (1955) *The Johari Window: A Graphic Model for Interpersonal Relations.* Berkeley: University of California Western Training Lab.

NHS England (2014) *Five Year Forward View.* Available at: www.england.nhs.uk/wp-content/uploads/2014/10/5yfv-web.pdf

NHS England (2016) *Leading Change, Adding Value: A Framework for Nursing, Midwifery and Care Staff.* Available at: www.england.nhs.uk/wp-content/uploads/2016/05/nursing-framework.pdf

NHS Improvement (2016) *Developing People – Improving Care.* Available at: www.nwacademy.nhs.uk/sites/default/files/resource_files/Developing%20People%20-%20Improving%20Care.pdf

NHS Plan (2001) *The NHS Plan: An Action Guide for Nurses, Midwives, and Health Visitors.* Available at: www.nursingleadership.org.uk/publications/agnmhv.pdf

NHS Professionals (2020) *The Importance of Resilience in the NHS Right Now.* Available at: www.nhsprofessionals.nhs.uk/joining-nhsp/latest-news/detail?Id=the-importance-of-resilience-in-the-nhs-right-now

NMC (Nursing and Midwifery Council) (2018) *The Code: Professional Standards of Practice and Behaviour for Nurses, Midwives and Nursing Associates.* Available at: www.nmc.org.uk/standards/code/

Oxford Dictionary (2016) Power. Available at: https://en.oxforddictionaries.com/definition/power

Roebuck, C. (2011) *Developing Effective Leadership in the NHS to Maximise the Quality of Patient Care: The Need for Urgent Action.* London: The King's Fund.

Rose, S. (2015) *Better Leadership for Tomorrow. NHS Leadership Review.* London: Department of Health. Available at: www.gov.uk/government/publications/better-leadership-for-tomorrow-nhs-leadership-review

Rothstein, M.G. and Burke, R.J. (2010) *Self-management and Leadership Development.* Cheltenham: Edward Elgar.

Rotter, J.B. (1990) Internal vs. external control of reinforcement. *American Psychologist*, 4: 490–3.

Skills for Care (2013) *Leadership Qualities Framework for Adult Social Care.* Available at: www.skillsforcare.org.uk/Support-for-leaders-and-managers/Developing-leaders-and-managers/Leadership-Qualities-Framework.aspx

Skills for Care (2021) Leadership and management. Available at: www.skillsforcare.org.uk/Leadership-management/Leadership-and-management.aspx

The King's Fund (2011) *The Future of Leadership and Management in the NHS: No More Heroes.* London: The King's Fund.

The King's Fund (2014a) *Culture and Leadership in the NHS.* London: The King's Fund.

The King's Fund (2014b) *Developing Collective Leadership for Health Care*. London: The King's Fund.

The King's Fund (2015) *The Practice of System Leadership: Being Comfortable with Chaos*. London: The King's Fund.

The *Shape of Caring Review* (*Raising the Bar*) (2015). Available at: www.hee.nhs.uk/sites/default/files/documents/2348-Shape-of-caring-review-FINAL.pdf

Turnbull-James, K. (2011) *Leadership in Context: Lessons from New Leadership Theory and Current Leadership Development Practice*. London: The King's Fund.

United Kingdom Government Coronavirus (covid-19) weekly report. Available at: https://coronavirus.data.gov.uk/details/deaths

West, M., Armit, K., Loewenthal, L., Eckert, R., West, T. and Lee, A. (2015) *Leadership and Leadership Development in Healthcare: The Evidence Base*. London: The King's Fund.

WHO (World Health Organization) (2009) *Human Factors in Patient Safety: Review of Topics and Tools*. Report for Methods and Measures Working Group. Geneva: WHO.

WHO (World Health Organization) (2022) Covid dashboard. Available at: https://covid19.who.int/

Yukl, G.A. (2012) *Leadership in Organizations*. London: Pearson.

4

PRACTISING VALUES AND ETHICS IN HEALTH AND CARE SETTINGS

GILLIAN ROWE

STANDARDS OF PROFICIENCY FOR NURSING ASSOCIATES (2018)

Relevant Platforms include:

Platform 1:1.1 Understand and act in accordance with the code of professional standards of practice and behaviour for nurses, midwives and nursing associates, and fulfil all registration requirements.

Platform 1:1.2 Understand and apply relevant legal, regulatory and governance requirements, policies, and ethical frameworks, including any mandatory reporting duties, to all areas of practice.

Platform 1:1.3 Understand the importance of courage and transparency and apply the duty of candour, recognising and reporting any situations, behaviours and errors that could result in poor health outcomes.

Platform 1:1.4 Demonstrate an understanding of, and the ability to, challenge or report discriminatory behaviour.

Platform 1:1.9 Communicate effectively with a range of skills and strategies with colleagues and people at all stages of life and with a range of mental, physical and cognitive and behavioural health challenges.

Platform 1:1.11 Provide, promote, and where appropriate, advocate for non-discriminatory, person-centred and sensitive care at all times. Reflect on people's values and beliefs, diverse backgrounds, cultural characteristics, language requirements, needs and preferences, taking into account any need for adjustment.

Platform 1:1.14 Demonstrate the ability to keep complete, clear, accurate and timely records.

Platform 1:1.15 Take responsibility for continuous self-reflection, seeking and responding to support and feedback to develop professional knowledge and skills.

Platform 3:3.5 Work in partnership with people, to encourage shared decision making, in order to support individuals, their families, and carers to manage their own care when appropriate.

Platform 3:3.9 Demonstrate the knowledge, skills and ability required to meet people's needs in terms of nutrition, hydration, and bladder and bowel health.

Platform 3:3.18 Demonstrate the ability to monitor the effectiveness of care in partnership with people, families and carers. Document progress and report outcomes.

Annex A Communication skills for providing and monitoring care 1.1–1.13, 2.4–2.9, 3.1.

Our lives begin to end the day we become silent about things that matter.

Dr Martin Luther King

This chapter will support your understanding of the role of values underpinning care in different settings and asks you to investigate your understanding of the practical application of the principles of values in care settings. You will also consider your own value base as you understand the theories that sustain ethical practice. You are required to evidence and demonstrate strong professional values during your period of training, and this chapter will support your learning.

Glossary

- **Anti-oppressive practice** Respects diversity and difference and affirms the autonomy of the people whose health you are working for
- **Code of conduct, code of ethics or code of practice** A guide to the standards of behaviour required in your day-to-day work, and a guide to ethical decision making
- **Confidentiality** Respecting the privacy of information that your patients (clients, service users) give you and ensuring that this information is shared, stored and used in ways governed by the Data Protection Act 1998/2018
- **Courage** Acting in accordance with your personal values, even if this makes you unpopular
- **Delegated duties** Tasks that you perform under the accountability of registered staff
- **Deontology** Ethical rules and laws
- **Diagnostic overshadowing** When a health professional assumes that the behaviour of a person is part of their ailment without exploring other factors
- **Empathy** The ability to understand and share the feelings of another
- **Reality ethics** Ethical principles based on virtues
- **Teleology** Seeking good outcomes or consequences
- **Values** A belief in the things we hold to be right and fair
- **Virtues** Characteristics valued as moral goods

INTRODUCTION

What are ethics and values and why do we have them? Philosophers have been pondering the question of how we live and moral responsibility for more than 25 centuries. Socrates said that 'the unexamined life is not worth living', meaning that we need to be reflective and examine our conscience. This is underscored by Dr Martin Luther King's quote (above), that we need to speak out when we see evidence of wrongdoing. You must act in the best interest of your patients at all times (NMC Code, section 16) and raise concerns when harm or risk of harm is present.

Working for health is a moral action, for which you need a moral imagination (Burke, 1790; Patel and Philips, 2021); therefore, you need to understand your own morals and values, those of your family, your culture and your community, where you as a person are coming from. You will at times be challenged by competing demands on your physical and emotional resources: trying to put aside your personal feelings when your patient's values challenge your own, trying to do your best when you do not have the equipment or staff you need to do your job properly. Trying to be ethical when you are exhausted requires inner reserves you may not know you possess. This is when you need your moral understanding and ethical framework to support you in your work. Activity 4.1 asks you to think about the values that you have and how you can explore these.

⚙ Activity 4.1

Think about the values that you have and how important they are to you, such as not being lied to or having your views respected, and think about how you would feel if they were ignored. You can read more about values in care on the SCIE/ Skills for Care website (www.scie.org.uk/).

REGULATION OF DELEGATED DUTIES

Many HCPs/HCAs are training for the NA role under the current apprenticeship scheme or are sponsored by their employer; while in training, you work under the supervision of registered nurses and NAs. Once you have qualified, the Nursing and Midwifery Council (NMC) licenses and regulates your work and provides you with the same code of practice as registered nurses. However, codes of practice share many features and so I have included reference to both the NMC Code and the Codes of Conduct for Healthcare Support Workers and Adult Social Care Workers in England, Scotland and Wales and used them to highlight how the codes collectively govern your work, especially when engaging in devolved nursing duties.

The characteristics of a profession include: using a technical language, accountability, responsibility, autonomy of action, work that is bound by a code of ethics, and a confidential relationship between the practitioner and client, and (according to Wickenden, 1952) rendering a specialised service based upon advanced specialised knowledge and skill.

Whichever role you have, accountability rests with the registered staff who supervise your work. They have to ensure that when you are delegated a task:

1. You have the skills and abilities and are competent to perform it.
2. That the delegation is appropriate and, in the patient's best interests, as all patients should expect the same standard of care, whoever delivers it.

Go Further 4.1

The RCN has an advice sheet called 'Accountability and delegation: What you need to know'. It can be found on the RCN website at: www.rcn.org.uk/Professional-Development/Accountability-and-delegation

A fact sheet from the NMC can be found at: www.nmc.org.uk/globalassets/sitedocuments/nmc-publications/delegation-and-accountability-supplementary-information-to-the-nmc-code.pdf

The main points from the NMC Delegation and Accountability documents are:

- Only delegate tasks and duties that are within the other person's scope of competence, making sure that they fully understand the instructions.
- Make sure that everyone you delegate tasks to is adequately supervised and supported so they can provide safe and compassionate care.
- Confirm that the outcome of any task delegated to someone else meets the required standard.

ETHICS IN CARE

We talk about ethics, morals, values and virtues as if the words are interchangeable. *Moralis* is a Latin word meaning morals and is concerned with actions; *ethics* is a Greek word that has a relationship with *ethnos* (ethnicity) and considers what is moral behaviour in any given society. Virtue is about moral excellence (from the Greek *arete* meaning excellence and the Latin *vir* meaning valour). The Greek philosopher Aristotle considered that if you have good virtues, you can only behave in a virtuous manner. Aristotle also said, 'a virtuous action is only moral when it is done with the desire to do the right thing'. The classical virtues are temperance, prudence, justice and courage. Values are principles and standards of behaviour, and these can be religious, political or ideological; they are beliefs and attitudes. Putting these principles into action is called a 'social good'. Rawls (1999) discusses the notion of social goods in relation to principles of justice. He considers that each person has an equal right to opportunity and to a share in society's goods.

Ethical philosophy considers how ethical decisions are made and how those decisions are put into practice; they are the why and how we as individuals and as a society work, and each individual society decides its own moral code. There are three main types of ethical enquiry: meta ethics, which examines various societies' attitudes to things; applied ethics, such as the ethical principles used by business or medical ethics; and normative ethics. Normative ethics are the ethics used in healthcare.

NORMATIVE ETHICS

These are two types: deontology and teleology.

DEONTOLOGY

Deon comes from *deus*, which means God; so deontological thinking is about duties and rules, such as the Ten Commandments in the Bible. All ethical work takes place within a framework; this might be legal, religious or cultural. Therefore, you need to follow the rules. The main theorist for deontological thinking is Immanuel Kant (1724–1804), who formulated the Categorical Imperative, which is 'Do not act on any principle that cannot apply to all men'. Therefore, when formulating a rule, it must apply to everyone, such as if lying is wrong, then it is wrong for everyone to tell lies for any reason, and you have a moral duty not to lie, even if that results in harm to someone. Deontologists do not consider the consequences of an act. The Categorical Imperative states that moral actions are right or wrong in themselves, without reference to circumstance, therefore truth telling is a moral duty. Kant considered that people should not be treated as 'a means to an end' – meaning they should be treated as autonomous individuals and an end in and of themselves.

📖 Scenario 4.1   Mrs Rivers

Mrs Rivers, aged 74, has just been diagnosed with stage 4 cancer of the bowel; there is evidence of metastasis to the liver. She has refused intervention and wishes to go home to die. She said that she wishes to enjoy what is left of her life but will seek hospice care and pain relief when she needs it. She has asked the nursing staff not to inform her family of her diagnosis as she feels they will pressure her to undertake chemotherapy and surgery. Mrs Rivers' daughter asks you to tell her what is wrong with her mother. She says her mother suffers from depression and is confused at times and is therefore not capable of making her own decisions. What would you do?

TELEOLOGY

Telos means 'end' and is the ethics of ultimate purpose; it considers what are the consequential effects of an action. This is broken down into three branches:

- **Act consequentialism**: argues that the morality of any action is dependent upon its consequences. Thus, the most moral action is the one that leads to the best consequences.
- **Rules consequentialism**: argues that focusing only on the consequences of the action in question can lead people to commit outrageous actions when they foresee good outcomes. Therefore imagine that an action was to become a general rule – if the following of such a rule would result in bad consequences, then it should be avoided even if it would lead to good consequences in this one instance. It is somewhat similar to deontology.
- **Utilitarianism**: devised by Jeremy Bentham (1748–1842) and derives from *utilis* (Latin), meaning useful. Bentham maintained that humans are driven by pleasure and pain, so he devised his hedonist (or felicific) calculus. The calculus determines that an action is right if it produces the greatest good for the greater number of people, and of any two actions, the most ethical one will produce the greater balance over harms. The drawback of the greatest good for the greater number of people is that minorities can be harmed in the process. Read Case Study 4.1 for an understanding of how this works in healthcare.

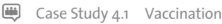 Case Study 4.1   Vaccination

Vaccination is a process that can protect the population from preventable contagious diseases. It is a demonstrably successful procedure; however, some people refuse to be vaccinated because they feel it is a harmful procedure (such as Covid-19 anti-vaxxers). If people were forced to be vaccinated, so that 100% of the population were vaccinated, then on statistical probability, some would be harmed. For instance, possibly 1 in every million persons vaccinated for smallpox will die as a result of an adverse reaction but 99.99% of vaccinated people will be protected against the disease (herd immunity). From 1967 to 1980, there was a global eradication programme to rid the world of this disease (WHO, 2016). There were 4.5 billion (4500 million) people on the planet in 1980 and over 80% of them were vaccinated; this means a death rate of (very) approximately 4000 adverse reaction deaths. Do you think this was a price worth paying for protection? Would it help to know that from 1900 to 1977, 300 million people globally died from smallpox (WHO, 2016)? How would a deontologist view this and compare that with how a teleologist would view this.

REALITY ETHICS

Bioscience ethicists devised reality ethics to help healthcare workers resolve ethical issues; the principles are based on virtues. In their classic book

Principles of Biomedical Ethics (currently in its 7th edition), Beauchamp and Childress formulated the following:

- Autonomy – respect for the individual and their right to choice making
- Beneficence – do only good and the principle of acting in the patient's best interests
- Non-maleficence – 'above all, do no harm', stated in the Hippocratic Oath (if you cannot make a situation better, do not make it worse)
- Justice – respect for, and recourse to, the law, which also emphasises fairness and equality

Beauchamp and Childress proposed seven principles in all; the other three are:

- Proportionality – balancing individual freedom against a wider social good
- Efficiency – the moral duty to use scarce health resources efficiently such as evidence-based medicine
- Health maximisation – maximising the health of the general population

We could also add to this list: veracity, truth telling and honesty.

CODES OF PRACTICE

Irrespective of whether you work in health or social care, your work is governed by codes of practice: the Nursing and Midwifery Council (NMC) Code of Professional Standards (revised, 2016, revised to include nursing associates, 2018), which covers health work; the Codes of Conduct for Healthcare Support Workers and Adult Social Care Workers in England, Scotland and Wales; the General Social Care Council Codes of Practice for Social Care Workers; and the Northern Ireland Social Care Council Code. The Core Standards for Assistant Practitioners can be found at www.nhsggc.org.uk/media/221012/hr_career_framework_app_11.pdf

---

Go Further 4.2

You can download the current version of the Code from the NMC website and the Code of Conduct from the Skills for Care website. It is important that you read and understand these as they govern your practice. You can find the NMC Code here: www.nmc.org.uk/globalassets/sitedocuments/nmc-publications/nmc-code.pdf and the Skills for Care code here: www.skillsforcare.org.uk/Documents/Standards-legislation/Code-of-Conduct/Code-of-Conduct.pdf

What these codes all have in common is a desire to promote ethical practice in your daily work:

- Respecting people
- Treating people with dignity
- Treating people fairly
- Supporting patients' choices
- Disclosing when something goes wrong

PERSON-CENTRED CARE (PCC)

Person-centred care places the patient first: it is important that we have an understanding of the patient and their needs, but equally important that we recognise that the patient is an expert in themselves. We should support the patient to express their needs by using appropriate communication skills and ensuring that meaningful dialogue takes place. PCC should be care led, not resource led, but the reality is that often we have to negotiate a plan of care that is effective and efficient, and that is acceptable to both the patient and to the care team. For social care workers and healthcare practitioners, this also means challenging commissioning agencies (such as adult social care) where the person's safety and wellbeing may be jeopardised by the way the service has been commissioned (UKHCA, 2021). We must ensure our work is ethical, this means ensuring the plan of care is fair, non-judgemental, respectful and non-prejudicial, and that we promote care practice that seeks to enhance the patient's wellbeing, health and welfare. We have a responsibility for the safeguarding of our patients; often patients are vulnerable, we must ensure that care giving is safe and patient protection is paramount.

ANTI-OPPRESSIVE PRACTICE

Before engaging in any intervention, seeking consent from the patient is critical. Any intervention without consent could be deemed an assault to the individual (read more about consent in Chapter 9, Essential Skills for Care). You need to ensure that the patient has been provided with enough information to give an informed and valid consent, so that they know what will happen and why. Birkenbach et al. (2012) considered the informed consent interaction as an 'info-suasive dialogue': how can you be persuasive without being coercive and thus undermining the patient's autonomy? The medical and nursing profession has a long history of paternalism (we are the experts, and we know what is best for you). There is a knowledge/power differential in healthcare work, but we must acknowledge that the patient is the expert about themselves, therefore the partnership or shared decision-making model is now adopted as the most ethical model when laying out the pros and cons of any intervention. The asymmetrical nature of power and knowledge means that you need to support a patient with decision making, and that the information needs to be presented in a manner that the patients can understand, retain, reflect and decide on, then communicate their choice.

Ethical congruence relates to your own understanding of your ethical self, the values that you have and how they are aligned with the values of the organisation for which you work. If you share the same ethical principles, you are more likely to sustain your working relationships.

What the Codes Say 4.1

The NMC Code states that you should (2.1) 'work in partnership with people to make sure you deliver care effectively', (2.3) 'encourage and empower people to share decisions about their treatment and care' and (2.5) 'respect, support and document a person's right to accept or refuse care and treatment'.

The Codes of Conduct for Healthcare Support Workers and Adult Social Care Workers in England, Scotland and Wales state (2.5): 'always gain valid consent before providing healthcare, care and support. You must also respect a person's right to refuse to receive healthcare, care and support if they are capable of doing so'; and (4.3) 'always explain and discuss the care, support or procedure you intend to carry out with the person and only continue if they give valid consent'.

Some patients may not be able to give valid consent at a time when they need to due to cognitive impairment, or they may lack the capability to give valid consent if their mind is impaired or disturbed. This impairment may be temporary or permanent. Patients need to be assessed using guidance from the Mental Capacity Act (2005, amended 2018). If someone is judged as not having capacity, health workers need to consider what is in the patient's best interests. Family members are usually consulted as they are likely to know the person's wishes if they have not made an Advance Decision Directive (this used to be known as a 'living will'). The main elements to choosing to intervene will be 'can this procedure wait until the patient is able to make their own decision?' and if not, then to try to identify what choices the patients would have made, taking into consideration their personal, religious and cultural beliefs. If no one suitable is available to help, an Independent Mental Capacity Advocate (IMCA) must be consulted.

Go Further 4.3

To deepen your knowledge, read about 'Planning for your future' and the Mental Capacity Act; this can be found at: https://digital.nhs.uk/data-and-information/publications/statistical/mental-capacity-act-2005-deprivation-of-liberty-safeguards-assessments/annual-report-2017-18-england

---

COMMUNICATING WITH PEOPLE WHO ARE COGNITIVELY IMPAIRED

Communication is the imparting or exchanging of information by speaking, writing, or using some other medium for the transmission of information (OED, 2021). We also communicate our thoughts and feelings, but people who are cognitively impaired have difficulty managing this. They may be a young child, have had a stroke (properly, a cerebrovascular event), have a learning disability (LD), dementia, hearing loss or may be mentally disturbed, any of which are barriers to communication. Healthcare staff may need to be creative in finding ways to make their message understood; you could try using sign language or Makaton with deaf or LD patients, pictograms, or talk to text systems. Patients may communicate by blinking, nodding their head or by moving or clenching a finger. The introduction of the hospital passport (All About Me Patient Passport), which is a downloadable form to be filled in before a hospital visit, supports communication with patients with cognitive impairments such as a learning disability. The passport will explain likes/dislikes and communication preferences. If a patient with an LD is admitted for a hospital stay, it is recommended that the passport is kept with the end of bed notes, so that all staff have access to it.

Ensure that the person you are speaking to can see you clearly and make eye contact, and that the communication is taking place in a quiet area so they can hear you. Keep your message short and to the point and if you are offering options, make sure that you state them clearly and one at a time.

We have all been in restaurants or cafes where the waiter/ess has reeled off a list of items so fast that you have had to stop them and ask them to repeat what they have said – it's annoying and makes you feel stupid. Sometimes it may be easier for the patient if you ask closed questions which require a yes or no answer, for example, Are you in pain: yes/nod/squeeze finger/blink/groan.

It might help to have a family member present who is used to communicating with the patient and can support the conversation, especially if it is regarding consent for treatment, or to help them to understand what the treatment is and how it is going to happen.

> ## What the Codes Say 4.2
>
> The NMC Code states (7.2) 'take reasonable steps to meet people's language and communication needs, providing, wherever possible, assistance to those who need help to communicate their own or other people's needs', (7.3) 'use a range of verbal and non-verbal communication methods, and consider cultural sensitivities, to better understand and respond to people's personal and health needs' and (7.4) 'check people's understanding from time to time to keep misunderstanding or mistakes to a minimum'.
>
> The Codes of Conduct for Healthcare Support Workers and Adult Social Care Workers in England, Scotland and Wales state (4.1) 'communicate respectfully with people who use health and care services and their carers in an open, accurate, effective, straightforward and confidential way'.

RIGHT TO CONFIDENTIALITY

> ### 🗨 Scenario 4.2   Mrs Rivers (continued)
>
> Mrs Rivers has told you that she does not wish her family to be told of her diagnosis as she feels that they will try to coerce her into accepting treatment. You feel that her family has a right to know and should be consulted, as Mrs Rivers has said she wishes to go home to die and will therefore need their support to do this. Would you encourage Mrs Rivers to tell her family?

The NHS Confidentiality Policy states that:

> All employees working in the NHS are bound by a legal duty of confidence to protect personal information they may meet during the course of their work. This is not just a requirement of their contractual responsibilities but also a requirement within the common law duty of confidence and data protection legislation – the European General Data Protection Regulation (GDPR) and Data Protection Act 2018 (DPA 2018) which implements the GDPR in the UK. Confidentiality is also a requirement within the NHS Care Record Guarantee, produced to assure patients regarding the use of their information. (NHS England, 2019)

Patients disclose all sorts of information to health workers; quite often, patients will disclose information that they have never shared with anyone before (when was the last time you had a conversation about how often you have a bowel movement?). Health workers expect patients to negate all conversational niceties and give them intimate information. More often than not the patient does but does so expecting you to fully respect their confidence and not share this information beyond the care setting.

What the Codes Say 4.3

The NMC Code states (2.4) 'respect the level to which people receiving care want to be involved in decisions about their own health, wellbeing and care' and (5.2) 'make sure that people are informed about how and why information is used and shared by those who will be providing care'.

The Codes of Conduct for Healthcare Support Workers and Adult Social Care Workers in England, Scotland and Wales state (5.1) 'treat all information about people who use health and care services and their carers as confidential' and (5.2) 'only discuss or disclose information about people who use health and care services and their carers in accordance with legislation and agreed ways of working'.

Dame Fiona Caldicott's report *A Guide to Confidentiality in Health and Social Care* (2013) was produced for the Health and Social Care Information Centre and it set out five rules regarding the use of confidential information in care settings:

- Rule 1: Confidential information about service users or patients should be treated confidentially or respectfully
- Rule 2: Members of the care team should share information when it is needed for safe and effective care
- Rule 3: Information that is shared for the benefit of the community should be anonymised
- Rule 4: An individual's right to object to their information not to be shared should be respected
- Rule 5: Organisations should put policies, procedures and systems in place to ensure the confidentiality rules are followed

Caldicott considers that 'Confidential information is given on a basis of trust and this is fundamental to safe and effective care.' Sharing information within the care team carries with it the notion of 'implied consent', that the patient has consented for information to be shared with the team in their best interests and for effective care to take place. Healthcare workers need to feel that the care team will also respect their patient's confidentiality and that anyone with access to confidential information is aware of their responsibilities.

📠   Scenario 4.3   Mrs Rivers (continued)

Mrs Rivers has told you that she does not wish her family to be told of her diagnosis. You need to inform your colleagues of her decision so that someone does not inform the family by accident. This information must be reported and recorded.

Reporting and escalating information to senior staff is crucial to team decision making. Without up-to-date information, mistakes can be made; equally, recording information is critical. Patient notes are legal documents, admissible in a court of law, therefore it is essential that they are accurate records of events. The box below explains how the codes describe this.

What the Codes Say 4.4

The NMC Code states (10.1) 'complete all records at the time or as soon as possible after an event, recording if the notes are written sometime after the event', (10.2) 'identify any risks or problems that have arisen and the steps taken to deal with them, so that colleagues who use the records have all the information they need' and (10.3) 'complete all records accurately and without any falsification, taking immediate and appropriate action if you become aware that someone has not kept to these requirements'.

The Codes of Conduct for Healthcare Support Workers and Adult Social Care Workers in England, Scotland and Wales state (4.4) 'maintain clear and accurate records of the healthcare, care and support you provide. Immediately report to a senior member of staff any changes or concerns you have about a person's condition.'

WHY WE RECORD PATIENT CARE

Recording patient care, whatever you do for and with your patient to meet their needs, is essential so the care team know what has taken place. The general rule is that 'if it's not recorded, it didn't happen' and this includes supporting patients with personal care and with nutrition and hydration. Age UK commissioned a report called *Hungry to be Heard* in 2006 and its follow-up, called *Still Hungry to be Heard*, in 2010. The original report found that older patients were either admitted to hospital malnourished and nothing was done about it or became malnourished in hospital because they didn't get the right food, or the help needed to eat it. The RCN carried out two surveys (2007 and 2010) and found that while staff understood that nutrition was important, they did not have the time to devote to patients' nutrition.

The RCN states that the following are barriers to adequate nutrition (see Table 4.1).

Table 4.1   Barriers to good nutrition and hydration

- poor understanding, from the person, their family and the staff caring for them
- unsuitable meal times
- not being able to address personal and cultural preferences
- poor motivation
- poor staffing
- medication
- ill health
- poor oral hygiene and dentition
- boring or inappropriate food
- lack of appropriate aids to support people to eat
- social isolation
- nil by mouth
- sensory loss
- delirium

For people with learning difficulties the situation is far worse. The report *Death by Indifference* (Mencap, 2007, 2012) revealed 74 deaths due to malnutrition or dehydration and Mencap alleges NHS institutional discrimination against people with learning difficulties. In 2014, 95 patients died of starvation or dehydration on a hospital ward and 15 died in care homes from the same cause; the figure was higher in 2015 (Office for National Statistics, 2017). It has been reported that ward doctors are prescribing water, to ensure patients are given drinks. Many trusts are making improvements and some trusts are training nursing associates as link nurses to ensure nutrition is supported and recorded. Nutritional support is now a key line of enquiry within the CQC inspection process.

Go Further 4.4

Read the *Hungry to be Heard* and *Death by Indifference* reports. They are challenging to read as they are evidence of poor care and neglect; however, they will help you to become a better care worker.

📠 Scenario 4.4   Mrs Rivers (continued)

Mrs Rivers has a poor appetite. The Trust runs a 'red tray' scheme and has protected meal times. It has been noticed that Mrs Rivers is losing weight, but

(Continued)

staff mark this down to her disease progression (cachexia) and she has not been proposed as a 'red tray' patient; do you think this is an example of diagnostic over-shadowing? You notice that when the catering staff bring the next meal trolley, they ask her if she is hungry and when she says 'no' they pass on to the next bed. When you check Mrs Rivers' notes, no food intake has been recorded since her admission. Do you think this is because she has not eaten or that it hasn't been recorded? Without accurate records, how can you be sure, and think about how this sits with non-maleficence and safeguarding principles?

WHAT ARE THE SIX CS?

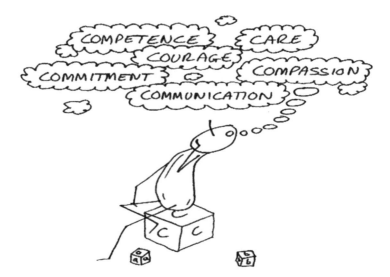

Figure 4.1   The six Cs

The changing nature of ethics in healthcare has moved from obliga-tion (deontology) to responsibility (consequentialism). An early exponent, Tronto (1993), said 'there is a pre-existing moral relationship between peo-ple; therefore, the question is, "How can I meet my caring responsibility?"' (p. 127) The dreadful events at Mid Staffordshire NHS Foundation Trust led some to believe that modern nurses suffered from moral blindness and were able to 'pass by on the other side' as they were not moved to alleviate their patients' suffering and accept their caring responsibility. The subsequent report by Robert Francis QC (Francis, 2013) made 290 recommendations, and the NMC acted against several nurses, who were struck off the regis-ter. One of the recommendations by Francis was to examine the way that student nurses are educated and to introduce value-based training. This initiated the 'six Cs' of care to underpin *Compassion in Practice* by Bennett and Cummings (2012). A further document, called *Compassion in Practice: Evidencing the Impact* was published 2016.

Care: 'Care is our business' means that we work at individual, family and population level. It means prevention, early intervention and health promotion as well as treatment of ill health.

- Compassion: means that we give care using sympathy, empathy, respect and dignity, which has been described as 'intelligent kindness'.
- Communication: this relates to communication skills with your patients, with your colleagues, with team members and the wider caring community. It also considers the communication you have with your patients and is central to 'No decisions without me'.
- Commitment: a commitment to care for your patients in the best way that you can.
- Competence: that you have the skills, knowledge and expertise to carry out your duties.

Last but not least:

- Courage: you have a duty of candour, so develop the personal strength to speak out and speak up for your patients and have the courage to embrace new ways of working for your patients. Also, have the courage not to accept second best for either your patients or for yourself.

Go Further 4.5

Read the *Compassion in Practice* report to deepen your understanding of how the six Cs can be applied to your practice.

You can find out more on the NHS England website: www.england.nhs.uk/wp-content/uploads/2016/05/cip-yr-3.pdf and the NHS Leadership Academy website: www.leadershipacademy.nhs.uk/category/6cs/

CONTINUOUS PROFESSIONAL DEVELOPMENT

📰 Scenario 4.5   Mrs Rivers (continued)

Mrs Rivers still hasn't told her family about her diagnosis. You are concerned that her daughter has said she suffers from depression; this isn't in her nursing notes, but you are aware that she is refusing food. You wonder if she would benefit from some grief counselling, but you do not have this training or skill. What is the most beneficial thing that you can do for this patient?

Knowing when you do not have a skill for an activity is important. If you can identify gaps in your training, you can then find the means to gain skills by asking your practice supervisor to find a training provider, if one is not available within the workplace.

What the Codes Say 4.5

The NMC Code states (6.2) 'maintain the knowledge and skills you need for safe and effective practice' and (22.3) 'keep your knowledge and skills up to date, taking part in appropriate and regular learning and professional development activities that aim to maintain and develop your competence and improve your performance'.

The Codes of Conduct for Healthcare Support Workers and Adult Social Care Workers in England, Scotland and Wales state (1.6) 'Strive to improve the quality of healthcare, care and support through continuing professional development'.

TRUTH TELLING

The almost seventh C is that of candour, the duty to tell the truth and speak out. The RCN guidance states 'Generally, the law imposes a duty of care on a healthcare practitioner in situations where it is "reasonably fore-seeable" that the practitioner might cause harm to patients through their actions or omissions'. The NMC and GMC have produced guidance on the Duty of Candour called *Openness and Honesty When Things go Wrong: The Professional Duty of Candour* (2015). Alasdair MacIntyre (2007 [1981]) discusses truth telling from a virtue perspective, considering honesty, courage and justice are virtues in practice.

📖 Scenario 4.6   Mrs Rivers (continued)

Mrs Rivers is deeply upset; she tells you that someone has shared her diagnosis with her son. As she suspected, he wants her to have treatment, and he is coming back this evening with his sister to have a family meeting to decide their way forward. Mrs Rivers said her wishes have not been respected and her confidentiality breached. She says she wants to discharge herself and go home as she no longer trusts the hospital staff.

ETHICAL CONTRADICTIONS

Mrs Rivers feels her rights have clearly been disregarded, and she is distressed as this is a conversation she wished to avoid for as long as possible.

The staff member who disclosed her diagnosis did not respect her autonomy. Autonomy is the individual's right to make decisions on their own behalf, whereas non-maleficence is the health worker's duty to do no harm. However, the staff member may consider that as the son asked for his mother's diagnosis, they felt they could not lie to him on deontological principles and that he had a right to know, and the principles of beneficence and non-maleficence have a place in evaluating truth telling and non-disclosure. The staff member who made the disclosure might argue that they acted for 'the greater good'; that the deontological principle of confidentiality should be overridden by teleological principles. It has been argued that respecting the autonomy of the individual does not imply a one-size-fits-all approach to truth telling. There may also be cultural considerations; in many cultures the family is informed before the patient, as they are considered as having primary decision-making responsibility.

What the Codes Say 4.6

The NMC Code states (4.1) 'balance the need to act in the best interests of people at all times with the requirement to respect a person's right to accept or refuse treatment', (5.5) 'share with people, their families and their carers, as far as the law allows, the information they want or need to know about their health, care and ongoing treatment sensitively and in a way they can understand' and (16.4) 'acknowledge and act on all concerns raised to you, investigating, escalating or dealing with those concerns where it is appropriate for you to do so'; also (17.1) 'take all reasonable steps to protect people who are vulnerable or at risk from harm, neglect or abuse'.

The Codes of Conduct for Healthcare Support Workers and Adult Social Care Workers in England, Scotland and Wales state (1.1) 'Be accountable by making sure you can answer for your actions or omissions'.

The codes have some contradictions. On the one hand, you need to respect the patient's autonomy on their right to accept or refuse treatment; on the other hand, you need to act in the best interests of all and share information, and you must be accountable for your actions or omissions. Mrs Rivers might argue that she is vulnerable to pressure from her family and is therefore at risk of abuse. She feels her daughter will ask to have her mental capacity assessed. If Mrs Rivers is found to lack capacity, do you think this would mitigate the breach of confidentiality?

Privacy is the right of individuals to keep information about themselves from being disclosed. Patients are in control of information about themselves. Patients should decide with whom, when and where to share their health information. Therefore, probably a disciplinary offence has taken place. The responsibility to maintain confidentiality is defended by the principle of beneficence, which asserts that health workers should act in ways that prevent harm and promote good to others. NHS Trusts' legal responsibility is explicitly stated in the Confidentiality Policy (NHS England, 2019): 'Patients, staff, members and the general public have a right to expect that NHS Trusts are a confidential environment in which their information will be treated with due care and respect, shared only with their consent, in their best interests or through a legislative duty.' All trusts and care providers will have their own version of the Confidentiality Policy and it is your responsibility to read and understand them.

WHISTLEBLOWING

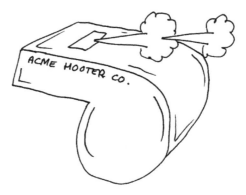

Figure 4.2   Whistleblowing

⚙ **Activity 4.2**

You were on duty the day the breach was committed, and you have a good idea who made the disclosure. You feel that action should be taken against the staff member, but it seems to have been 'brushed under the carpet', and your manager seems deaf to your comments. How would you deal with this?

The Public Disclosure Act (1998) and the Public Interest Disclosure Act (2014, amended 2018) (PIDA) support staff who 'whistleblow' on poor practice. In the past, employees were reluctant to raise concerns about wrongdoing because they feared that they would not be listened to or that they would be putting their jobs at risk. The above Acts allow employees to voice authentic concerns about misconduct and malpractice without receiving penalties such as dismissal, victimisation, or denial of promotion, facilities or training opportunities. Certain types of disclosures qualify for protection if they are made in good faith, and if the disclosure tends to show that the misconduct is happening now, happened in the past or will likely happen in the future. The staff member who made the disclosure probably did so believing they were acting in the family's best interests, and probably would, given the same set of circumstances, do the same thing again. Before taking any complaints out of the organisation, you need to discuss your concerns with your manager to give them the opportunity to address them. However, the 'deaf effect' (Mannion and Davies, 2015), which occurs when 'the decision-maker does not hear, ignores or overrules a report of bad news', can lead to frustration and hostility by the whistleblower, who may then pursue an external course of action. Recent research by the *BMJ* found that organisational inefficiencies can negatively impact the benefits of speaking up about bad patient care (Rauwolf and Jones, 2019). The law allows for disclosure to be made to a third person, known as a 'prescribed person'. Under the Public Interest Disclosure Act, the NMC is named as a prescribed person in the law (NMC, 2021). Further details can be found at www.nmc.org.uk/standards/guidance/raising-concerns-guidance-for-nurses-and-midwives/whistleblowing/

Go Further 4.6

Read this article to help you understand whistleblowing in the NHS: Mannion, R. and Davies, H.T. (2015) Cultures of silence and cultures of voice: the role of whistleblowing in healthcare organisations. *International Journal of Health Policy and Management*, 4(8): 503–5. Available at: http://doi.org/10.15171/ijhpm.2015.120.

Also, read 'The Public Disclosure Act from NHS and Social Care Perspectives', available at: www.england.nhs.uk/contact-us/privacy-notice/how-we-use-your-information/public-and-partners/if-you-whistleblow-to-nhs-england/, and social care whistleblowing can be reported to CQC; their policy document is available at: www.cqc.org.uk/sites/default/files/20200420_Whistleblowing_quick_guide_final_update.pdf

---

All employers should have a 'whistleblowers' procedure, which must be adhered to if you are to be protected. Please be warned that undertaking whistleblowing is not for the faint-hearted. Although you are protected by law, sometimes the law is not enough, and whistleblowing has affected careers and obstructed job opportunities; it is an act of courage to speak out. Francis (2015: 30) stated: 'When an NHS worker speaks up, they are making a vital contribution to the quality and safety of patient care. This is true not just of doctors, nurses, and other qualified healthcare professionals, but of all NHS workers regardless of position.'

> ### Go Further 4.7
>
> You can read the executive summary of the Francis Report online: www.gov.uk/
> government/publications/report-of-the-mid-staffordshire-nhs-foundation-trust-
> public-inquiry

NHS VALUES

When the NHS was founded in 1948 (The National Health Service Act 1946), Aneurin Bevan stated it was based on three core principles: these were that it met the needs of everyone, that it should be free at the point of delivery, and that it was based on clinical need, not ability to pay. This was one of the five giants that Bevan said needed slaying (the others were want, squalor, ignorance and idleness). There was an emerging consensus that access to healthcare should be a human right, not something available only to the wealthy, or given on application by philanthropic organisations. Bevan's plan was that everything should be free at the point of delivery but prescription, dental and optical charges were introduced quite quickly as the budget could not sustain the demands on it. Whilst care is not currently being rationed, those working within the NHS must be mindful of costs and ensure that wastefulness is contained, and that practice is evidence-based for effectiveness. The impetus for a national health service, paid for through general taxation and free at the point of delivery arose from postwar social solidarity and shared sacrifice; that solidarity has been eroded over time. All governments since 1979 have sought to limit the cost of the NHS with below inflation budget increases (1.4% average) and now it is dreadfully underfunded; nearly 50% of NHS beds have gone (Ewbank, 2017) despite an increasing population. The cost of privatisation and PFI agreements eats into the budget leaving the frontline depleted. Governments of all political flavours look to the USA and an insurance-based model for future health delivery, and despite reassuring rhetoric, it would seem that UK politicians are too captured to protect the NHS founding principles.

The NHS constitution is based on the founding principles and has stated values that you must support within your working day. These values are:

- Working together for patients, and that patients come first in everything we do
- Compassion
- Respect and dignity
- Improving lives
- Commitment to quality of care
- Everyone counts

Health workers must understand the Equality Act 2010 and how it protects people from discrimination based on age, gender reassignment, sex, race, religion or belief, pregnancy and maternity, marriage and civil partnership, sexual orientation and disability. These are called protected characteristics. The Act also considers discrimination on grounds of disability. This is defined by Section 6(1) of the Equality Act as: 'A person has a disability for the purposes of this Act if they have a physical or mental impairment which has a substantial and long-term adverse effect on their ability to carry out normal day-to-day activities.' While the NHS tries to ensure it complies with the Act, unfortunately some individuals practise discrimination either by intention or by default. This can happen in a number of ways. Muslims need to pray five times a day, they might need support to access a faith room, but no one is free to take them. Practising Jews who celebrate the sabbath do not use electricity (they cannot use lifts or tea making facilities) or phones. So other forms of contact need to be arranged.

Sometimes the care given falls short of the standards demanded when a patient receives care of worse quality because of stereotyping or prejudice: street homeless people tend to receive poor care, as do people who self-harm. These groups of people are seen as authors of their own misfortune or attention seekers and therefore not genuine. GPs have been known to refuse to take on high-cost patients with chronic conditions, or to delist patients with poor mental health when they persistently fail to attend appointments.

ETHICAL DECISION MAKING

In order to make ethical decisions, you need some tools, the best-known being David Seedhouse's ethical grid. It is a four-layer diagrammatic grid containing ethical connections that need to be considered. In the centre is the person (autonomy). Layer 2 considers the virtues of truth telling, beneficence (do only good) and non-maleficence (do no harm). Layer 3 could be considered teleological, as it considers what is good for the person, the family and society, and layer 4 could be considered deontological as it considers laws, codes and risks. Seedhouse (2008: 209) states:

> The Ethical Grid is a tool, and nothing more than that. Like a hammer or screwdriver used competently, it can make certain tasks easier, but it cannot direct the tasks, nor can it help decide which tasks are the most important. The Grid can enhance deliberation, it can throw light into unseen corners and can suggest new avenues of thought, but it is not a substitute for personal judgement.

The grid can provide some coherence when mulling over the best way forward through a moral maze. The grid is helpful when making multi-professional team decisions for empowering patients with complex needs, as it can facilitate patient choice making to support them to manage their own care needs. The grid also can be used in the context of overcoming barriers within primary care, community services and hospitals by providing person-centred care and the coordinated health services people need. This supports the *Next Steps on the Five Year Forward View* (2019; see Further reading) which is about breaking down barriers to care provision.

Seedhouse also considers where any agent stands in terms of ownership of the decision-making process, using his 'rings of uncertainty'. For a full explanation of using the grid and rings, read David Seedhouse's book, *Ethics: The Heart of Health Care* (see Further reading).

CHAPTER SUMMARY

- You have been introduced to the study of ethics in healthcare, to understand that there is more than one way of determining the right moral action.
- Deontology considers what the rules are, what the law says you should do; teleology asks what you are trying to achieve, and how you can secure the best outcomes for patients and their families.
- Reality ethics considers the application of virtuous practice: doing only good, not making things worse, acting fairly and being honest. I have included excerpts from the various codes of practice; these give you a framework to work within, to guide your work and to give you support when you are challenged to justify your practice.
- You have looked at the tools you might use to make sure you have considered all the stakeholders when making an ethical decision that affects patients, their families and the wider community. Remember that your work must take place within these frameworks in order to be ethical.

FURTHER READING

All these codes, articles and books are mentioned in the text and will help you to deepen your understanding of ethics in your working practice. The codes are regularly updated and freely available on the internet.

CODES

- The NMC Code of Practice for Nurses, Midwives and Nursing Associates
- The Codes of Conduct for Healthcare Support Workers and Adult Social Care Workers in England, Scotland and Wales

- The British Association of Social Workers Code of Ethics
- HCPC Standards of Conduct, Performance and Ethics

REPORTS

- Francis, R. (2013) *The Mid Staffordshire NHS Foundation Trust Public Inquiry* (Chaired by Robert Francis QC). Report of the Mid Staffordshire NHS Foundation Trust. London: HMSO.
- *Next Steps on the Five Year Forward Review*: www.england.nhs.uk/publication/next-steps-on-the-nhs-five-year-forward-view/

VIDEOS

- Ethics in Nursing UK: www.youtube.com/watch?v=HxZwIRUlpA8
- Nursing and Midwifery Council (NMC) Standards (2018): Accountability: www.youtube.com/watch?v=iMaVr1M-slA
- LGBTQ+ | Non-binary | Gender Fluid in Nursing: www.youtube.com/watch?v=HUfPdo-K4RA

BOOKS

- Armstrong, A. (2010) *Nursing Ethics: A Virtue-based Approach*. Basingstoke: Palgrave.
- Banks, S. (2012) *Ethics and Values in Social Work* (Practical Social Work Series). London: Palgrave/BASW.
- Melia, K. (2013) *Ethics for Nursing and Healthcare Practice*. London: Sage.
- Seedhouse, D. (1998, 2008) *Ethics: The Heart of Health Care*. Chichester: John Wiley.

JOURNAL ARTICLE

- Mannion, R. and Davies, H.T. (2015) Cultures of silence and cultures of voice: the role of whistleblowing in healthcare organisations. *International Journal of Health Policy and Management*, 4(8): 503–5.

REFERENCES

Age UK (2006) *Hungry to be Heard: The Scandal of Malnourished Older People in Hospital*. London: Age UK. Available at: www.dignityincare.org.uk/_assets/Resources/Dignity/CSIPComment/Hungry_to_be_Heard.pdf

Age UK (2010) *Still Hungry to be Heard: The Scandal of People in Later Life Becoming Malnourished in Hospital*. London: Age UK. Available at: www.ageuk.org.uk/bp-assets/globalassets/london/documents/campaigns/still-hungry-to-be-heard.pdf

Beauchamp, T. and Childress, J.F. (2013) *Principles of Biomedical Ethics* (7th edn). Oxford: Oxford University Press.

Bennett, V. and Cummings, J. (2012) *Compassion in Practice: Nursing, Midwifery and Care Staff. Our Vision and Strategy.* London: Department of Health and NHS Commissioning Board. Available at: www.england.nhs.uk/wp-content/uploads/2012/12/compassion-in-practice.pdf

Birkenbach, A., Singer, H. and Litan, R. (2012) An empirical analysis of aftermarket transactions by hospitals. *Journal of Contemporary Health Law and Policy*, 28(1): 23–38.

Burke, E. (1790) *Reflections on the Revolution in France.* London: Penguin Classics.

Caldicott, F. (2013) *A Guide to Confidentiality in Health and Social Care: Treating Confidentiality with Respect.* Leeds: Health and Social Care Information Centre. Available at: http://content.digital.nhs.uk/media/12822/Guide-to-confidentiality-in-health-and-social-care/pdf/HSCIC-guide-to-confidentiality.pdf

Ewbank, L. (2017) Hospital bed numbers – can the downward trend continue? Available at: www.kingsfund.org.uk/blog/2017/09/hospital-bed-numbers

Francis, R. (2013) *The Mid Staffordshire NHS Foundation Trust Public Inquiry* (Chaired by Robert Francis QC). Report of the Mid Staffordshire NHS Foundation Trust. London: The Stationery Office.

Francis, R. (2015) *Freedom to Speak Up: An Independent Review into Creating an Open and Honest Reporting Culture in the NHS.* Available at: http://freedomtospeakup.org.uk/wp-content/uploads/2014/07/F2SU_web.pdf

MacIntyre, A. (2007 [1981]) *After Virtue: A Study in Moral Theory* (3rd edn). Indiana: University of Notre Dame Press.

Mannion, R. and Davies, H.T. (2015) Cultures of silence and cultures of voice: the role of whistleblowing in healthcare organisations. *International Journal of Health Policy and Management*, 4(8): 503–5.

Mencap (2007) *Death by Indifference: Following up the* Treat Me Right! *Report.* Available at: www.mencap.org.uk/sites/default/files/2016-06/DBIreport.pdf

Mencap (2012) *Death by Indifference: 74 Deaths and Counting. A Progress Report 5 Years On.* London: Mencap. Available at: www.mencap.org.uk/sites/default/files/2016-08/Death%20by%20Indifference%20-%2074%20deaths%20and%20counting.pdf

Next steps on the NHS Five Year Forward View (2019). Available at: www.england.nhs.uk/publication/next-steps-on-the-nhs-five-year-forward-view/

NHS England (2016) Compassion in Practice: Evidencing the Impact. Available at: www.england.nhs.uk/publication/compassion-in-practice-evidencing-the-impact/

NHS England (2019) Confidentiality Policy. Available at: www.england.nhs.uk/wp-content/uploads/2019/10/confidentiality-policy-v5.1.pdf

NMC (Nursing and Midwifery Council) (2021) *Raising Concerns.* Available at: www.nmc.org.uk/standards/guidance/raising-concerns-guidance-for-nurses-and-midwives/

NMC and GMC (Nursing and Midwifery Council and General Medical Council) (2015) *Openness and Honesty When Things go Wrong: The Professional Duty of Candour.* Available at: www.nmc.org.uk/standards/guidance/the-professional-duty-of-candour/

OED (Oxford English Dictionary) (2021) Communication. Available at: https://languages.oup.com/google-dictionary-en/

Office for National Statistics (2017) *Deaths from Dehydration and Malnutrition, by Place of Death, England and Wales, 2014 to 2015*. Available at www.ons. gov.uk/peoplepopulationandcommunity/birthsdeathsandmarriages/deaths/ adhocs/009065deathswheremalnutritionwastheunderlyingcauseofdeathorwas- mentionedanywhereonthedeathcertificatepersonsenglandandwales2001to2017

Patel, M. and Philips, C. (2021) COVID-19 and the moral imagination. *The Lancet*, 397(10275): 648–9. https://doi.org/10.1016/S0140-6736(21)00151-3

Rauwolf, P. and Jones, A. (2019) Exploring the utility of internal whistleblowing in healthcare via agent-based models. *BMJ Open*, e021705. https://doi.org/10.1136/ bmjopen-2018-02170

Rawls, J. (1999) *A Theory of Justice*. Cambridge, MA: Harvard University Press.

RCN (Royal College of Nursing) (2007) Nutrition and hydration. Available at: www. rcn.org.uk/clinical-topics/nutrition-and-hydration

RCN (Royal College of Nursing) (2019) Nutrition essentials. Available at: www.rcn. org.uk/clinical-topics/nutrition-and-hydration/nutrition-essentials

Seedhouse, D. (2008) *Ethics: The Heart of Health Care*. Chichester: John Wiley.

Tronto, J. (1993) *Moral Boundaries: A Political Argument for an Ethic of Care*. London: Routledge.

UKHCA (United Kingdom Homecare Association) (2021) Code of Practice. Available at: www.dignityincare.org.uk/_assets/Resources/Dignity/OtherOrganisation/ UKHCA_Code_of_Practice.pdf

Wickenden, W. (1952) Professional organisations and professional schools. *Journal of Engineering Education*, 23: 52–62.

World Health Organization (2016) Smallpox. Available at: www.who.int/csr/ disease/smallpox/en/

5

APPLIED HEALTH SCIENCES

GILLIAN ROWE AND AMI JACKSON

STANDARDS OF PROFICIENCY FOR NURSING ASSOCIATES (2018)

Relevant Platforms include:

Platform 2:2.4 Understand the factors that may lead to inequalities in health outcomes.

Platform 2:2.5 Understand the importance of early years and childhood experiences and the possible impact on life choices, mental, physical and behavioural health and wellbeing.

Platform 2:2.6 Understand and explain the contribution of social influences, health literacy, individual circumstances, behaviours and lifestyle choices to mental, physical and behavioural health outcomes.

This chapter will introduce you to the psychology and sociology of health, and it has content links with Chapter 14, Protecting Children and Vulnerable Adults. You will develop an understanding of psychological theory and sociological factors and how these can impact on an individual's health and life chances. The first part will focus on developing an understanding of underpinning psychological theories in relation to health and illness and will examine the role of psychology as an explanation of development through the life span. The second part will identify sociological theories and theorists that explain inequality in health and life chances.

When caring for individuals, it is important to understand where they stand in relation to the social and psychological determinants to health, in order that we do not prejudge people when care giving. The NMC Code states 'Avoid making assumptions and recognise diversity and individual choice' (1.3, NMC Code, 2018), the more you understand about someone's life chances, the better you will be as a caregiver.

Within this chapter, you will encounter scenarios from practising nursing associates and trainee nursing associates in order for you to understand how the theories of applied sciences can be translated into practice; also provided are model answers at the end of the chapter. These scenarios are taken from NA and TNA work experience and therefore the rules of patient confidentiality have been adhered to.

INTRODUCTION

This chapter is intended to equip you with an understanding of the psychology of health and illness and how sociological factors impact on the health of an individual, family and society. Every human being is different. We all grow and change over time physically, mentally, emotionally and socially. So, what makes us who we are and what determines what sort of person we become? What determines the lives we lead? Look at Table 5.1 and consider what has determined who you are.

Table 5.1 Nature or nurture? What determines who we are – genetics or the environment we are born into?

Nature	Nurture
We all agree we inherited our physical characteristics from our parents – but did we also inherit our behaviour and personality?	Refers to environmental influences. This can include any factors from before, during and after birth as well as factors during our upbringing such as nutrition, cultural expectations, education, family. What did you inherit from your environment?

DEVELOPMENT ACROSS THE LIFE SPAN

THE ARGUMENTS

Some theorists think that development occurs continuously where individuals gradually add more of the same type of skills. Others argue that development takes place discontinuously as individuals change rapidly with new understanding at specific times. Figure 5.1 demonstrates this.

In order to understand psychological theory, this part of the chapter is grouped by psychological themes to give you a basic understanding of who the theorist is and how their theory fits within the main paradigms. Psychology for health is a relatively new branch of psychology and this means new interpretations of established theory. The interaction between the mind and body, a person's health beliefs and coping mechanisms, all contribute to the success (or otherwise) of an intervention and recovery. Research (Blot and Tarone, 2015; Doll and Peto, 1981) has shown

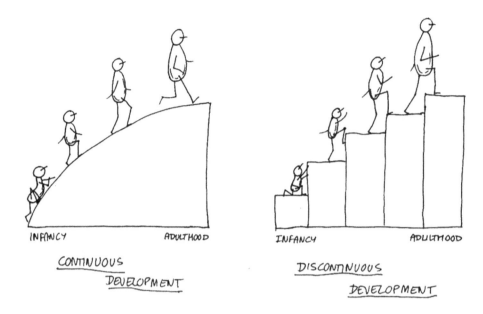

Figure 5.1   Theories of development

that health behaviours have a contributing effect on the likelihood of developing cancer. Smoking tobacco causes 30% of all lung cancers and poor diet is responsible for 35% of other cancers (such as bowel cancer). Therefore, if someone's coping mechanism for psychological stress is to smoke and eat junk food, there is a statistical probability of them developing cancer. Heart disease can develop because of high cholesterol in the cardiovascular system, the burden of overnutrition being a leading contributory source. As one eminent cardiac surgeon said, 'the chance of developing heart disease is 50% genes and 50% burger'.

BEHAVIOURISM

KEY THEORISTS

John B. Watson, Ivan Pavlov, Burrhus Frederic Skinner, Albert Bandura, Edward Thorndike

KEY POINTS OF BEHAVIOURIST THEORY

This theory posits the notion that we are born as a clean slate (*tabula rasa*) and that there is no such thing as free will, as all behaviour is learned from our environment as a response to stimulus and therefore it is considered deterministic. Theorists believe that this mechanism is common to animals and that the behaviour of humans and animals can be compared. Experiments by Watson and Rayner (1920) on 'Little Albert' to condition him to be frightened of rats were successful and prompted further research. Behaviourists are credited with making psychology a scientific discipline as experiments are conducted under laboratory conditions; however, critics argue that the experiments are conducted in artificial circumstances and do not reflect 'real-world' experiences. Behavioural therapy is used with autistic children and has been proven useful for people who are phobic.

CONDITIONING

KEY THEORISTS

Ivan Pavlov (classical), B.F. Skinner (operant)

KEY POINTS OF CONDITIONING THEORY

1. Classical conditioning forms an association between two stimuli.
2. Operant conditioning forms an association between a behaviour and a consequence.

There are four possible consequences to any behaviour. They are:

a. Something Good can start or be presented.
b. Something Good can end or be taken away.
c. Something Bad can start or be presented.
d. Something Bad can end or be taken away.

PSYCHODYNAMIC THEORY

KEY THEORISTS

Sigmund Freud, Erik Erikson

KEY POINTS OF THE PSYCHODYNAMIC APPROACH

We move through a series of stages during our life span in which there is an apparent conflict between biological drives and social expectations. The way in which this conflict is resolved is the main determining factor in our ability to learn, get along with others and cope with anxiety. There is a presumption that unconscious forces of which we are unaware manifest themselves in the things we say and do. The psychodynamic approach conflicts with behaviourism by suggesting that behaviour and feelings are affected by unconscious motives and that all behaviour has an unconscious cause. This has a relationship with our upbringing and may have been laid down before we were able to speak. Freud is considered as the 'father of psychology' although it could be argued that Charles Darwin first described adaptive behaviours in his work on evolution. Table 5.2 explains Freud's theory of personality and Table 5.3 lists Erikson's stages of development and complexes.

Freud considered that the Ego operates mainly in conscious and pre-conscious levels, although it also contains elements of the unconscious because both the Ego and the Super Ego evolved from the Id. Figure 5.2 encapsulates the theory.

FREUD'S STAGES OF DEVELOPMENT

- Oral stage
- Anal stage
- Phallic stage

Table 5.2   Freud's theory of personality: *The Ego and the Id* (2010 [1923])

The Super Ego	The set of moral controls given to us by outside influences. It is our moral code or conscience and is often in conflict with the Id
The Ego	The conscious self, the realist who mediates between the Super Ego and the Id
The Id	The unconscious self, the part of the mind containing basic drives and repressed memories. It is amoral, has no concern about right and wrong and is only concerned with itself

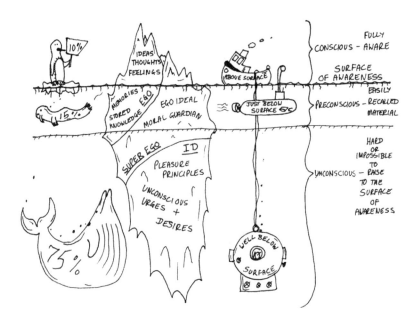

Figure 5.2   Freud's iceberg theory

In order to develop psychologically, the child must resolve the Oedipus/ Electra conflict:

Oedipus complex = male child's desire for sexual involvement with his mother

Electra complex = female child's desire for sexual involvement with father

Freud considered that both lead to a deep-seated feeling of guilt starting at a very young age. Erik Erikson (1994 [1959]) took Freud's ideas further. He believed that the Ego developed through a set of stages, at the end of which there was a crisis which needed to be resolved for the individual to move on to the next stage. Erikson's stages (Table 5.3) argue that psychological maturity depends on how well the conflict is resolved.

Table 5.3   Erikson's stages

Infant: Basic Trust vs Mistrust: responsive care vs neglect

Toddler: Autonomy vs Shame: independence vs forced action

Preschool: Initiative vs Guilt: initiative vs control

School-age Child: Industry vs Inferiority: sense of self vs bullying

Adolescent: Identity vs role confusion: self-identity vs no clear identity

Young Adult: Intimacy vs Isolation: meaningful relationships vs self-isolation

Middle-aged Adult: Generativity vs Self-absorption: having children and productive work vs selfishness

Older Adult: Integrity vs Despair: life accomplishment vs life dissatisfaction

Freud's theories of development ended at adolescence; however, Erikson considered that there are eight life stages. Critics of Erikson's stages point out that this is a very Western-centric viewpoint that does not translate globally and that it is misogynistic as it does not take women's life experiences into account.

👥 Scenario 5.1   Student Voice

Heather S – Nursing associate

Robert, a 45-year-old male, was admitted to hospital with multiple infected wounds to his arms, legs and back. Robert had a long history of injecting drug use; this was deemed to be the cause of the wounds on his body. Robert was experiencing heroin and alcohol withdrawal at the time of his admission. The Clinical Institute Withdrawal Assessment for Alcohol (CIWA) was used to manage alcohol withdrawal

(Continued)

---

which indicated chlordiazepoxide dosage. The patient was started on methadone once his alcohol withdrawal had subsided, as the doctors decided there was a risk of complications if both medications were commenced at once.

Robert was transferred to my ward, and following a review by the medical team, bilateral amputation of both his arms and legs was considered the most viable option. Robert declined this; therefore, vacuum assisted closure (VAC) treatment was deemed the most appropriate intervention once his withdrawal symptoms had subsided. Initially, Robert was very reluctant to engage with the ward staff and had several episodes of verbal aggression and refused care interventions during his first week on the ward.

I cared for Robert and worked with registered nurses to provide nursing care interventions such as personal care, monitoring his physical health condition, and ensuring he received the appropriate medications to reduce the symptoms of withdrawal and his level of pain. During this time, I was able to slowly build a therapeutic relationship with Robert, and he became comfortable with me and the team.

The treatment Robert received resulted in a 3-month hospital stay, and during this time, he discussed his life prior to being admitted to hospital. Robert talked about struggling in school and receiving no encouragement from his parents. He explained that he had been using heroin since his late teens as it was deemed the family 'norm'. He had witnessed his father using heroin, his mother misusing alcohol, and his older brother also using heroin. Robert had been to prison many times during his adult life, and he had struggled to maintain a drug-free life after each prison term.

Questions

1.   Thinking about nature vs nurture and learned behaviours, which of the theoretical models best apply to Robert? How can Robert be supported to make healthy changes. Read the rest of the chapter and return to this scenario, which other theories apply?

2.   Have you dealt with patients in this situation?

Please see the model answer at the end of the chapter.

THE COGNITIVE APPROACH

KEY THEORISTS

Jean Piaget, Edward Tolman

KEY POINTS OF THE COGNITIVE APPROACH

The cognitive approach conflicts with behaviourist theory as it focuses on internal processes rather than external behaviour. Cognitivism sometimes makes comparisons between humans and computers processing information.

It considers that behaviour can be largely explained in terms of how the mind operates, that is, the information processing approach. Piaget stated in *The Construction of Reality in the Child* (1954) that he believed intelligence is fixed at birth and that children actively seek to understand the world they live in. He believed they learn through experience and developed what he called 'schemas' to make sense of the world around them.

Piaget believed that children pass through four stages of cognitive development (Table 5.4).

Table 5.4 Piaget's theory of cognitive development

Birth to 2 years	Sensorimotor stage: children learn assimilation and accommodation
Ages 2 to 4	Preoperational stage: not able to abstractly conceptualise, needs concrete objects
Ages 7 to 11	Concrete operations: able to abstractly conceptualise
Ages 11 to 15	Formal operations: capable of deductive and hypothetical reasoning

Tolman (1948) believed individuals do more than merely respond to stimuli, that they act on beliefs, attitudes, changing conditions, and they strive towards goals. Tolman is virtually the only behaviourist who found the stimulus–response theory unacceptable; because reinforcement was not necessary for learning to occur, he felt behaviour was mainly cognitive.

SOCIAL LEARNING THEORY

KEY THEORISTS

Albert Bandura, Lev Vygotsky, Jean Lave

KEY POINTS OF SOCIAL LEARNING THEORY

Social learning theory is considered a bridge between behavioural and cognitive theory. Bandura (1977) considered that children learn through modelling significant others' behaviours. He used the 'Bobo doll experiment' (1961–3) to prove this. This theory examines how social influences, personal factors and behaviours interact. The theory explains how we might choose to adopt the behaviours of a role model. Bandura went on to develop the theory of 'Social Cognitive Learning' (1986), which is called triangulate reciprocal determinism: behaviour, personal factors and environment. Self-efficacy is a core factor in the triangulate mechanism. Self-efficacy is about self-appraisal and self-belief, and this influences beliefs about what a person can (or cannot) achieve (Figure 5.3).

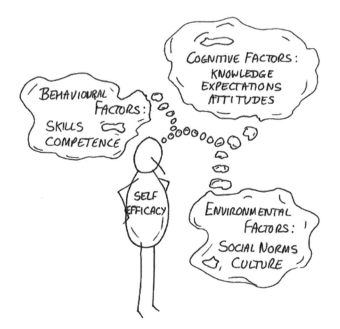

Figure 5.3   Self-efficacy

HUMANISM

KEY THEORISTS

Carl Rogers, Abraham Maslow

KEY POINTS OF THE HUMANISTIC APPROACH

Humanism studies the whole person; therefore, it is considered holistic. The theory states that behaviour is connected to feelings and self-concept. A humanist looks at behaviours through the eyes of the individual doing the behaviour to understand their motives and drives. Humanism rejects behaviourism as it considers the theory to be deterministic and mechanistic. Humanists also consider it lacks understanding regarding promoting personal agency as it does not acknowledge free will. Both Rogers and Maslow believed that people could overcome adversity and achieve fulfilment and satisfaction, which was named 'self-actualisation'. Humanism also rejects the scientific method and promotes qualitative methods such as writing reflective journals based on thinking and feeling. When constructing the hierarchy of needs (1943), Maslow studied those he believed were successful and productive. Kenrick et al. (2010) consider the hierarchy pyramid to be 'one of the most cognitively contagious ideas in the behavioural sciences'. Maslow determined that once one need was satisfied, a person could then move up the pyramid. It should be stated that everyone has their own personal take on the pyramid, an idea of what constitutes *for them* notions of achieving each level, and each person will have a different view of what self-actualisation means.

📖 Scenario 5.2   Student Voice

Lindsay S – Nursing associate

Mr Smith is a 39-year-old married man with young children. He has recently lost his father suddenly due to a heart attack (myocardial infarction). Mr Smith makes an appointment with his GP for a well man check.

I began talking to Mr Smith about his reasons for attending his well man check. Mr Smith said, 'I am extremely anxious about my health, I have recently lost my father due to a heart attack.' I sensed Mr Smith's anxiety and loss and felt it was important to listen and give him time to talk and build trust.

Mr Smith told me that he currently smokes, he has smoked for a long time and started at an early age; most of family were smokers. He also disclosed that recently due to the stress of juggling work and dealing with his father's death and financial affairs, he has been drinking a lot more alcohol. Mr Smith did not know what alcohol units were and what these meant but did identify that he had been drinking more than usual, he thinks as a coping mechanism to deal with his stresses.

I explained to Mr Smith the benefits of undertaking his health check. The health check is a preventative screening tool for health ailments such as heart conditions, kidney disease and diabetes using a QRISK2 score. The health check is also used as a platform for behaviour change discussion.

We talked about the risk factors of heart disease, how they are modifiable relating to lifestyle choices such as smoking, increased alcohol intake, poor diet and lack of exercise, and non-modifiable relating to family history, age and sex.

We discussed how obesity and blood pressure can impact on heart health. I checked Mr Smith's height, weight and blood pressure. His BMI was in a healthy range.

When asked about his diet, Mr Smith identified that he felt his diet could be better and identified that he had been eating a lot of convenience foods such as take away type foods and other foods high in sugars, fats and salts. We discussed healthy foods and how he could adjust his diet by doing some simple food swaps and preparing and batch cooking foods that can be frozen or refrigerated and easily accessed when required.

Questions

1. Thinking about Mr Smith and Maslow's hierarchy, Mr Smith has recognised he has a problem with smoking and drinking and that he needs to make changes in his behavioural habits. What advice would you give to Mr Smith to support his health?

Please see the model answer at the end of the chapter.

ATTACHMENT THEORY

See also Chapter 14, Protecting Children and Vulnerable Adults, which gives more detail on attachment theory.

KEY THEORISTS

John Bowlby, Mary Ainsworth, Cindy Hazan, Philip Shaver

KEY POINTS OF ATTACHMENT THEORY

Attachment theory is based on the idea that our first relationship with our primary carer (usually the mother) shapes the way we relate to others throughout our lives. It covers two important aspects of attachment formation and although it is a single theory, it is convenient to look at it in two parts:

1. The way in which children form attachment bonds and the nature of these bonds.
2. What happens if these bonds are not formed properly, i.e. the effects of deprivation and privation on a child.

Children have an instinctive need to attach to one person and are biologically 'pre-programmed' to make such an attachment; the attachment process keeps the child safe. There is a critical period, from 7 months to 3 years, during which the baby is most likely to form this attachment bond. If it is not formed by the age of about 3, it is unlikely to form at all and the child may never attach to anyone. This can have a considerable impact on the ability to form successful relationships in later life. The main characteristics of attachment are shown in Table 5.5. Schaffer (1996) described attachment as 'A long-enduring, emotionally meaningful tie to a particular individual'.

Table 5.5   The characteristics of attachment

Attachments are selective - they are directed towards specific individuals who are preferred above all others
They involve the desire to be near the person they are attached to
They provide comfort and security and are particularly important when the child is upset, ill, or tired
They involve separation protest - the child becomes upset if they are separated from the person to whom they are attached

SIGNS OF ATTACHMENT

- Separation protest: Becomes distressed if their primary caregiver leaves the room and they cannot see her/him. They will cry and, if they are mobile, will crawl towards the door through which she/he left.

- Stranger anxiety: Very wary of strangers. If a stranger tries to interact with them while they are with their primary carer, they will ignore them or look away. If they are approached by a stranger when they are within the vicinity of the primary carer, they will move towards her/him quickly. If they are unable to crawl, they will put out their hands for her/him. Mary Ainsworth used the 'Strange situation experiment' to determine five types of attachment, which are detailed in Chapter 14.

Adult ageing was considered by Daniel Levinson (1986), who developed a 'seasons of life' model of development as a different explanation to Erikson's, although it is still a stage model. All stage models (see Figure 5.4) are open to the criticism that they do not apply to all people everywhere.

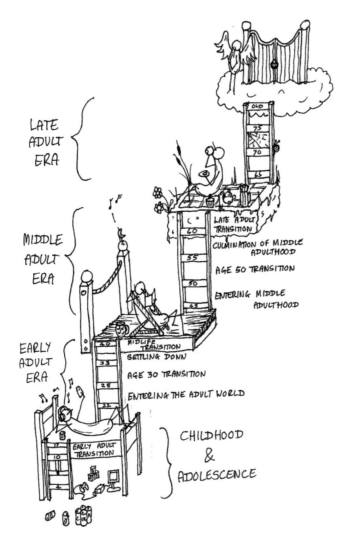

Figure 5.4　The stage model of development

These theories have a relationship with George Vaillant's (2002) 'Adult Tasks' theory and Bernice Neugarten's (1974) 'Social Clock' theory. The midlife crisis is considered a time of re-evaluation that leads to questioning long-held beliefs and values. This may be the result of factors such as divorce, change in jobs, moving home, loss of parents/caring for parents. Typically beginning in the mid-40s, the crisis often occurs in response to a sense of mortality, as middle-aged adults realise that their youth is limited and that they have not accomplished all of their desired goals in life. Not everyone experiences stress or upset during middle age: other middle-aged adults prefer to reframe their experience by thinking of themselves as being in the prime of their lives rather than in their declining years, especially now that longevity has increased in the Western world. As the population ages, an interesting phenomenon is appearing, namely the migration of the age at which someone is considered old. People were considered officially old when they reached retirement age, however the Baby Boomers are now not only working into their 70s but are becoming more active within their communities and developing creative businesses. Neugarten tied the Social Clock to women's biological clock, but improvements in reproductive science have extended the child-bearing years, and social changes mean that women do not fear becoming an 'old maid' – many actively embracing the singleton life.

OTHER THEORIES OF AGEING

The role and status of old people varies enormously from one society to another, as does the age at which a person is viewed as 'old'. In the UK and other industrial countries, retirement from work is an important transition point in the process of growing old. Two conflicting theories explain attitudes to ageing. Disengagement theory argues that elderly people begin to disengage from their previous social roles as they realise that they will die soon. The theory was developed by Elaine Cumming and Warren Earl Henry in their 1961 book *Growing Old* and was one of the first theories of ageing developed by sociologists. This process benefits society by avoiding the potential disruption that would be caused by key members dying suddenly.

Subsequently, the theory has been largely disproven by the 'activity theory of ageing', which proposes that older adults are happiest when they stay active and maintain social interactions. The theory was developed by Robert J. Havighurst (1963) as a response to the disengagement theory of ageing. The process of successful ageing is greatly facilitated when older people pursue hobbies and relationships and generally lead a more active lifestyle. George L. Maddox and Robert Atchley developed the 'continuity theory' (Atchley, 1989), which considers that internal structures of continuity remain constant over a lifetime and include elements such as personality traits, ideas and beliefs. It helps people make future decisions by providing them with a stable foundation. External structures of continuity help maintain a stable self-concept and lifestyle and include relationships and social roles.

ELISABETH KÜBLER-ROSS AND THE STAGES OF GRIEF

When someone is confronted with the knowledge of approaching death, reactions can depend on the age of the person and the reason for death. Western society tends to be 'death denying', and often, reluctant to acknowledge someone is dying, important conversations are not said, or said too late.

The dying person may visit 'the stages' (see Table 5.6 below) before death, and after the death their family may also experience the stages while mourning their loss. Elisabeth Kübler-Ross (1969) proposed five stages in approaching death (Table 5.6), although not everyone follows the sequence through the stages and not all people experience all the stages. Grieving is a process and each person will experience it differently; there is no set time for visiting each stage and many return to some stages during the mourning process.

There are criticisms of Kübler-Ross' stage theory. Kastenbaum and Costa (1977) deny any evidence that the stages exist and suggest her data-gathering methodology is flawed, and Corr et al. (2007) considered the stages reductionist and therefore unhelpful as they reject the person's ability to employ their own coping strategies.

Table 5.6   Kübler-Ross's stages of approaching death

Denial ('It must be a mistake')
Anger ('It isn't fair!')
Bargaining ('Let me/them live longer and I'll be a better person')
Depression ('I've lost everything important to me')
Acceptance ('What has to be, has to be')

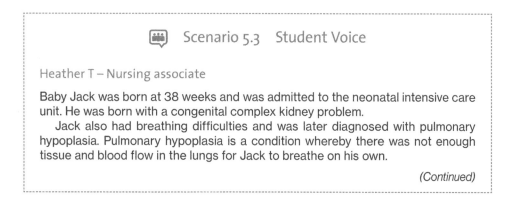

🗨 Scenario 5.3   Student Voice

Heather T – Nursing associate

Baby Jack was born at 38 weeks and was admitted to the neonatal intensive care unit. He was born with a congenital complex kidney problem.

Jack also had breathing difficulties and was later diagnosed with pulmonary hypoplasia. Pulmonary hypoplasia is a condition whereby there was not enough tissue and blood flow in the lungs for Jack to breathe on his own.

(Continued)

Jack was intubated and placed on high flow ventilation with a plan to closely monitor his progress for the next 24 hours before any further decisions were made. Jack's parents were given the devastating news that their baby was requiring a lot of intervention and support with his circulation and blood pressure and that his condition was deteriorating.

As Jack's prognosis was poor, his parents prepared themselves with the support of the team for the inevitable outcome. They wished to have Jack christened; arrangements were made for this to happen a few hours later. Jack's parents were supported to dress him in their choice of outfit and take him out of the incubator for cuddles. He had many tubes and monitoring wires in place, but nursing staff facilitated this safely. The christening was carried out and I felt hugely privileged to share this very emotional experience with the family.

Questions

1. Elisabeth Kübler-Ross explores the stages of approaching death, where do you think Jack's parents are in this process?

2. Reflect upon a time in practice that you have experienced caring for a deteriorating patient and their family. Can you link Kübler-Ross's theory to any of the aspects of your situation?

3. What could you do as a nursing associate to care for both Jack and his parents during this time?

See Heather's model answer at the end of the chapter.

WHAT IS PSYCHOLOGY FOR HEALTH?

Health psychology, often synonymous with behavioural medicine and medical psychology, is the application of psychological theory and research to health, illness and healthcare. Clinical psychology focuses on mental health and neurological illness; health psychology is concerned with the psychology of a range of health-related behaviour. Understanding psychological theory supports the care practitioner to understand the patient/client and make choices regarding interventions. Table 5.7 looks at the approaches examined in this chapter in relation to psychology for health.

Table 5.7   Psychology for health

Psychological theory provides the basis of psychological approaches for intervention
The **behavioural** approach looks at observed behaviour
The **cognitive** approach listens to the client
The **humanistic** approach listens to the client and gives the client choices
The **psychodynamic** approach interprets what the person says and does

The biopsychosocial model of health was developed by George Engel (1977) as a means to move the stale medical vs social model of health debate forward (see Chapter 13, Introduction to Mental Health and Wellbeing, for further detail on the models of health). The biopsychosocial theory posits that each one of these factors is not sufficient to bring about health or psychological illness, but the interaction between them determines the course of one's development. The biological influences on mental health and mental illness are varied, and include genetics, infections, physical trauma, nutrition, hormones and toxins. The psychological component looks for potential psychological causes for a health problem, such as lack of self-control, emotional turmoil and negative thinking.

Social and cultural factors are conceptualised as a set of stressful events (e.g. losing one's job) that can differentially impact mental health depending on the individual and the social context in which they live. Despite its usefulness, there are issues with the biopsychosocial model including the degree of influence that each factor has, the degree of interaction between factors, and variation across individuals and life spans.

The biopsychosocial model states that the workings of both the body and the environment affect the mind, and the workings of the mind can affect the body and environment (see Figure 5.5). Thus, this theory posits that each one of these factors is not sufficient to bring about health or illness, but the interaction between them is what determines health outcomes.

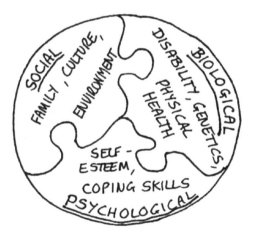

Figure 5.5   The biopsychosocial model

UNDERSTANDING AND EXPLAINING SOCIAL PHENOMENA

The Oxford English Dictionary states that 'Sociology is the scientific or academic study of social behaviour, including its origins, development, organisation, and institutions.' It is a social science that uses various methods of empirical investigation and critical analysis to develop a body of knowledge about social order, social disorder and social change. The origins of sociology lie in the eighteenth century when advances during 'The Enlightenment' led people to believe there was a rational explanation to the problems facing society. Auguste Comte (1798–1857) coined the name 'sociology', the science of society: ideas about society are conceptual, and research and evidence then lead to theoretical development, which is why it is a science.

Stated basically, the medical model assumes that the body is a machine that breaks down now and then and it is the role of medicine to repair it, reducing the role of medical and nursing staff to that of mechanic and technician. The social model examines the world that the body exists in and social science seeks to understand how culture, experience and society explain health and illness.

WHAT ARE PARADIGMS?

Paradigms are used to explain ideas, rather like looking at something through a particular lens or perspective. Paradigms are broad perspectives or viewpoints that allow social scientists to have a variety of tools to describe the behaviour of society and be able to create hypotheses and theories. The notion of paradigms was developed by Thomas Kuhn (1962) to explain a set of changing circumstances or changes in knowledge resulting in changing circumstances.

PARADIGMS IN SOCIOLOGY

Sociology has many perspectives, but this chapter will focus on three major paradigms and will apply them to the sociological enquiry into health.

THE CONFLICT PARADIGM

KEY THEORISTS

Karl Marx, Fredrick Engels, Ivan Illich

KEY POINTS OF SOCIAL CONFLICT THEORY

Key elements in this perspective are that society is structured in ways to benefit a few at the expense of the majority, and factors such as wealth, property, race, sex, gender, class and age are linked to social inequality. To a social conflict theorist, this is all about dominant group vs minority group relations. Conflict is considered an engine for change to challenge an unequal social order and bring about equilibrium in resources and power.

Feminist theorists such as Abbott and Wallace (1990), Rege (2003) and Millett (2000) argue that none of the perspectives consider the roles and voice of women, and they critique systems designed by and for (mainly white, middle-class) men. Feminists focus on gender, disadvantage and health. The feminist perspective considers that health is paternalistic, especially in relation to the physiology and control of reproduction. Black women activists such as bel hooks (2001) call this 'intersectionality', where wealth, power and white privilege meet together to form an oppressive exclusive social system.

CONFLICT THEORY AND HEALTH

This theory argues that people from disadvantaged social backgrounds are more likely to become ill and to receive inadequate healthcare. Paul Farmer (1999) said that 'Inequality itself constitutes our modern plague – inequality is a pathogenic force.' Ivan Illich (1976) considered that medicine itself could be a force for ill and developed the theory of medical iatrogenesis. He considered this to take three forms (Table 5.8).

Table 5.8   Illich's three forms of medical iatrogenesis

Clinical	Social	Cultural
The damage done to patients through ineffective, unsafe and flawed treatments. He recommended that all treatments should be proven using evidence-based medicine. It could be argued that adverse psychological treatments and therapies come under this heading.	The medicalisation of social conditions such as sadness, age-related declines.	Removing from people the ability to trust their own instincts regarding their health, and the ridicule of traditional ways of dealing with, and making sense of, death, suffering and sickness. This reduces or encourages people to lose their autonomous coping skills. This might include homely remedies such as wearing a copper bracelet to ward off joint pain or using lay knowledge such as that described by Stacey (1994: 106): 'Not taking your child to the cold draughty health clinic on a pouring wet winter day is health giving rather than health denying, that's the intelligent use of lay knowledge.'

Conflict theory considers that health should be a natural right and such things that promote health (safe employment, dry home, decent food, access to clean water, access to healthcare, etc.) are human rights and not commodities only available to those who can afford them.

THE FUNCTIONALIST PARADIGM (THE POSITIVIST APPROACH)

KEY THEORISTS

Auguste Compte, Emile Durkheim, Talcott Parsons

KEY POINTS OF FUNCTIONALISM

Society consists of a system of interdependent institutions and organisations held together by shared values and common symbols (family, education, economy, polity and religion) that function for the survival of the society, and functionalism is always oriented towards what is good for the whole of society. Functionalism considers society at the macro level and examines its core institutions and how they promote stability and productivity. Critics such as Gramsci consider that this stability is at the cost of progress and change, and he names this 'cultural hegemony', which explains domination or rule maintained through ideological or cultural means.

FUNCTIONALISM AND HEALTH

Parsons considered that shared values led to common expectations, thus the individual replicates the norms of the society they have lived in, and this is considered to underpin socialisation and social control. Socialisation is supported by the positive and negative sanctioning of role behaviours that do or do not meet these expectations. Parsons (1951) considered that ill health is a social phenomenon or 'an unmotivated deviance' rather than a physical/mental disorder, stating that health is 'The state of optimum capacity of an individual for the effective performance of the roles and tasks for which s/he has been socialised.'

Parsons (1951) considered 'the sick role' and explained that in order to meet society's expectations, the sick person needed to perform functions within the sick role and therefore had certain rights and obligations (see Table 5.9 for an explanation of the sick role), and in the process makes health professionals agents of social control, for instance by writing fit notes (previously sick notes) to allow time off work to be ill.

If the sick person does not comply with the strictures of the role, then they are said to be 'malingering', and therefore are not deserving of our sympathy. This attitude can have consequences, such as assuming anorexia is a self-seeking behaviour rather than a serious mental health issue with the highest mortality rate of any psychiatric disorder. This model does not function for people with chronic conditions who will not recover their health.

Table 5.9   The obligations of the sick role

Rights	Obligations
The sick person is exempt from 'normal' social roles relative to the nature and severity of the illness	The sick person should try to get well. The first two aspects of the sick role are conditional upon the third aspect
The sick person is not responsible for their condition, an individual's illness is usually thought to be beyond their own control	The sick person should seek technically competent help, and cooperate with the physician
A morbid condition of the body needs to be changed and some curative process apart from the person's will power or motivation is needed to get well	

THE SYMBOLIC INTERACTIONIST PARADIGM

KEY THEORISTS

George Herbert Mead, Charles Horton Cooley, Howard Becker, Ervine Goffman, Emile Durkheim

KEY POINTS OF THE INTERACTIONIST PARADIGM

This paradigm considers that reality is socially constructed through our interactions with one another. Morality, ethics and values are not a given; we create them through our interactions with others. Therefore, it must follow that health and ill health must be social constructs and that society determines them. Social action is influenced by a person's beliefs, attitudes, perceptions and negotiations of meanings. Language plays a role in the interactions, and individuals are called 'social actors'. Through interaction we act out the roles that make up our day-to-day life. Mead (1934) separates the 'I' and 'Me' (Figure 5.6) in his 'theory of the social self' in our interactions, and these make up our concept of self and are situated within a social context. Scenario 5.4 explains this concept.

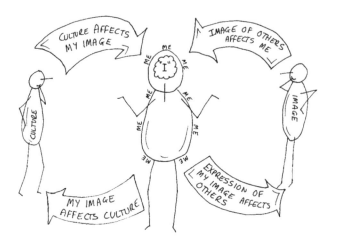

Figure 5.6   Mead's I and me

🗨️   **Scenario 5.4**

You have tripped and fallen over and the pain in your knee makes you want to cry ('I'). However (the social context), you do not want to look like a wimp in front of your friends ('Me'), so you just swear instead (social context) or laugh it off if swearing is unacceptable.

Howard Becker (1963) said that society creates rules, and by doing this anyone who acts outside of these rules is a deviant; he also considered notions of deviancy to be social constructions that could therefore be negotiated. This has a relationship with labelling theory (Becker, Goffman). Durkheim (1951 [1897]) explains that society's attitude will label some behaviours as deviant, such as 'committing' suicide. Social stigma labels the families of social deviants (criminals, gays, transgender, mentally ill) as part of that deviancy. Once you have been labelled as deviant, it is hard to escape the role society has created for you. Goffman (1963) calls this role 'the resident alien'. Cooley (1930 [1902]) examined self-image and said we see ourselves through the eyes of other people, and that we incorporate their views of us into our own self-concept. He said this is made of three components (see Table 5.10) and this can lead to self-doubt and feelings of insecurity. Cooley determined that our self-view is a reflection of how others see us.

Cooley's three components:

Table 5.10

1	We imagine how we must appear to others
2	We imagine and react to what we feel their judgement of our appearance must be
3	We develop our self through the judgements of others

Source: Adapted from Yeung and Martin (2003)

ETHNICITY

The UK is considered a multicultural society, so we need to think about cultural differences in social meanings of illness and healthcare delivery. Not giving sufficient consideration to cultural beliefs and needs can lead to isolation of ethnic groups and misunderstandings about healthcare needs. Marginalising ethnic groups can lead to false health assumptions, such as is happening for black Anglo-Caribbean men. Gypsy, Roma and Traveller (GRT) communities experience a life expectancy of minus 20 to 28 years compared with settled populations. The GRT community also has greater child mortality and reduced take up of vaccinations. As this group is socially excluded, they have multiple barriers to accessing healthcare; this would include the inability to register with a GP surgery or dental clinic. The GRT community face prejudice and discrimination by all sectors of society and as a result are poorly educated and face communication, language and cultural issues. They are often quite fearful of contact with health professionals based on historical institutional abuses (Rowe et al., 2021).

THE SOCIAL DETERMINANTS OF HEALTH

The social determinants of health are the intersections where people, their environment, their working lives, education and family circumstance meet and create an individual's life chances. A child's opportunity for health begins before they are born; children growing up in deprivation, poor or interrupted schooling and poverty have poorer outcomes throughout their life span. Health is more than an individual's personal health status but has a strong relationship with familial, political, social, economic, cultural, commercial, industrial and environmental factors; therefore, health goes beyond treating disease in individuals but provides a case for requiring the moral, social and economic resources for investing in action that creates and maintains health. In 1948, the United Nations Universal Declaration of Human Rights (Article 25) stated that good health is a basic human right. There is an economic case to be made for promoting health in society: healthier people are more productive in work and contribute to society as active participants.

People with ill health or disabilities are more likely to be unemployed or to earn a lower income; they are also more likely to be employed in work that has further health impacts such as irregular work and consequent irregular income in zero-hours contracts or jobs that stress the musculoskeletal system. Sir Michael Marmot, writing in *The Health Gap* (2015: 53) explains, 'Most of us cherish the notion of free choice, but our choices are constrained by the conditions in which we are born, grow, live, work and age.' A burden of Covid infections and deaths fell on those who were in occupations that could not be furloughed or who could not work from home: workers in schools, retail, factories, public transport, health and social care. Many workers could not afford to self-isolate and government support was difficult to negotiate. Covid's disruption to employment, childcare and school routines has had severe economic impact on families and single parent families.

People who grow up in poverty are more likely to engage in behavioural risks which have health impacts, and have low paid, low skilled work which will have physiological and psychological impact. People who have limited expectations tend to be less future orientated and so engage in risk-taking behaviours.

CHAPTER SUMMARY

- This chapter has given you an introduction to the sociology of health. You have gained an understanding that health and disease are essentially contested (that is, there is no one single agreement on what this means).
- By gaining an understanding of your patients' lives, their psychological roots and their social backgrounds, you will also have a better understanding of how people behave and react as they do when they come into contact with the caring services and how they cope with illness, pain and the demands of everyday life.
- The scenarios given by trainee nursing associates in this chapter show how theory is used to help understand your patients' lived experiences.

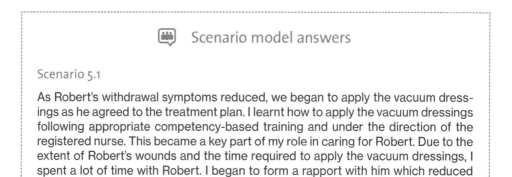

Scenario model answers

Scenario 5.1

As Robert's withdrawal symptoms reduced, we began to apply the vacuum dressings as he agreed to the treatment plan. I learnt how to apply the vacuum dressings following appropriate competency-based training and under the direction of the registered nurse. This became a key part of my role in caring for Robert. Due to the extent of Robert's wounds and the time required to apply the vacuum dressings, I spent a lot of time with Robert. I began to form a rapport with him which reduced his previous reluctance to engage with staff.

Although Robert had received treatment for minor drug-related wounds in the past, he said he had neglected to seek help for over a year as he had cared for his older brother whose health had quickly deteriorated. Following the death of his brother, he had become very depressed and further neglected himself, which had led to his current condition. Robert asked me to refer him to the hospital's mental health team, something he had previously declined, as he felt this would help him deal with his depression and addictions.

Robert had experienced psychological and physical neglect as a child as his parents were emotionally unavailable to him due to their own addictions. His social family norm was a strong predisposing factor to Robert's own drug and alcohol abuse. Attitudinal tolerance is dependent on social milieu and the individual's parent–child relationship. Children who suffer long-term anxiety will turn to drugs for their anxiolytic effect. Drugs also give a (temporary) boost to self-confidence. Robert clearly has self-belief and self-efficacy issues.

Robert had responded well to the treatment, and his wounds had healed enough for him to not require the vacuum dressings anymore, and he was able to engage with the ward's physiotherapy team. This enabled him to complete his own personal care and, following daily therapy sessions, he was eventually able to walk unaided. I discussed Robert's future with him as we approached him becoming medically fit enough to be discharged from hospital.

Robert was worried about returning to his previous home as he felt he would struggle to remain drug and alcohol free in his previous environment and feared it would affect the progress he had made in both his physical and mental health. I discussed with Robert the possibility of a rehabilitation placement to continue his progress. Robert felt this would be the best option for him and I began his discharge planning, liaising with the hospital's discharge team and Robert's newly allocated social worker. Robert was discharged from hospital to a rehabilitation centre, with a support plan from the community mental health team, and a referral to the district nurse for wound management to continue their healing.

Scenario 5.2

I used a motivational interview approach to empower Mr Smith, by asking him 'are there any behaviours within your lifestyle that you feel would increase your risk of heart disease? If so, which would be your priority to address first?' This approach allowed the discussion to be led by Mr Smith, promoting self-empowerment with lifestyle choices. Maslow considered that needs motivate behaviour and are hierarchical in nature. Maslow's theories are the basis of the Transtheoretical Model Stages of Change developed by Prochaska and Velicer in 1997, and that stages of change arise from readiness to change.

I was able to input all the information from the patient into a QRISK2 score tool to identify his risk of developing a cardiovascular disease, which was 4.7%. I then calculated QRISK again as a non-smoker, which showed Mr Smith how his risk score was reduced to 1.9%. Mr Smith was shocked at how much he could reduce risk just by stopping smoking.

This allowed Mr Smith to prioritise his goals. He identified that he wanted to stop smoking, when asked were there any obstacles that he felt would prevent him

(Continued)

from reaching his goal, he identified that he was quite stressed with juggling work and the death of his father.

I signposted Mr Smith to the GP to discuss time off work for stress, gave him a referral to the stop smoking service and gave him contact details for bereavement counselling.

Scenario 5.3

Jack's parents talked and sang to him constantly, reassuring him how much they loved him. They were understandably emotional, and this was an important part of accepting the situation they found themselves in. They made some memories to treasure which I feel helped them begin to go through the grieving process. They took photographs, hand and footprints, and a lock of his hair for the memory box provided by the hospital.

The following day the consultant team discussed Jack's current medical situation with his parents. After much discussion a joint decision was made to withdraw treatment later that afternoon. Jack's parents were offered time to contact their relatives to come and see Jack, but they declined this.

A few hours later Jack was moved to a private room with his parents where extubation took place while he was having cuddles with them. Jack was given medication to keep him calm and comfortable; he passed away peacefully in his Mum and Dad's arms. The family spent time with him before leaving him in the care of the nurses. They were able to visit him and spend time with him for a few days after death. The parents were introduced to the bereavement support team before Jack died, to help establish a relationship and rapport to provide support.

📖 FURTHER READING

WEBSITES

- The SocioWeb: www.socioweb.com
- UK Data Archive: www.data-archive.ac.uk
- British Sociological Association: www.britsoc.co.uk
- Office for National Statistics: http://ons.gov.uk/ons/taxonomy/index.html?nscl=Health+and+Social+Care
- Online resources for the social determinants of health: https://ctb.ku.edu/en/table-of-contents

BOOKS

- Beckett, C. and Taylor, H. (2012) *Human Growth and Development*. London: Sage.
- Crawford, K. (2010) *Social Work and Human Development* (3rd edn). London: Sage.
- Giddens, A. and Sutton, P. (2013) *Sociology* (7th edn). Cambridge: Polity Press.

- Gleitman, H., Gross, J. and Reisberg, D. (2007) *Psychology* (7th edn). London: Norton.
- Illich, I. (1976) *Limits to Medicine: Medical Nemesis – The Expropriation of Health*. London: Boyers Publishing.
- Nettleton, S. (2013) *The Sociology of Health and Illness* (3rd edn). Cambridge: Polity Press.
- Sudbury, J. (2009) *Human Growth and Development*. London: Routledge.

VIDEOS

- Intro to Psychology crash course: www.youtube.com/watch?v=vo4 pMVb0R6M
- What is Sociology? Crash Course Sociology: www.youtube.com/ watch?v=YnCJU6PaCio
- Social Determinants of Health: Claire Pomeroy at TEDxUCDavis: www. youtube.com/watch?v=qykD-2AXKIU

REFERENCES

Abbott, P. and Wallace, C. (1990) *An Introduction to Sociology: Feminist Perspectives*. London: Routledge.

Atchley, R.C. (1989) A continuity theory of normal aging. *The Gerontologist*, 29(2): 183–90.

Bandura, A. (1977) *Social Learning Theory* (Prentice-Hall Series in Social Learning). Englewood Cliffs, NJ: Prentice-Hall.

Bandura, A. (1986) *Social Foundations of Thought and Action: A Social Cognitive Theory*. Englewood Cliffs, NJ: Prentice-Hall.

Becker, H. (1963) *Outsiders*. New York: Macmillan.

Blot, W. and Tarone, R. (2015) Doll and Peto's quantitative estimates of cancer risks: holding generally true for 35 years. *Journal of the National Cancer Institute*, 107(4). doi: 10.1093/jnci/djv044.

Burke, E. (1790) *Reflections on the Revolution in France, and on the proceedings in certain societies in London relative to that event*. London J.Dodsley (British Library copy)

Cooley, C.H. (1930 [1902]) *Human Nature and the Social Order*. New York: Scribner.

Corr, C., Doka, K. and Kastenbaum, R. (2007) Dying and its interpreters: a review of selected literature and some comments on the state of the field. *Omega: The Journal of Death and Dying*, 39: 239–59.

Cumming, E. and Earl Henry, W. (1961) *Growing Old*. New York: Basic Books.

Doll, R. and Peto, R. (1981) The causes of cancer: quantitative estimates of risks of cancer in the United States today. *Journal of the National Cancer Institute*, 66(6): 1191–308.

Durkheim, E. (1951 [1897]) *Suicide: A Study in Sociology*. New York: The Free Press.

Engel, G. (1977) The need for a new medical model: a challenge for biomedicine. *Science*, 196(4286): 129–36.

Erikson, E. (1994 [1959]) *Identity and the Life Cycle*. New York: Norton.

Farmer, P. (1999) *Infections and Inequalities: The Modern Plagues*. Berkeley: University of California Press.

Freud, S. (2010 [1923]) *The Ego and the Id*. Seattle: Pacific Publishing Studio.

Goffman, E. (1963) *Stigma*. London: Penguin.

Havighurst, R.J. (1963) *Adjustment to Retirement: A Cross-national Study*. Assen: Van Gorcum.

hooks, b. (2001) Black women: shaping feminist theory. In K. Bhavnani (ed.), *Feminism and 'Race'*. Oxford: Oxford University Press. pp. 33–9.

Illich, I. (1976) *Limits to Medicine: Medical Nemesis – The Expropriation of Health*. London: Boyers Publishing.

Kastenbaum, R. and Costa, P. (1977) Psychological perspectives on death. *Annual Review of Psychology*, 28: 225–49.

Kenrick, D., Griskevicius, V., Neuberg, S. and Schaller, M. (2010) Renovating the pyramid of needs: contemporary extensions built upon ancient foundations. *Perspectives on Psychological Science*, 5(3): 292–314.

Kübler-Ross, E. (1969) *On Death and Dying*. New York: Simon & Schuster.

Kuhn, T. (1962) *The Structure of Scientific Revolutions*. Chicago: University of Chicago Press.

Levinson, D. (1986) *The Seasons of a Man's Life: The Groundbreaking 10-Year Study That Was the Basis for Passages*. London: Random House.

Marmot, M. (2015) *The Health Gap: The Challenge of an Unequal World*. London: Bloomsbury Press.

Maslow, A. (1943) Theory of human motivation. *Psychological Review*, 50(4): 370–96.

Mead, G.H. (1934) *Mind, Self and Society: From the Standpoint of a Social Behaviorist* (ed. C.W. Morris). Chicago: University of Chicago Press.

Millett, K. (2000) *Sexual Politics*. Urbana: University of Illinois Press.

Neugarten, B. (1974) Time, age, and the life cycle. *American Journal of Psychiatry*, 136: 887–93.

Oxford English Dictionary (2022) Definition of sociology. www.oed.com/

Parsons, T. (1951) *The Social System*. London: Routledge & Kegan Paul.

Piaget, J. (1954) *The Construction of Reality in the Child*. New York: Basic Books.

Prochaska, J.O. and Velicer, W.F. (1997) The transtheoretical model of health behavior change. *American Journal of Health Promotion*, 12(1): 38–48. doi:10.4278/0890-1171-12.1.38

Rege, S. (2003) *Sociology of Gender: The Challenge of Feminist Sociological Knowledge*. Thousand Oaks, CA: Sage.

Rowe, G., Gee, D. and Jackson, A. (2021) *Health Promotion for Nursing Associates*. London: Learning Matters/Sage.

Schaffer, H.R. (1996) *Social Development*. London: Wiley.

Stacey, M. (1994) The power of lay knowledge: a personal view. In J. Popay and G. Williams (eds), *Researching the People's Health*. London: Routledge.

Tolman, E.C. (1948) Cognitive maps in rats and men. *Psychological Review*, 55(4): 189–208. https://doi.org/10.1037/h0061626

Vaillant, G. (2002) *Aging Well: Surprising Guideposts to a Happier Life from the Landmark Study of Adult Development*. Cambridge, MA: Harvard University Press.

Watson, J. and Rayner, R. (1920) Conditioned emotional reaction. *Journal of Experimental Psychology*, 3: 1–14.

Yeung, K. and Martin, J. (2003) The looking glass self: an empirical test and elaboration. *Social Forces*, 81(3): 843–79.

PART TWO

BIOSCIENCES AND ESSENTIAL KNOWLEDGE AND SKILLS FOR CARE

6

BIOSCIENCE

GILLIAN ROWE

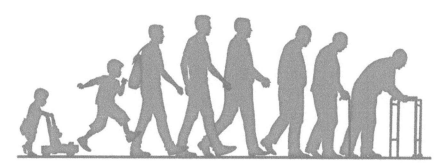

Figure 6.1   The stages of life

This chapter introduces you to the basic anatomy and physiology (A&P) of body systems and asks you to consider the effects of ageing on the systems and the body as a whole. You will use that knowledge to consider the processes involved in wound healing. This chapter links to Chapter 7, Genomics and Pathophysiology, and Chapter 8, Prevention and Control of Infection, and A&P revision resources are given to support your learning. Although this chapter does not have a glossary, you will learn plenty of new anatomy and physiology terms through the text and accompanying illustrations. The NMC Code (2018) tells you to 'maintain the knowledge and skills you need for safe and effective practice' and for that you need a good understanding of how the human body works.

INTRODUCTION

A good understanding of the anatomy and physiology of the human body is a prerequisite for health and social care workers: you wouldn't take your car to a mechanic who has no idea what happens under the bonnet, would you? You need to also understand the changes in the body as it ages, and the impact that ageing has on the various body systems and their functions. When caring for ill people, you need to know what is normal and what is abnormal to assist with the diagnostic process. This chapter gives some basic knowledge and indicates where you can go for further information. Remember to watch YouTube channels from reliable sources (NHS, The Khan Academy, Bozeman Science for example) to support your learning.

The body is made of trillions of cells, all with their own shape and function. The study of cells is called cytology – the prefix cyto refers to cells.

Every living thing contains cells; there are two major types: prokaryotic (bacteria) and eukaryotic (plants and animals). Plant and animal cells share some similarities, but there are also differences between them.

Cells are the smallest functional units in the body and the building blocks of the organs. Cells contain organelles: these do the cell's work. The cell's internal functions are the same as the body's functions: organelles grow, eat, breathe, excrete, work, reproduce and die. There are approximately 200 different types of cells within the human body, all with a specific function which is directly related to its shape. Non-sexual cells are called somatic, sexual cells are called gametes. Figure 6.2 is a diagram of the cell and contents.

Anything in the cell is called intracellular, things outside of the cell are extracellular. The cell is surrounded by a bilipid plasma membrane, and the cell keeps its shape by the use of a gel substance called cytoplasm. Materials move through cytoplasm by diffusion. Figure 6.3 shows detail of the bilipid layer.

The membrane is made up of a double layer of phospholipids, proteins and cholesterol. Phospholipids have a phosphate head and a lipid tail.

1. Phosphate heads are water-attracting or hydrophilic
2. Lipid tails are water-repelling or hydrophobic

Phospholipids in water spontaneously form a bilayer: phosphate heads to the outside and lipid tails to the inside of the bilayer. Figure 6.4 shows detail of the bilipid layer.

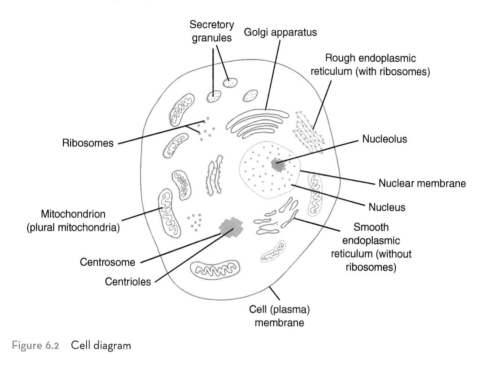

Figure 6.2 Cell diagram

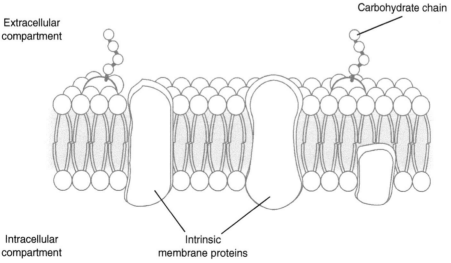

Figure 6.3 Bilipid plasma membrane

In the fluid mosaic model, the double layer of lipids is thought to be quite fluid, with globular proteins 'floating' in this layer. The function of the membrane is to control the flow of substances in and out of the cell. Water passes through aquaporins. Carbon dioxide, ammonia and oxygen move freely through the layers. However, some substances need to be transported by protein transporters which act as 'gates' through the layers. Ions (charged particles) and glucose need to be transported through these channel proteins by facilitated and active transport.

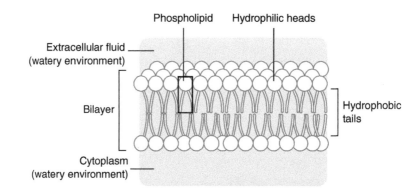

Figure 6.4   Bilipid layer

Transport proteins span the bilipid layer. They transport by acting as a hydrophilic channel or by shape shifting or actively transporting substances by hydrolysing adenosine triphosphate (ATP). Transport protein carrier action resembles enzyme substrate reactions and, in many ways, carriers behave like enzymes, except that the transported solute molecule is not modified or changed.

Cholesterol molecules disturb the packing of phospholipids; this regulates membrane fluidity which is important for membrane stability. Incidentally, alcohol disrupts the fluidity of the cell membrane and disturbs the function of membrane proteins.

Glycoproteins are proteins with a carbohydrate chain attached. They have a role in cellular recognition and the immune response. They may also act as 'docking stations' for hormone and neurotransmitter vesicles. These too stabilise the membrane structure by anchoring to the cytoskeleton.

Glycolipids are lipids with a carbohydrate attached; their role is to maintain the stability of the cell's membrane. They also have a role in cellular recognition and immune response and play an important part in ensuring the cells adhere together to form tissues.

Macromolecules include receptor proteins which 'dock' extracellular molecules and by binding, activate secondary messengers inside the cell for cellular responses (such as hormone excretion). Oligosaccharides help with cell-to-cell recognition and can help alter the chemical and physical properties of proteins.

The structural framework of the cell is called the cytoskeleton, and this determines the cell's shape, locomotion type and cell division; intermediate filaments provide structural support against mechanical stress. Microfilaments direct the movement of the cell organelles and support cell division; microfilaments are made of actin, the same protein that skeletal muscle cells are made from. Microtubules are involved in cell movement and external to the cell are cilia and flagella.

The nucleus is the cell's command and control centre: it instructs the cell to grow, divide, mature and die. The nucleus is surrounded by the nuclear envelope and contains nucleoplasm, which protects the cell's deoxyribonucleic acid (DNA) and keeps it separate from the rest of the cell. The nucleolus is a dense region of ribonucleic acid (RNA) and creates the ribosomes.

The main organelles (little organs) in a cell are as follows:

- Ribosomes, which create proteins and are attached to the rough endoplasmic reticulum or can be free floating
- The endoplasmic reticulum (ER), which helps to process proteins made in the cell and to transport them around and out of the cell
- The Golgi apparatus, which modifies the proteins made in the ER and prepares them for export out of the cell
- Lysosomes and Peroxisomes, which recycle worn out components, kill invading bacteria, and remove toxic materials; lysosomes destroy proteins and peroxisomes contain oxidative enzymes which destroy lipids.

Another important organelle, mitochondria, named by Carl Benda in 1898, are still giving up their secrets, especially in cell division and proliferation regulation. Red blood cells do not have mitochondria, liver cells have approximately 2000. Mitochondria contain compartments, each with a specialised function. Best known is the production of the cell's energy adenosine triphosphate (ATP), or sometimes called phosphorylation of ADP (adenosine diphosphate). However, they also have a role in cell death (apoptosis), calcium signalling, regulation of cellular metabolism, steroid synthesis and hormone signalling. Mutations in any of these functions can lead to mitochondrial diseases.

Figure 6.5 shows the Krebs cycle, which is the mechanism for energy production and internal respiration. Confusingly, it is also known as the citric acid cycle, and the tricarboxylic acid cycle (TCA cycle). Cellular respiration is complex, and you will need to watch some YouTube videos to gain a good understanding of the process, as this is essential knowledge.

Also discovered by Krebs in association with Kurt Henseleit in 1932, is the urea or ornithine cycle. This is the biochemical reaction that produces urea (which the body tolerates) from ammonia (which is toxic), which is a by-product of amino acid catabolism. Urea cycle disorders mean that absence of any of the enzymes needed for conversion will lead to death, usually within 48 hours of birth.

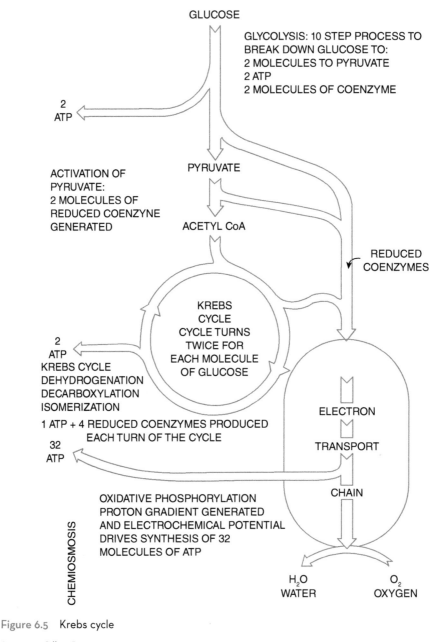

Figure 6.5   Krebs cycle

Source: © Gillian Rowe

Materials move through the cell and within the cell using diffusion, osmosis, filtration, active transport, exocytosis and endocytosis. Box 6.1 explains the various transport mechanisms.

Box 6.1   Transport mechanisms

1. **Diffusion** is the movement of particles (solutes) from a region of higher solute concentration to a region of lower solute concentration

2. **Osmosis** is the diffusion of solvent or water molecules through a selectively or semi-permeable membrane

3. **Filtration** uses pressure differential to move substances through a membrane

4. **Active transport** moves substances against a concentration gradient from a region of lower concentration to a region of higher concentration. This requires a carrier molecule and uses energy in the form of ATP

5. **Endocytosis** is the formation of vesicles to transfer particles from outside to inside the cell

6. **Exocytosis** is the movement of vesicles from the inside of the cell to the outside of the cell

---

Somatic cells reproduce by mitosis – that is direct replication – so that the daughter cells are identical to the parent; unlike sexual reproduction, no DNA is exchanged; any DNA damaged should be corrected or the cell destroyed. However, the correction process is suspended during replication to prevent fusion of telomeres at the end of the DNA's strand and transcription errors can occur.

Genomics is the study of genomes, which are the genetic components of chromosomes. Genes are an inherited functional subunit of DNA within a chromosome. The human genome is thought to contain approximately 25,000 genes. Further detail of genomics can be found in Chapter 7, Advanced Health Science: Genomics and Pathophysiology.

THE AGEING AND FAILING CELL

Cells that fail to function due to injury, anoxia, toxic reaction, malnutrition, infection or inflammation will be destroyed (apoptosis and necrosis). Cellular ageing leads to structural and functional declines which leave the cell susceptible to decreased capacity to recover from injury.

A cell's size can change: shrinking cells (atrophy) can lead to shrinking tissues and organs, for instance, muscles shrink from lack of stimulation and use, especially in old age or due to debilitation and disability. The atrophying muscle cell contains fewer mitochondria and endoplasmic reticulum. Atrophy as a result of chronic malnutrition can lead to autophagy where lysosomes engulf the cells to harvest proteins. It should be noted that autophagy is not just a survival mechanism but also a means of rejuvenating cells by clearing out and recycling cellular products; however within the ageing process, this becomes less effective. Thus, harmful products can accumulate. It is considered that failure to remove proteins from neurons in the central nervous system has a role in Alzheimer's disease.

Cells can enlarge (hypertrophy) again, such as skeletal and cardiac muscles owing to the demands of exercise. This expansion is due to increased numbers of organelles present in the cell. Cellular hypertrophy can occur in response to disease (pathologic hypertrophy) such as cardiac hypertrophy in response to myopathy.

Cell death due to trauma or injury leads to proliferation of cells (hyperplasia). Damaged cells release signals that stimulate production and regeneration; for instance, the liver can repair itself by regeneration, and to a limited extent, the kidneys can self-repair. Hyperplasia can also take place under the effects of hormones, such as relining the endometrium after the menstrual flow. Dysplasia refers to abnormal cells (not necessarily cancerous) and metaplasia refers to replacement cells which are similar but not the same. A good example of this is ciliated epithelial cells in the bronchus being replaced by squamous epithelial cells: the new cells are not ciliated, nor do they secrete mucus, so they are not as effective at removing pollutants from the airway. These cells grow as a stress response, usually to the irritants in tobacco. When the individual gives up smoking, normal ciliated cell production resumes.

CELLS TO TISSUES

Tissues are groups of cells that have the same structure and function as a unit. Intercellular matrix fills the gaps between cells and may contain substances particular to the tissue function. There are four main types of tissue:

Epithelial: Usually pink, they cover all the hollow organs and line the body cavities. These cells are tightly packed together with little intercellular matrix and are attached to connective tissue via a basement membrane. This membrane is created by proteins and carbohydrates donated by the epithelial and connective tissues. Epithelial tissue performs many functions including secretion, absorption, excretion, filtration, diffusion, protection and sensory reception. Epithelial cells come in a variety of shapes: simple and stratified squamous, cuboidal and columnar shapes; they are also arranged in single or multiple layers. Some epithelial cells are ciliated, with a hair-like protuberance, and these can work together such as in the bronchi to waft pollutants caught in mucus up (the mucus escalator) or to propel sperm. See Figure 6.6 for detail of the different types of epithelial tissue structures.

Connective: This tissue binds structures together, it forms a framework which supports the organs of the body; it stores fats; it also transports substances which protect against disease and helps to repair damaged tissue. Connective tissue can be loose (adipose), fibrous, elastic, cartilage and bone.

Muscle: Muscle tissue can contract (shorten) and the types are: skeletal, cardiac and smooth. Cardiac muscle is mononucleated and myogenic; smooth muscle is mononucleated; and skeletal muscle is striated and multinucleated. The contractile proteins are actin and myosin and move by sliding filament theory.

Nervous: This tissue is found in the brain, spinal cord and the nerves; it has a command and control function as it coordinates movement, monitors the internal environment, gains information from the senses, and creates memories and emotions. Cellular communication is via an impulse by electrical stimulation. Glial cells are the most abundant cells in the central nervous system but they do not transmit impulses; instead they act as support units providing support and insulation for neurons, nutrients and protection from infection.

ANATOMY AND PHYSIOLOGY OF THE BODY SYSTEMS

THE DIGESTIVE SYSTEM

The digestive system (Figure 6.8) is the process whereby nutrition and hydration is ingested, digested, absorbed, assimilated and, finally, excreted. The alimentary (or gastrointestinal) canal has several functional adaptations, such as the stomach (Figure 6.9) and the lining of the small intestine to provide the right pH environment for the breakdown and absorption of food (Figure 6.8) and to enable the action of enzymes to complete the process of digestion (see Figure 6.10). There is further detail on the alimentary system in Chapter 7.

Understanding the function of enzymes is crucial to your understanding of the system. Enzymes function best at 36–37°C, which is why homeostasis maintains your body at this constant. If your temperature is lower, fewer reactions occur; if it is higher, enzyme proteins become denatured (this means change shape) and cannot function through the lock and key mechanism (see Figure 6.10).

Go Further 6.1

Check out the following online document to find out more about enzymes: http://biologymad.com/resources/EnzymesRevision.pdf

---

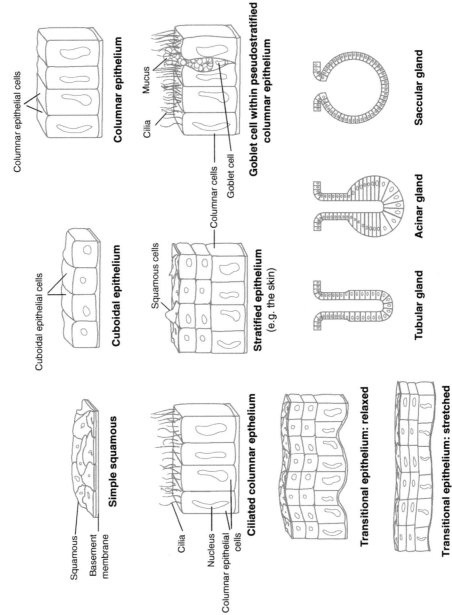

Figure 6.6 Epithelial tissue

Columnar epithelial cells

Columnar epithelium

Cilia Mucus

Columnar cells

Goblet cell

Goblet cell within pseudostratified columnar epithelium

Saccular gland

Cuboidal epithelial cells

Cuboidal epithelium

Squamous cells

Stratified epithelium
(e.g. the skin)

Acinar gland

Tubular gland

Squamous

Basement
membrane

Simple squamous

Cilia

Nucleus

Columnar epithelial
cells

Ciliated columnar epthelium

Transitional epithelium: relaxed

Transitional epithelium: stretched

Homeostasis a self-regulating process that allows the body's systems to maintain stability while adjusting to changing external conditions. It uses negative feedback to maintain temperature, fluid, oxygen and carbon dioxide and glucose regulation. See Figure 6.7 for examples.

When the immune system responds to attack by producing eicosanoids, these elevate the temperature (producing fever) via an inflammatory response. The immune system is at odds with the digestive system as homeostatic mechanisms try to reduce temperature. You can see this when charting the temperature of someone with an infection: the immune system pushes the temperature up and homeostasis tries to bring it down, hence the spikes on the chart.

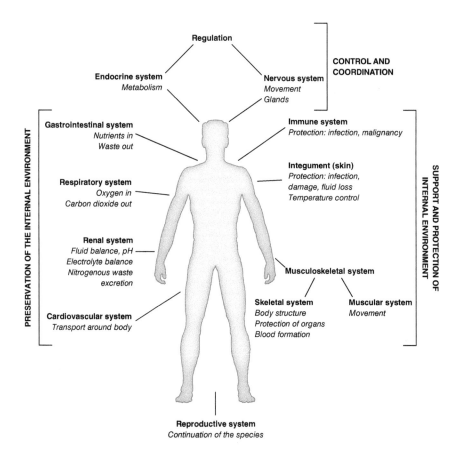

Figure 6.7   Body systems in homeostasis

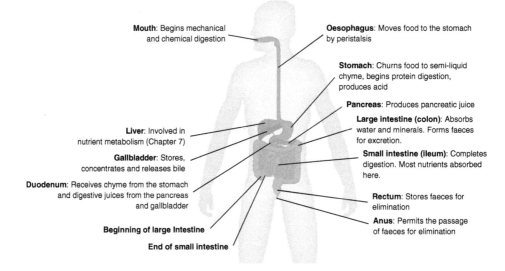

Mouth: Begins mechanical and chemical digestion

Oesophagus: Moves food to the stomach by peristalsis

Stomach: Churns food to semi-liquid chyme, begins protein digestion, produces acid

Pancreas: Produces pancreatic juice

Large intestine (colon): Absorbs water and minerals. Forms faeces for excretion.

Liver: Involved in nutrient metabolism (Chapter 7)

Small intestine (ileum): Completes digestion. Most nutrients absorbed here.

Gallbladder: Stores, concentrates and releases bile

Duodenum: Receives chyme from the stomach and digestive juices from the pancreas and gallbladder

Rectum: Stores faeces for elimination

Anus: Permits the passage of faeces for elimination

Beginning of large Intestine

End of small intestine

Figure 6.8   Components of the digestive system

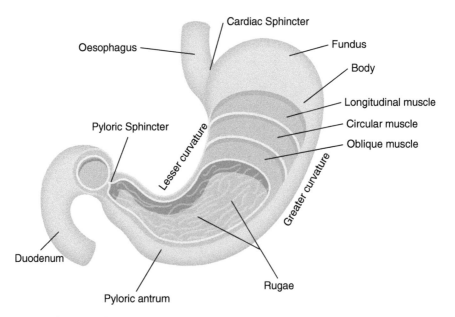

Cardiac Sphincter

Oesophagus

Fundus

Body

Longitudinal muscle

Circular muscle

Oblique muscle

Pyloric Sphincter

Lesser curvature

Greater curvature

Duodenum

Rugae

Pyloric antrum

Figure 6.9   The stomach

ENZYMES

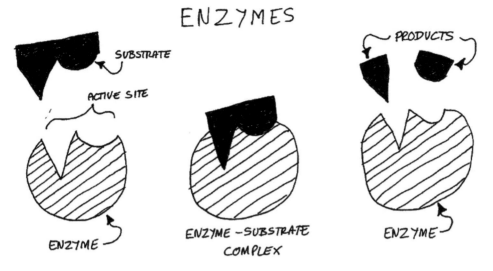

Figure 6.10   Enzymes' lock and key mechanism

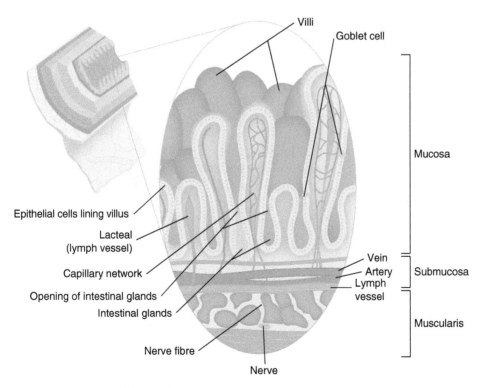

Figure 6.11   Structure of the small intestine

Once the enzymes have broken food into its constituent particles, absorption takes place through the gut lining. Finger-like projections called villi vastly increase the surface area to speed up the process; sugars and proteins are absorbed by the capillaries and sent to the liver via the hepatic portal system and fats are absorbed via the lacteals of the villi (see Figure 6.11). At this stage fat is in the form of chylomicrons and enters the circulatory system via the lymphatic system at the thoracic duct and empties into the subclavian vein.

The large intestine has only minor absorptive function other than reclaiming water and salts (anyone who has had diarrhoea will know how effective it is); it does, however, absorb vitamins which are created by bowel flora, such as vitamin K, vitamin B12, thiamine and riboflavin. This vitamin creation is essential for those with a poor diet, but the producing bacteria can be killed by antibiotics. Compacted waste is then excreted.

THE LIVER

The liver is a large organ (classed as a gland) which sits on the right side of the body tucked under the rib cage. Dark red in colour, it has two lobes, which are separated by the falciform ligament, a band of tissue that keeps it anchored to the diaphragm, and it has the gallbladder sitting underneath (Figure 6.12). Glisson's capsule, a fibrous tissue, covers the outside of the liver and together with the peritoneum, protects the liver from damage. The importance of the liver cannot be overstated as it carries out over 500 metabolic functions. It is the only organ that can self-repair (given time), although the primary cause of liver damage is alcohol excess. The liver is fed by the hepatic portal system, the portal vein from the digestive system and the hepatic artery; these end in capillaries in the lobules which house the hepatocytes; blood is returned to the heart via three hepatic veins. The main functions of the liver are:

- Storage of vitamins and minerals: vitamins A, D, E, K and B12, copper and iron stored as ferritin
- Production of bile, which is stored in the gallbladder; this breaks down fats
- Storage of glucose as glycogen
- Blood filtration
- The liver contains high numbers of Kupffer cells, which are involved in immunological activity and are part of the mononuclear phagocyte system
- Synthesis of angiotensinogen, which raises blood pressure by narrowing blood vessels
- The production of albumin, which is a common protein in blood serum; albumin helps transport fatty acids and steroid hormones

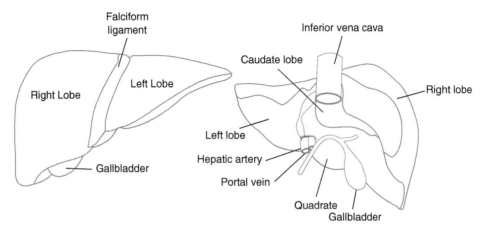

Figure 6.12   The liver

THE YOUNG CHILD'S DIGESTIVE SYSTEM

Prior to birth, the foetus's digestive system is considered sterile; once born, the baby is rapidly colonised by micro-organisms, some from the mother's microbiota, others from the environment. At birth, the baby's stomach is approximately the size of a walnut, which is why they need frequent feeding. From their mother's breast milk, they absorb nutrients and immunoglobulins; the child's digestive system is then colonized by *Bacteroides*, *Bifidobacteria* and *Lactobacillus* to support their developing immune system. These bacteria also reduce the amount of gas created during milk digestion. Children born by Caesarean section and/or fed formula tend to be colonized by *Clostridium* as well as *Bacteroides*, *Bifidobacteria* and *Lactobacillus*, which can cause diarrhoea and be life threatening if the child is receiving antibiotics, as the drugs can kill off beneficial gut flora. Babies' digestive systems strengthen over the first 6 months allowing them control over reflux; until then, they need adult support to release trapped wind.

Some babies may be born with a pyloric stenosis, preventing milk passing from the stomach into the intestine; these babies will projectile vomit if overfed. Ultrasound will reveal if surgical intervention is required.

EFFECTS OF AGEING ON THE DIGESTIVE SYSTEM

As the person ages, taste bud replacement lessens (which is why older people claim modern food is tasteless), slowing peristalsis increases constipation and the likelihood of developing haemorrhoids. Absorption slows, which taken with loss of taste buds, difficulties with chewing and constipation can lead to older folks suffering from loss of appetite and poor nutrition. Some drugs are absorbed through the lining of the colon and the condition of the ageing gut will have an impact on how effective their uptake is.

Go Further 6.2

Read through this online document about the digestive system: www.lamission. edu/lifesciences/lecturenote/aliphysio1/digestion.pdf

---

THE REPRODUCTIVE SYSTEM

Reproduction is crucial for the survival of any species and ours is no different. It could be argued that the basic purpose of our species is to reproduce. The equipment that differentiates men and women biologically is our reproductive organs. They become functional after the onset of puberty and the male system continues to function until death, but in women the reproductive system is functional only until menopause. The male system ends at successful intercourse whereas women's reproductive role extends until childbirth.

The functions of the male reproductive organs (Figure 6.13) are the production of male gametes (spermatozoa), the transportation of sperm to the female reproductive tract and production of the male sex hormone testosterone, which controls the secondary male sexual characteristics (body and facial hair, male physique, vocal chords).

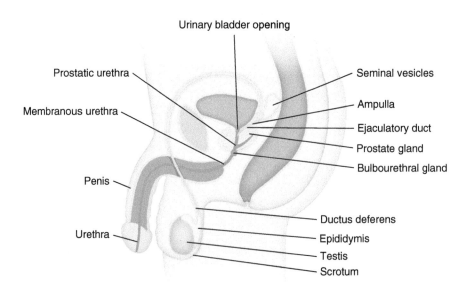

Figure 6.13   The male reproductive system

The functions of the female reproductive organs (Figure 6.14) are to produce eggs (ova), transport the ova to the uterus (via the fallopian tubes) and provide an environment for a growing foetus. If the ova are not fertilised, the lining of the uterus is shed (menstruation). The ovaries also produce the hormones oestrogen and progesterone under the direction of the follicle stimulating hormone, produced by the pituitary gland. Under the influence of human chorionic gonadotrophin, oestrogen and progesterone produced in the ovary (corpus luteum) maintain pregnancy until the placenta is mature enough to produce its own hormones.

Both the vagina and the uterus are potential spaces, this means that they are able to stretch to accommodate the growing baby and to allow passage of the baby into the world. As the baby grows, so does the uterus. The developing foetus is supported by nutrition and oxygen from its mother via the placenta and umbilical cord (see Figure 6.15). Whilst they do not share blood supply, products pass through the mother's blood and diffuse (or are actively transported) across the placental barrier to the child. Carbon dioxide and waste products are passed back to the mother using the same system.

As the birth approaches, oestrogen levels peak, causing intrauterine ripples called Braxton Hicks (false labour), this causes the endometrium to create receptors for oxytocin (see Figure 6.16) which are secreted by the foetal cells. The hypothalamus gland also cascades oxytocin, and this produces rhythmic contractions in the uterus. Relaxin is produced by the placenta and this increases the flexibility of the pelvic ligaments. As the contractions gain in force, the mucus plug gives way (the show), the cervix is fully dilated, and the baby is delivered.

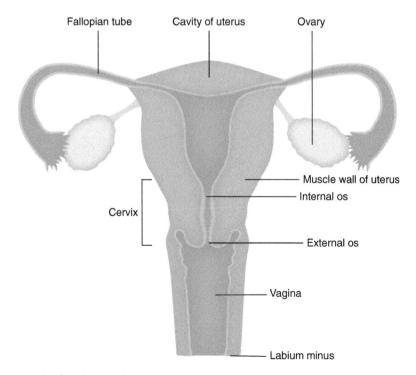

Figure 6.14   The female reproductive system

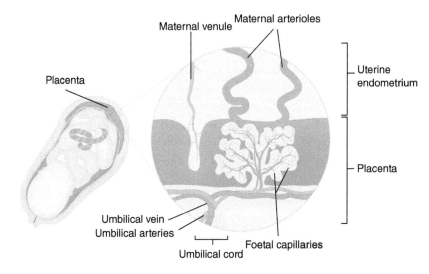

Figure 6.15   Pregnancy

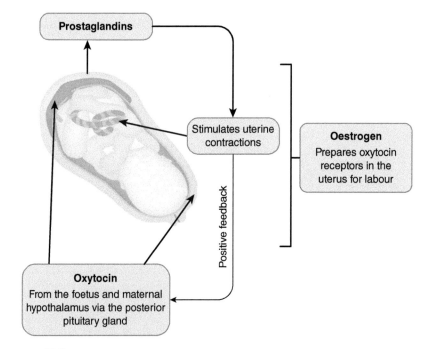

Figure 6.16   Birth

Hormonal interactions prepare the mother's body for lactation – the placenta produces human placenta lactogen (HPL) and prepares the breasts for lactation; HPL triggers the hypothalamus to excrete prolactin releasing hormones (PRH), which then stimulate the pituitary gland to make prolactin (Figure 6.17). While this process is going on (about 36 hours), the mammary glands produce colostrum, an essential vitamin-rich pre-milk which contains antibodies, antimicrobial factors and growth hormones to protect and stimulate the new baby.

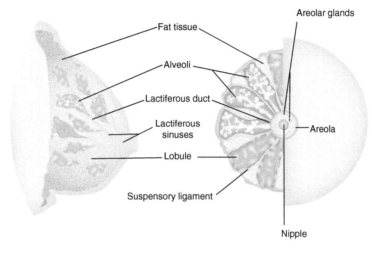

Figure 6.17   Lactation

THE NEWBORN BABY

When the baby is successfully delivered, s/he has approximately 300 bones; some of these will fuse together and ossify over time eventually reducing to 206 bones. The segments of the skull have gaps called fontanelles, the posterior fontanelle closes quite quickly (around 2 months); the anterior fontanelle closes at approximately 1 year. Sometimes the fontanelle bulges when babies cry but should return to a slightly convex shape when held upright, if the bulging continues and the child is feverish, this could indicate brain swelling and needs to be escalated to the medical team. By a month old, the baby should be recognising faces, which indicates clear vision, and will be startled by loud noises, which indicates good hearing. Around 8 weeks old, the baby should be able to lift their head when placed on their stomach, evidencing growing motor control. At 12 weeks old, they should begin to reach for objects, evidencing coordination between the brain, eyes and hands. These developmental milestones indicate that the baby is developing normally.

EFFECTS OF AGEING ON THE REPRODUCTIVE SYSTEM

Men retain their ability to reproduce into extreme old age; however, the rate of sperm production slows although sperm numbers remain the same. There may be an increase in chromosomal abnormalities. The skin pouches that hold the testicles continue to grow under the effect of declining testosterone, leading to sagging; also, the prostate gland enlarges.

Women undergo menopause at ages 45–55, although the use of hormone replacement therapy can push this age back until well into the 60s. At menopause, the production of oestrogen in the ovaries decreases by about 95% and there is a rapid decline in oocytes. Breast tissue loses elasticity leading to sag and the vaginal walls become thinner and lose elasticity, leading to an increased risk of prolapse.

Go Further 6.3

Read the following chapter notes on the reproductive system: www.gallantsbio-corner.com/uploads/9/1/3/5/9135671/sexnotes.pdf

Information on childhood development www.nhsggc.org.uk/kids/child-development/

THE URINARY SYSTEM

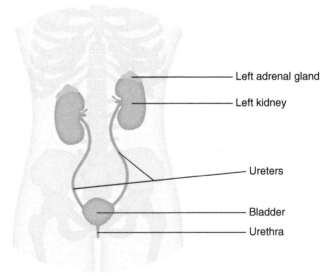

Figure 6.18   The urinary system

Adult humans consist of 60% fluid, although content varies with age: a newborn has about 80% water whereas in elderly people it can be as low as 50%. Table 6.1 shows how fluid is distributed throughout the body.

Table 6.1   Body fluid

The greatest part of the fluid is found in the cells (known as intracellular fluid)	about 25 litres
The rest is extracellular fluid (outside the cells and is made up of interstitial or tissue fluid), fluid that bathes the cells and is in the spaces between the cells	about 10 litres
Blood plasma (in blood vessels known as intravascular fluid)	about 3 litres
Urine and fluid in bowel	about 1.5 litres

The urinary system comprises of two kidneys, two ureters connected to one bladder and one urethra which is the outgoing tube (see Figure 6.18). The function of the urinary system is the elimination of waste metabolites and the control of the salt/water balance (osmoregulation). The kidneys (see Figure 6.19) filter all the circulating blood in the body 300 times a day. The function of the kidneys can be summarised as:

- Filtration
- Absorption
- Elimination

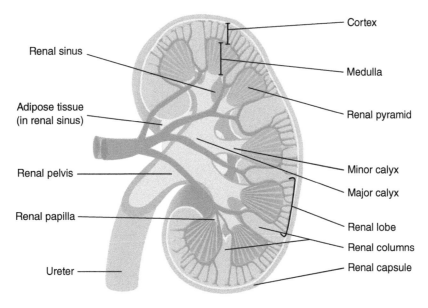

Figure 6.19   The kidneys

Kidneys clean blood and tissue fluid by removing excess water and urea which are excreted in urine. Urea, which gives urine its name, is a nitrogen-containing substance produced in the liver via the ornithine cycle to remove excess amino acids. Glucose and mineral products are reabsorbed for reuse in the body.

The functional renal unit is the nephron (Figure 6.20), which eliminates wastes from the body, regulates blood volume and blood pressure, controls levels of electrolytes and metabolites, and regulates blood pH. Each nephron begins with a cup-shaped structure, the Bowman's capsule. This encloses the glomerulus, which is a cluster of capillaries. Blood passing through the Bowman's capsule undergoes ultrafiltration, solutes (including urea) and water from the blood are forced out of a blood vessel into the Bowman's capsule by hydrostatic pressure (Starling's force). The glomerular filtration rate (GFR) is the amount of blood filtered by the kidney's glomerulus into the Bowman's capsule per unit of time. The blood pressure in the wide glomerular afferent capillaries becomes selectively higher, red and white blood cells and plasma proteins are too big to be passed through the filtrate and are returned to the circulatory system. The solute is then passed to the proximal convoluted tubule, here around 70% of the water and salt, and 100% of the glucose and amino acids in the filtrate are reabsorbed by active transport using ATP, thus the medulla tissue has high salt concentration. The proximal tubule regulates the pH (acidity) of the filtrate by exchanging hydrogen ions in the interstitial fluid for bicarbonate ions in the filtrate. The filtrate then passes into the loop of Henle; the descending limb has low permeability to urea and Na+ ions (sodium), but high permeability to water, therefore water can be drawn out of the filtrate and back into blood. The ascending limb actively transports Na (sodium), K (potassium) and Cl (chloride) ions out of the filtrate into kidney tissue. The distal convoluted tubule (DCT) is also responsible for the regulation of K, Na, Cl,

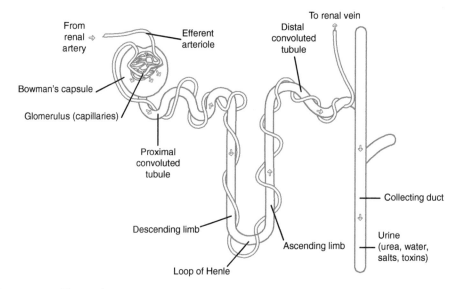

Figure 6.20   The nephron

pH and water. The DCT regulates pH by absorbing bicarbonate and secreting protons (H+ [hydrogen] ions) into the filtrate; the collecting ducts then pass through the salty tissue of the medulla and so water is reabsorbed by osmosis into the blood vessels (vasa recta).

Regulation of water is a homeostatic mechanism which controls the movement of water in and out of cells by osmosis and by receptor cells in the blood informing the hypothalamus in the brain if blood is too thick. The brain responds through the pituitary gland by producing antidiuretic hormone (arginine vasopressin) which prevents dehydration by conserving body fluids through reabsorbing dilute urine and triggering the sensation of thirst. Too much fluid in the body (hypovolaemia) can be caused by congestive cardiac failure (oedema), kidney failure, liver disease (ascites), acquired brain injury, or through iatrogenic causes such as saline intravenous fluid overload.

Go Further 6.4

For further detail of the urinary system visit: www.pearsonhighered.com/content/dam/one-dot-com/one-dot-com/us/en/higher-ed/en/products-services/course-products/amerman-1e-info/pdf/amerman-sample-chapter24.pdf

---

EFFECTS OF AGEING ON THE URINARY SYSTEM

Kidney tissue decreases along with a concomitant loss of renal nephrons, the blood vessels supplying the kidneys can suffer from atherosclerosis (hardening) with risk of aneurysm. The bladder muscles can weaken leading to incontinence, the loss of muscle tone can lead to a displaced urethra, and in men the enlarged prostate can cause flow pressure issues and retention. Retention in both men and women can lead to urinary tract infections (UTIs) which are difficult to resolve. The use of in-dwelling catheters is now discouraged unless absolutely essential as they are known to promote UTIs and subsequent kidney disease.

THE INTEGUMENTARY SYSTEM

Skin is the body's boundary between the internal and external world: it is the first line of defence of the immune system as it contains a whole biome of commensal (helpful) bacteria; it contains nerve endings that inform the brain about the external world; it protects against dehydration (by waterproofing), against overheating (sweat glands) and against sunburn (melanin) (see Figure 6.21). The integumentary system is the largest system of the body; in an adult, on average, the skin has a surface of 1.5 to 2 square metres (22 square feet or about the same area of a single sized bed) and would weigh (approximately) 9.7 kg (or 20 lb). The thickness of the skin varies, being thinnest in your eyelids and thickest on the soles of your feet. The skin has three layers (Table 6.2).

The skin is an organ of regulation in that it aids homeostatic mechanisms of thermoregulation and osmoregulation. It acts as a reservoir for the synthesis of vitamin D. Skin is also an organ of sensation – cold, heat, touch and pain. Wounds to the skin affect all the skin functions, especially burns or wounds that lead to scarring.

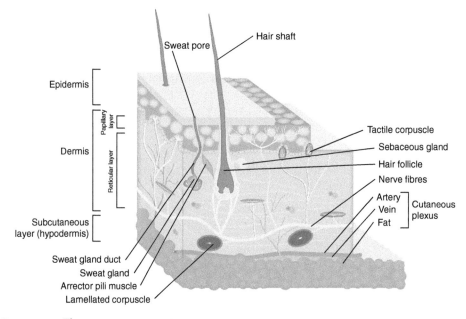

Figure 6.21   The integumentary system

Table 6.2   The layers of the skin

The epidermis	A sheet of dead cells that forms a protective barrier made of squamous cells which originate in the basal layer of the dermis and move up to the epidermis. The epidermis also contains Langerhans cells, keratinocytes and melanocytes and the hair follicles
The dermis	Contains sebaceous glands (which secrete sebum which is made of cholesterol, fatty acids and waxy esters), arrector pili muscles, blood vessels, nerve endings, sweat glands and lymphatic channels
The subcutaneous fatty layer	Nerve fibres and Pacinian (lamellar) corpuscles that sense vibratory pressure

THE CHILD'S SKIN

Young children have sensitive skin, which can be easily damaged. Babies can develop nappy rash if they are left in wet nappies; they can also be allergic to certain nappy brands and develop allergy rashes. Washing products can also trigger allergy rashes. Babies sometimes develop cradle cap (infantile sebor-rhoeic dermatitis): this is harmless although a little unsightly. Also affecting the newborn are milk spots (erythema toxicum and milia) which can appear anywhere on the body; again, these are harmless and will clear up over time. Babies may also develop birthmarks which are a congenital benign irregularity. Some are classed as pigmented, such as moles, and some are classed as vascular, these include port wine stains and macular stains (salmon patches). There are also skin lesions known as naevi. Nearly all of these birthmarks are harmless although some port wine stains can be prominent on the face and may be removed surgically or by laser for cosmetic reasons.

Other childhood skin conditions include acne vulgaris, ringworm, impetigo, urticaria, roseola, and the childhood infectious diseases such as measles, scarlet fever, chicken pox, slapped cheek, and hand, foot and mouth disease, all of which have rashes. Meningitis is most common in babies, young children, teenagers and young adults. It is characterised by rapid onset fever and a rash that does not fade when a glass is rolled over it; the child might be photophobic, vomit and have joint pain especially in the neck. Meningitis is classed as a medical emergency.

EFFECTS OF AGEING ON THE INTEGUMENTARY SYSTEM

Skin becomes more fragile with age. It loses collagen and elastin (elastosis); solar elastosis is the weather-beaten appearance of older people who work outdoors. Melanocyte production slows and the skin becomes translucent. Large pigmented spots appear on skin exposed to the sun (liver spots). The blood vessels of the dermis become more fragile leading to frequent bruising (senile purpura). The sebaceous glands produce less sebum resulting in the skin drying as oil production decreases. The subcutaneous layer retains less fat, which reduces insulation and means that older people feel the cold and are at greater risk of hyperthermia. Fat loss and mobility-limiting musculoskeletal disorders increase the risk of decubitus (pressure) ulcers for ageing skin. If this is complicated by type 2 diabetes, wound healing time rises by a factor of 4.

> ### Go Further 6.5
>
> A good chapter to read for further detail on the integumentary system can be found at: www.lamission.edu/lifesciences/AliAnat1/Chap%203%20-%20Integumentary%20System.pdf

THE CARDIOVASCULAR SYSTEM

The cardiovascular (CV) system is comprised of the heart and vascular tubing (blood vessels). There is further detail on the CV system in Chapter 7. Figure 6.22 shows the thoracic cavity and the position of the heart and lungs.

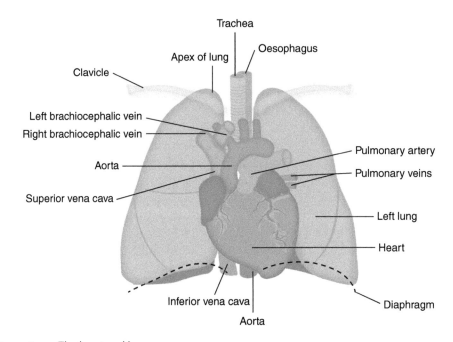

Figure 6.22   The heart and lungs

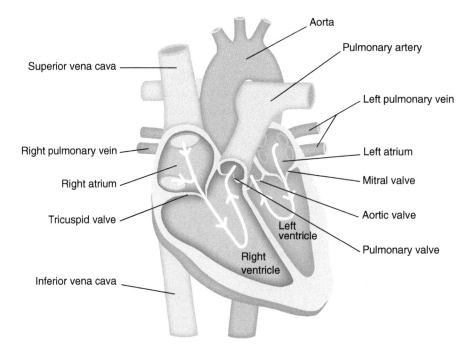

Figure 6.23   The blood flow of the heart

THE CARDIAC SYSTEM

The heart is a double pump: the upper chambers (atria, meaning waiting area from the Latin *atrium*) contract first, forcing blood into the two lower chambers, the ventricles (Figure 6.23). Ventricular force is higher as the blood has further to go and this is evidenced by the anatomy of the heart, where ventricular muscle is very thick compared to the upper heart. Blood is prevented from back flow by valves between the chambers and at the end of the blood vessels (see Figure 6.23).

The heart is powered by action potentials initiated at the sinoatrial node (cardiac pacemaker) and conducted to the left atrium via Bachmann's bundle causing atrial contraction; the signal then travels to the atrioventricular node which propagates the current through the Bundle of His to the Purkinje fibres which causes ventricular contraction (see Figure 6.25). The resting heart rate (sinus rhythm) is between 60 and 100 beats per minute (bpm) and can exceed 200 bpm at exercise.

Blood pressure is regulated by the renin-angiotensin-aldosterone system (RAAS), this also regulates fluid balance. When blood volume or sodium (Na) levels in the body are low, or blood potassium (K) is high, cells in the kidney release the enzyme renin. Renin converts angiotensinogen, which is produced in the liver, into the hormone angiotensin I. The angiotensin converting enzyme (ACE1) (found in epithelial cells, especially in the lungs) metabolises angiotensin I into angiotensin II. Angiotensin II causes

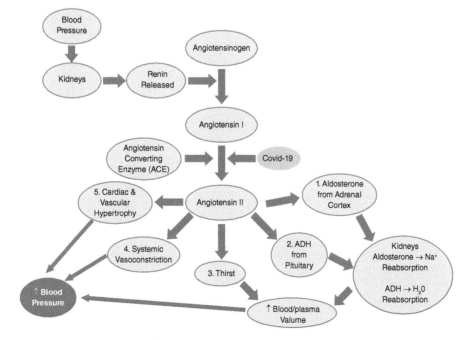

Figure 6.24   RAAS system and Covid

blood vessels to constrict (vasoconstriction) and blood pressure to increase. Angiotensin II stimulates the release of the hormone aldosterone in the adrenal glands, this causes the renal tubules to retain Na and water and to excrete K. ACE2 reduces angiotensin II and aldosterone raises blood volume (by vasodilation), blood pressure and Na levels in the blood to restore the balance of Na, K and fluids. See Figure 6.24 for a diagrammatic understanding of the RAAS system. You will note the ingress of SARS-CoV-2 at ACE2; the text below explains the implication of this.

ACE2 has a significant role in the development of SARS-CoV-2, as it is a protein on the surface of many cell types, such as epithelial cells. The nose, mouth and lungs are lined with epithelial tissue and therefore contain large amounts of ACE2. ACE2 is the site of the virus binding mechanism, which then prevents ACE2 from performing its function to regulate angiotensin II signalling. Thus, the reduction of ACE2 will increase tissue susceptibility to inflammation, cell death and organ failure, especially in the heart and the lungs.

THE VASCULAR SYSTEM

Deoxygenated venous blood is returned to the right side of the heart, oxygenated blood from the lungs is cycled via the left side of the heart. Venous blood travels through veins, back flow is prevented by lumen (which can become less effective with age and occupation, becoming varicose). Arterial blood travels

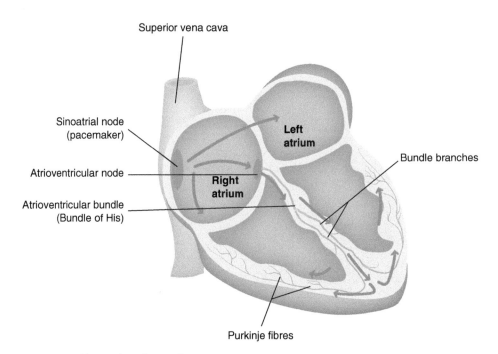

Figure 6.25   The cardiac electrical system

through arteries, the largest of which is the aorta (see Figure 6.23). Arteries have a thick muscular wall which allows for expansion to accommodate the 70–90 millilitres of blood ejected with each left ventricular contraction. See Figure 6.26 to examine the structural difference between arteries and veins.

Vessels become smaller the further away they are from the heart (arterioles, venules) until they become hair-like single-cell-thick capillaries, which is where gas (and nutrient/waste) exchange takes place, with oxygen diffusing out and carbon dioxide diffusing in (internal respiration).

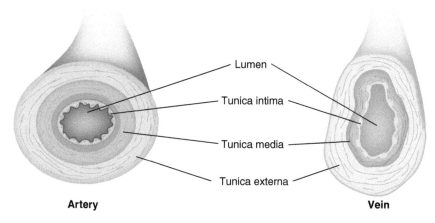

Lumen

Tunica intima

Tunica media

Tunica externa

Artery   **Vein**

Figure 6.26   Structure of arteries and veins

Blood is made up of (approximately) 55% plasma and 45% cells (erythrocytes, leucocytes and platelets). The volume of blood occupied by the cells is called the haematocrit. Plasma is made up of 92% water, 7% plasma proteins (albumin, globulin, fibrinogen: the clotting factors) and 1% dissolved solutes. The average adult has 5–6 litres of blood. Red blood cells are biconcave (saucer shaped) to give greater surface area for oxygen to attach to the haemoglobin. Table 6.3 explains the function of blood.

Table 6.3   The function of blood

Transportation	Gases, nutrients and waste, hormones and heat
Regulation	Temperature, osmoregulation, blood pH
Protection	Clotting factors to prevent blood loss; micro-organisms such as white cells and antibodies

The circulatory system has a relationship with the lymphatic system. Tissue fluid (lymph) is collected into blind-ended lacteals and is a return route to the blood, via lymph vessels that drain into the subclavian veins.

THE CHILD'S CARDIOVASCULAR SYSTEM

Very young children have a rapid heartbeat (compared to an adult), usually approximately 190 bpm; this gradually slows as the child grows. Children can be born with congenital cardiac disorders such as hole in the heart, which are holes in the heart's dividing septum. This can be atrial septal defect (ASD) or ventricular septal defect (VSD). Many small ASDs close on their own as the heart grows during childhood, and do not require surgical intervention; however larger ASDs can cause complications if not diagnosed and treated. Extra blood flowing into the right atrium through an ASD can cause the atrium to stretch and enlarge leading to arrhythmias, right side cardiac failure, pulmonary hypertension and, possibly, a stroke. A baby born with a VSD may have a single hole or several and may have other congenital cardiac malformations. Small VSDs will often close by themselves but large VSDs can cause symptoms in infants and children; these can lead to arrhythmias and heart failure. Septal defects may be genetic or environmental. Some diseases can predispose to developing septal defects such as Down syndrome, nearly half of Down's babies have a heart defect.

Ventricular tachycardia is diagnosed when children experience tiredness, shortness of breath, light-headedness and chest pains on exercise; this would be revealed by an electrocardiogram (ECG) or ECG stress test. Sometimes it is necessary to make a cardiac recording over several days, so the child might wear a halter monitor with three or four recording leads. Treatment includes a pacemaker, surgery and medication.

THE EFFECTS OF AGEING ON THE CARDIOVASCULAR SYSTEM

Most of the changes that affect the ageing heart and circulatory system are as a result of disease. By late adulthood, cardiac output decreases, and cholesterol increases leading to blood vessel walls thickening and hardening (arteriosclerosis), which reduces elasticity in the arteries and increases blood pressure (hypertension). More blood is left in the ventricles, decreasing ejection fraction to below 70%, and the heart rate may slow due to loss of pacemaker cells, leading to loss of capacity at the major organs. Heart murmurs increase as the cardiac valves become less flexible. Functional blood volume decreases and baroreceptors that monitor blood pressure when you change position become less sensitive, which can cause orthostatic hypotension.

Go Further 6.6

Download the following PDF which details the cardiovascular system and blood circulation: www.biologymad.com/resources/Ch%206%20-The%20Circulatory%20System.pdf

Visit the British Heart Foundation website to read about cardiovascular diseases, current research and preventative measures: www.bhf.org.uk

THE RESPIRATORY SYSTEM

The respiratory system (Figure 6.27) provides the route for entry of oxygen into the body and a route for excretion of carbon dioxide. Breathing warms or cools and moistens the atmospheric air and it cleans atmospheric air using mucus and cilia to trap airborne particles.

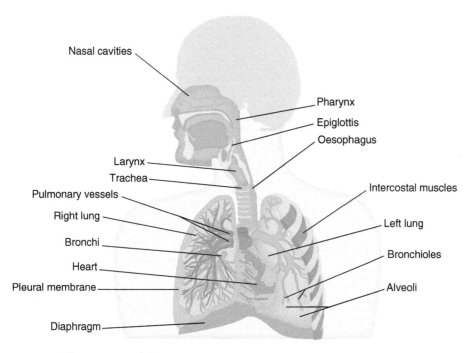

Figure 6.27   The structure of the respiratory system

The human lungs are a pair of large, spongy organs optimised for gas exchange between our blood and the air. They are lobular, with three on the right side and two on the left (space needed to accommodate the heart). Our bodies require oxygen in order to survive and the lungs provide us with vital oxygen while also removing carbon dioxide before it can reach hazardous levels. Air is drawn in through the mouth or nose and passes through the nasal or buccal cavity, pharynx and larynx, drawn down through the trachea into the right and left bronchus and thence to the alveoli (Figure 6.28). Table 6.4 details other functions of the respiratory system. Figure 6.28 explains the mechanics of breathing.

Gas exchange takes place in the alveoli of the lungs. Inspired atmospheric air contains 78% nitrogen, 21% oxygen, 0.04% carbon dioxide and variable amounts of water vapour. Expired air contains 78% nitrogen, 14% oxygen, 4% carbon dioxide and is saturated with water vapour. Once oxygen has diffused into the bloodstream it binds to oxyhaemoglobin molecules (HbO_2) in the red blood cells. The actual number of O_2 molecules binding depends upon the partial pressure (PO_2) of oxygen. See Figure 6.29 for detail of gas exchange.

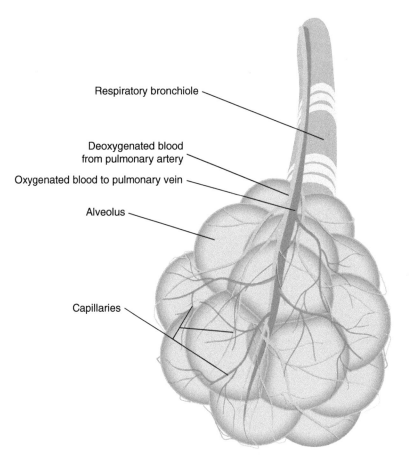

Respiratory bronchiole

Deoxygenated blood from pulmonary artery

Oxygenated blood to pulmonary vein

Alveolus

Capillaries

Figure 6.28   The alveolus

Table 6.4   Other functions of the respiratory system

Hearing	The auditory tube extends from the nasopharynx to the middle ear and protects the tympanic membrane
Protection	Lymphatic tissue protecting the tonsils (pharyngeal and laryngeal), cough reflex, mucus escalator to trap and remove particles
Speech	The thoracic cavity acts as a resonating chamber for volume, pitch and intonation

Control of breathing is coordinated in the brain as respiratory rate has a relationship with the heart rate. The respiratory centre is in the medulla oblongata, which is responsible for inspiration, basic respiratory rhythm and forced expiration. The pneumotaxic centre in the pons varolii is responsible for inhibition of inspiration (Figure 6.30), which results in expiration. The mechanical action of breathing is under control of the central nervous system. Innervation of the diaphragm is by the phrenic nerve (which originates from the C3, C4 and C5) and innervation of the external intercostal muscles is by the intercostal nerves (which originate from the thoracic portion of the spinal cord T1–T12) (see Figure 6.29).

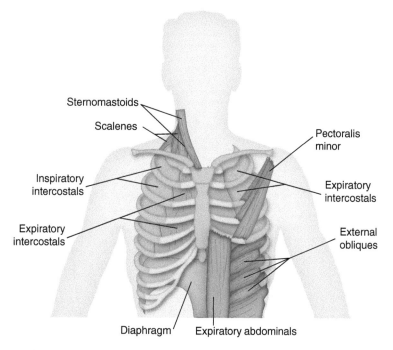

Figure 6.29   The mechanics of breathing

THE CHILD'S RESPIRATORY SYSTEM

Children are born with a limited lung capacity and have around 50–70 million alveoli – adult lungs have approximately 300 million alveoli. In the first 6 months, the baby's alveoli will develop quite rapidly, then growth slows. Some children are born with genetic conditions such as cystic fibrosis; others can rapidly develop asthma, which can be a combination of genetic influences and atmospheric pollution. Lung development may be retarded in low birth weight or premature babies, who could then develop respiratory distress syndrome. Children's lungs are especially susceptible to airborne pollution with a long period of vulnerability. Exposure to neurotoxins,

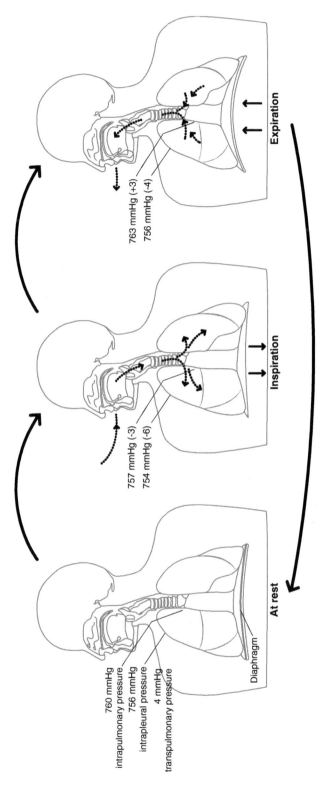

760 mmHg
intrapulmonary pressure
756 mmHg
intrapleural pressure
4 mmHg
transpulmonary pressure

Diaphragm

At rest

757 mmHg (-3)
754 mmHg (-6)

Inspiration

763 mmHg (+3)
756 mmHg (-4)

Expiration

Figure 6.30   Internal and external respiration

such as hydrocarbons (from car exhausts) in the air can have long-term effects on the cardio-respiratory system due to oxidative stress.

Research conducted by ZOE and King's College London into the impact of SARS-CoV-2 (Covid-19) on children found that the common symptoms were fatigue, headache, a sore throat and loss of smell (anosmia). They also found that most children recovered within 28 days of symptom onset and a positive Covid test. A small number of children had prolonged symptoms (long Covid) but recovered within 56 days (Molteni et al., 2021). This research also shows that the risk of severe illness and death from Covid-19 is extremely low in children and teenagers. The risk of PIMS-TS, a rare inflammatory syndrome in children caused by Covid-19, is very low and generally only affects young people with multiple health conditions and complex disabilities.

The Pfizer-BioNTech vaccine has been authorised for children and (as of July, 2022) is given in two doses, a smaller dose for children under age 11.

THE EFFECTS OF AGEING ON THE RESPIRATORY SYSTEM

The air spaces in the alveoli become enlarged and lose their elasticity, meaning that there is less area for gases to be exchanged across. The lungs become stiffer (lose compliance), muscle strength and endurance diminish, and the chest wall becomes rigid. The strength of the respiratory muscles (the diaphragm and intercostal muscles) decreases. This change is closely connected to the general health of the person. There is an increase in mucus production and a decrease in the activity and number of cilia. Older people cough more to remove airborne particles and to clear the lungs of phlegm. The body becomes less efficient in monitoring and controlling breathing. All of these changes mean that an older person might have more difficulty coping with increased stress on their respiratory system, such as pneumonia, than a younger person would.

Older people have been particularly affected by coronavirus SARS-CoV-2 (Covid-19), with most deaths (74%) occurring in people over the age of 65 globally (see Figure 6.31 for England which reflects the global figures). While research is ongoing to determine why older people are at greater risk of severe illness, it would seem from previous research that prior to SARS-CoV-2, human coronaviruses and influenza viruses were known to impact older people disproportionately. Comorbidities such as hypertension, diabetes, obesity, cardiovascular disease and respiratory system disease clearly have an adverse impact. As Covid-19 is transmitted through aerosol transmission of respiratory droplets (Tang et al., 2021), the virus enters the lungs where it infects alveolar epithelial cells called pneumocytes. This can lead to acute respiratory distress syndrome (ARDS) due to pathophysiological changes that characterise the ageing respiratory system. Other age-related changes to the immune system then begin to take effect, increasing the risk of death.

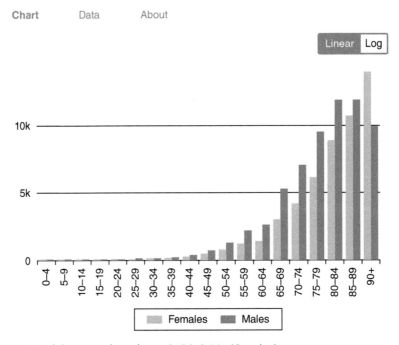

Chart   Data   About

Linear | Log

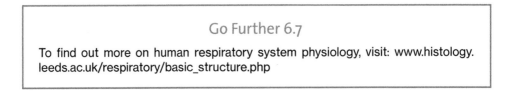

Figure 6.31   Death by age and sex due to SARS-CoV-2 (Covid-19)

© ons.gov.uk/datasets open commons licence

Go Further 6.7

To find out more on human respiratory system physiology, visit: www.histology. leeds.ac.uk/respiratory/basic_structure.php

---

THE NERVOUS SYSTEM

The nervous system is multifunctional: it allows you to speak, hear, feel, sense, taste, see, smell, think, create, respond, move, have morals, experience pain and pleasure, learn and remember. It has two main parts: the central nervous system (the brain and spinal cord) and the peripheral nervous system (autonomic, somatic, sympathetic and parasympathetic nervous systems) (see Figure 6.32).

THE CRANIAL CAVITY (SEE FIGURE 6.33)

- The cerebrum is divided into two hemispheres housing the motor and sensory cortex. It is responsible for the control of both voluntary and involuntary actions.

- The right side of the brain controls the left side of the body (and vice versa).
- The basal ganglia are responsible for fine control of complex movements.
- The thalamus relays sensory inputs and redistributes them to the appropriate sensory areas.
- The hypothalamus has links to the pituitary gland and controls the autonomic nervous system, appetite and homeostatic mechanisms.

THE CENTRAL NERVOUS SYSTEM (CNS)

The spinal cord runs from the brain to the lumbar region and is protected by the vertebrae. It contains cerebrospinal fluid which circulates within membranes (meninges) around the outside of the CNS and also inside a canal within the CNS. Both the brain and spinal cord contain white matter which contains axons and dendron, and grey matter which is mainly the cell bodies of neurons. The brainstem links the spinal cord to the brain and attaches to the medulla oblongata which controls and coordinates three vital centres: the cardiovascular centre, the respiratory centre and the reflex centres for vomiting, coughing, sneezing and swallowing.

THE PERIPHERAL NERVOUS SYSTEM

This has several parts: there are nerves that control the involuntary (autonomic) activities of the body, such as the heart beat or digestion, and nerves that control voluntary activities of the body, such as musculoskeletal movement. The autonomic nervous system controls the sympathetic system, better known as 'fight or flight': the effects on the smooth muscles of the airways, blood vessels, cardiac muscle and various glands are rapid; the parasympathetic nervous system resets the body to default after the excitement has calmed down.

NERVE STRUCTURE AND FUNCTION

Nerve cells are called neurons and they come in three shapes and sizes, depending on their function (see Figure 6.34 and Table 6.5). Sensory neurons send messages moving away from a central organ or point and relay messages from receptors (such as in the skin) **to** the brain or spinal cord. Interneurons are relay neurons and relay messages from sensory neurons to motor neurons. Motor neurons send messages towards a central organ or point and relay messages **from** the brain or spinal cord to the muscles and organs.

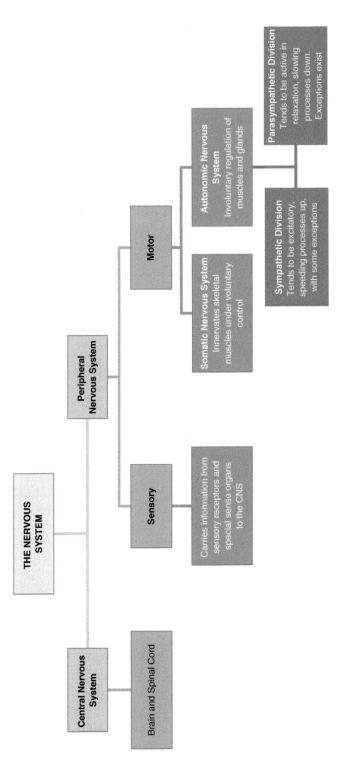

Figure 6.32   The nervous system

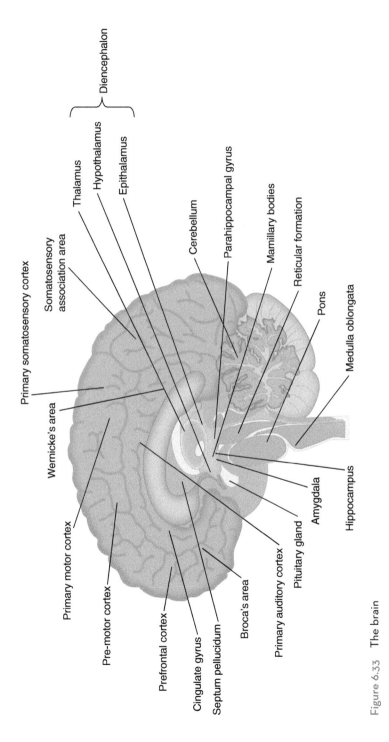

Figure 6.33 The brain

Primary somatosensory cortex

Somatosensory association area

Thalamus

Hypothalamus

Epithalamus

Diencephalon

Cerebellum

Parahippocampal gyrus

Mamillary bodies

Reticular formation

Pons

Medulla oblongata

Wernicke's area

Primary motor cortex

Pre-motor cortex

Prefrontal cortex

Cingulate gyrus

Septum pellucidum

Broca's area

Primary auditory cortex

Pituitary gland

Amygdala

Hippocampus

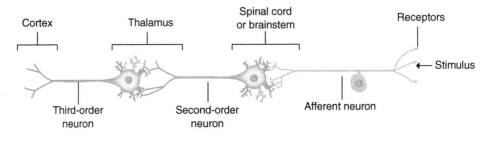

Figure 6.34   A sensory neuron

Table 6.5   Neurons

	Sensory neuron	Interneuron	Motor neuron
Length of fibre	Long dendrites and short axon	Short dendrites and short or long axon	Short dendrites and long axons
Location	Cell body and dendrite are outside of the spinal cord	Entirely within the CNS	Dendrites and the cell body are located in the spinal cord; the axon is outside the spinal cord
Function	Conducts impulse to the spinal cord	Interconnects the sensory neuron with appropriate motor neuron	Conducts impulse to an effector (muscle or gland)

Each neuron has a cell body and axons and dendrites. Messages are relayed along the branches by action potentials which are controlled by the Schwann cells and the nodes of Ranvier. These are protected by a wrapping of myelin sheath. Neurons are complex and do not reproduce once damaged, they cannot heal or be repaired, although science is doing its very best to overcome this. Neurons and nerve endings do not actually touch each other; there is a slight gap called a synapse (see Figure 6.35). Messages need to pass across the synapse, and they do this via hormones called neurotransmitters, which travel across the synapse and lock into receptor sites and thus pass on the action potential.

Pre-synaptic neuron = neuron sending impulse

Post-synaptic neuron = neuron receiving impulse

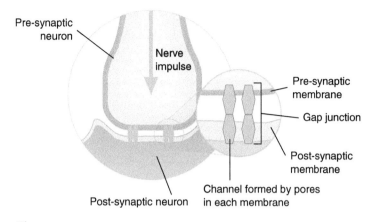

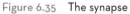

Pre-synaptic neuron

Nerve impulse

Pre-synaptic membrane

Gap junction

Post-synaptic membrane

Channel formed by pores in each membrane

Post-synaptic neuron

Figure 6.35   The synapse

Go Further 6.8

This process is quite complex; you might improve your understanding of this by watching Bozeman Science or Khan Academy YouTube videos.

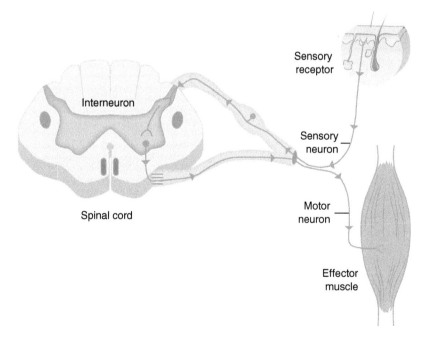

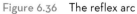

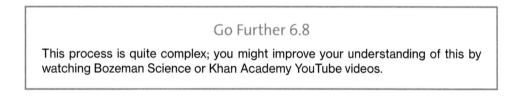

Interneuron

Sensory receptor

Sensory neuron

Motor neuron

Spinal cord

Effector muscle

Figure 6.36   The reflex arc

Nerves are made up of hundreds of neurons somewhat analogous to an electrical cable made up of hundreds of filaments. They form the nerve pathways; some are simple reflexes, which are innate, such as blinking or knee jerk (Figure 6.36), and some are learned responses and require conscious thought; these are very complex as different responses can result from a single stimulus.

THE CHILD'S NERVOUS SYSTEM

Babies are born with an immature nervous system which matures over the first few years of life. Babies can be born with neural tube deficits, these include spina bifida, anencephaly and encephalocele. These might be caused by maternal folate deficiency, anti-epileptic medication or genetics. Many spina bifida babies also have hydrocephalus (water on the brain) which requires a shunt to drain the fluid. Anencephaly babies are usually stillborn or die shortly after birth. Damage to the brain and spinal cord is quite rare, this includes neonate stroke, hemiparesis, porencephaly, cerebral palsy and brain tumour. The most common is epilepsy, which has multiple causes. Learning disability can be caused by anoxia during delivery or by childhood meningitis, or it might be genetic such as Down syndrome or cerebral palsy. Children with a learning disability can have quite complex needs.

EFFECTS OF AGEING ON THE NERVOUS SYSTEM

With ageing there is a loss of nerve/brain cells which do not regenerate, and coupled with lessening production of neurotransmitters this leads to increases in reaction time. Receptors become less sensitive, which results in reduced sense of touch and sensitivity to pain. Changes in memory and increased forgetfulness may be the result of disease processes such as dementias, but cognitive decline generally depends on the individual. Keeping intellectually active can slow decline, although research (studies too numerous to mention individually) shows that older adults perform less well on tasks involving encoding, retention and retrieval of information.

Go Further 6.9

Read more on the nervous system: www.blackwellpublishing.com/intropsych/pdf/chapter3.pdf

---

THE IMMUNE SYSTEM

You have on average about 100,000 bacteria on every square centimetre of your skin. These dine on the 10 billion flakes of skin that you shed every day, plus all the oils and minerals that you secrete. There are trillions more inside your body – in your nose, in your gut (more trillions) – they can reproduce in less than 10 minutes, so in 24 hours one can become 280,000 billion. However, we cannot live without bacteria: they process waste, synthesise vitamins and go to war against invading microbes. Table 6.6 introduces you to the words we use to describe types of infective agents.

Table 6.6   Infective agents

Vector	Living organisms that can transmit infectious diseases between humans or from animals to humans
Pathogen	An infective agent such as a bacteria, virus, fungus or parasite
Antigen	A chemical constituent of a pathogen, which the immune system recognises as a threat

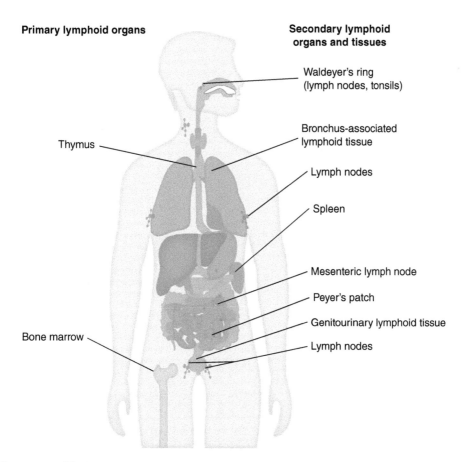

Figure 6.37   The immune system

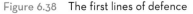

You can find more detail about the immune system in Chapter 8 on the prevention and control of infection.

The immune system (Figure 6.37) works across the body systems because bacteria, fungi, viruses and parasites enter through orifices such as the mouth, nose, ears, genitals, eyes and skin pores and through wounds, cuts and abrasions and can affect every part of the body. The immune system can override homeostasis and is known as the 'command and control' system (see Figure 6.38). There are three parts to the immune system, we will look at them in turn.

THE FIRST LINES OF DEFENCE

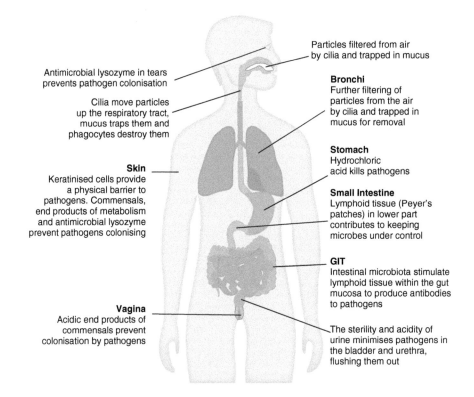

Figure 6.38 The first lines of defence

- The skin: prevents pathogens entering the body and has a biome of helpful commensal bacteria.
- The nose and bronchi: contain sticky mucus that traps pathogens; they are coughed up and swallowed. Macrophages (phagocytes) swim in the fluid that surrounds the alveoli; these eat and destroy invading microbes. When they have achieved their task, they too are swept up the bronchi via the mucus escalator.

- Blood: contains histamines to invoke the inflammatory response.
- Tears and saliva: contain the killer enzyme lysozyme.
- The stomach: gastric acid has a pH of 1.5, this kills many pathogens.

THE SECOND LINE OF DEFENCE: THE NON-SPECIFIC OR INNATE SYSTEM

The second line of defence is the non-specific immune system. This can kill or limit the spread of pathogens, but it is not an efficient killer of specific invaders as it does not learn to recognise one particular antigen from another. This line of defence uses engulfing cells called phagocytes, which are cells that eat invading organisms (think Pac-Man). These are the link between the non-specific and specific immune system. Once a phagocyte has engulfed the invader, it becomes an antigen-presenting cell, which then stimulates the mediated system.

Inflammation is one of the first responses of the immune system to infection. The symptoms of inflammation are redness and swelling, which are caused by increased blood flow into a tissue (which is what actually causes the pain). Inflammation is produced by the mast cells eicosanoids and cytokines (such as pyrogens), which are released by injured or infected cells. Eicosanoid prostaglandins produce fever and the dilation of blood vessels associated with inflammation. Leukotrienes attract leucocytes: these are the main defence in the bloodstream; they float through the stream until they detect the chemical signals of an invader, then travel to the cells to mount an inflammatory response (chemotaxis). They are either granular or agranular depending on the presence of small grain-like vesicles in their cytoplasm. Table 6.7 gives the different types of leucocytes.

Table 6.7   Leucocytes

Monocytes	Turn into macrophages and engulf invaders
Neutrophils	Attack and kill bacteria and fungi
Eosinophils	Kill parasites such as flatworms and flukes
Eicosanoids	Prostaglandins which cause fever
Basophils	Release histamine during allergic reactions

CYTOKINES

These are chemical messengers that carry communication between cells and include:

- Interleukins that are responsible for communication between white blood cells, and
- Interferons that have antiviral effects, such as shutting down protein synthesis in the host cell.

These cytokines and other chemicals recruit immune cells to the site of infection and promote healing following the removal of pathogens.

The complement system is a biochemical cascade that attacks the surfaces of foreign cells. It contains over 20 different proteins and is named for its ability to 'complement' the killing of pathogens by antibodies. Complement is the major humoral component of the nervous system/ innate immune response (see Figure 6.39).

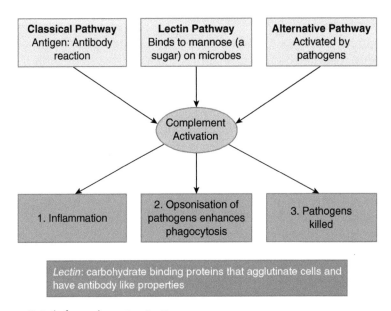

Figure 6.39   Detail of complement activation

THE THIRD LINE OF DEFENCE OR THE ADAPTIVE RESPONSE SYSTEM

Lymphocytes are specialised attack cells which respond to both external and internal (for instance cancer) invaders. They are an improvised response to a specific invader and are created in the bone marrow. They are capable of remembering invaders. This defence system is slower to react as it must determine the nature of the attack and formulate a response. Although mature lymphocytes look pretty much alike, they are extraordinarily diverse in their functions. Figure 6.40 gives a schematic overview of the function of the three systems.

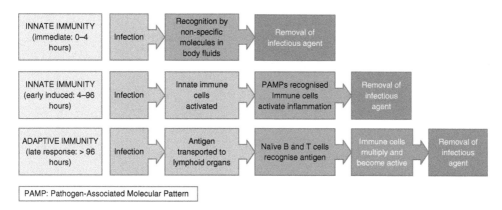

Figure 6.40   Schematic of the three systems

HUMERAL (LYMPHATIC) IMMUNE SYSTEM

• B lymphocytes (B-cells)

Each B-cell is specific for a particular antigen. What this means is that each is able to bind to a particular molecular structure. This response is carried out by antibodies, which are also known as immunoglobulins. These come in different types: IgG is the most common, followed by IgM, IgA (in mucus) and IgE (in the inflammatory response). These are made of molecules of protein that derive from B-lymphocytes. They circulate in the body fluids (hence humeral: from the old concept of humours) and are transported by the lymphatic system and stored in the lymph nodes. Blood plasma contains 15 different proteins collectively known as complement (see above). These are activated by immunoglobulins, and when activated the complement proteins interact with the humeral immune response.

• B-cells

Antibodies: The humeral antibody system produces antibodies that bind to antigens and identify the antigen complex for destruction (lyse). Antibodies act on antigens in serum and lymph. B-cell antibodies may either be attached to B-cell membranes or free floating in the serum and lymph. The plasma cells live for only 4–5 days but can be reproduced at a rate of 2000 antibody molecules per second.

Although the general structure of an antibody is similar, a small region at the tip is variable (hypervariable region). Each of these variants binds to a different target (antigen). The unique part of the antigen recognised by the antibody is called an epitope; these epitopes bind with their antibodies and tag them for attack and destruction. Table 6.8 describes how antibodies work. Figure 6.41 shows you the difference between a virus and a bacteria: each offers the immune system different challenges to break through their defences.

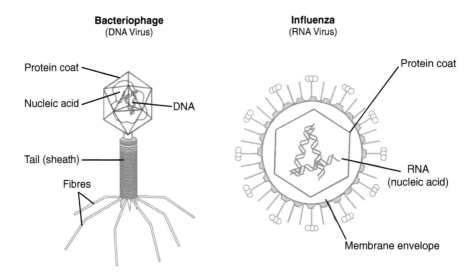

Figure 6.41   Bacteriophage and influenza virus

Table 6.8   How antibodies work

Antibodies produced in the lymph nodes link antigens together causing agglutination (clumping together) of pathogens
Precipitation of antibody molecules that react with soluble antigens (complement)
Activates systems that cause lysis of pathogens (T-cells)
Opsonise (coats) pathogens: identifying them as foreign cells to phagocytes

- T-cells or the mediated system

T-cells are so called because they migrate to the thymus gland to mature. Immunity is given by specific activated T-lymphocytes which destroy (lyse) infected cells, cancerous cells or foreign cells (such as those in transplanted organs). These can be helper, cytotoxic (killer), suppressor or memory T-cells. The mediated system acts on antigens appearing on the surface of individual cells. T-cells produce T-cell receptors, which recognise specific antigens bound to the antigen-presenting structures on the surface of the cell. When a T-cell is presented with an antigen, its receptor binds to the antigen, and it is stimulated to divide and reproduce. Killer T-cells (cytotoxic) only recognise antigens coupled to Class I MHC (major histocompatibility complex) molecules. Helper T-cells produce a growth factor called an interleukin; this proliferates the killer T-cells.

Killer T-cells are activated when their T-cell receptor (TCR) binds to this specific antigen in a complex with the MHC Class I receptor of another cell. Recognition of this MHC–antigen complex is aided by a co-receptor on the T-cell called CD8. The T-cell then travels throughout the body in search of cells where the MHC I receptors bear this antigen. When an activated T-cell contacts such cells, it releases cytotoxins, such as perforin, which form pores in the target cell's plasma membrane, allowing ions, water and toxins to enter. T-cell activation is tightly controlled and generally requires a very strong MHC–antigen activation signal, or additional activation signals provided by the helper T-cells. Helper T-cells have no cytotoxic activity and do not kill infected cells or pathogens directly. They instead control the immune response by directing other cells to perform these tasks.

•   Natural killer lymphocytes

These are similar to killer cells as they break down target cells, but they do not need to interact with other lymphocytes or antibodies.

•   Suppressor T-cells

These regulate the overall response of the killer cells and B-cells. They protect uninfected cells and act as a restraining influence when the response is no longer required.

MEMORY CELLS: THE ADAPTIVE IMMUNE SYSTEM

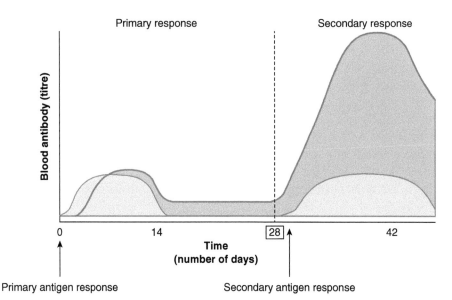

Figure 6.42   Secondary immune response

Memory cells are a part of the acquired immunity system; once the body has been exposed to a disease and survived, a large group of B-cells and T-cells (memory cells) remains capable of producing a secondary immune response should the pathogen reappear in the body. This is called naturally acquired immunity. A secondary immune response is more powerful than the primary response, producing antibodies so quickly that the disease should never get a chance to develop (see Figure 6.42).

The characteristics of the immune systems are summarised in Table 6.9.

Table 6.9   Summary of the immune systems

Innate immune system	Adaptive immune system
Response is non-specific	Pathogen and antigen-specific response
Exposure leads to immediate response	Delay between exposure and response
Cell-mediated and humoral components	Cell-mediated and humoral components
No immunological memory	Immunological memory

WHEN IT ALL GOES WRONG

When the immune system is functioning normally, it distinguishes 'self' from 'non-self' but sometimes the immune system mistakes its own cells for pathogens, resulting in an autoimmune disease. The immune system attacks the tissue of the body, such as in multiple sclerosis, which results from the destruction of the myelin sheath of nerve fibres.

THE CHILD'S IMMUNE SYSTEM

Babies are born protected by their mother's immune system and develop their own by passive immunity with the help of breast milk which contains immunoglobulins and lactobacillus, which are protective. However, they are only protected from ailments their mother has been exposed to. The baby's immune system is not fully formed, and so very young children are at increased risk of infection; this is due to neonatal antigen-presenting cells having a reduced pattern recognition. This also has an impact on vaccine effectiveness, so young children need regular boosts to their vaccination. As the child grows, and has survived encounters with pathogens, the immune system strengthens and accumulates immunological memory.

THE EFFECTS OF AGEING ON THE IMMUNE SYSTEM (IMMUNOSENESCENCE)

The immune system becomes less able to distinguish self from non-self (see above). Therefore, autoimmune disorders become more common (such as arthritis). There are fewer white cells and macrophages, and T-cell function slows.

This impacts on complement production, which explains why cancer is more common in older people and why they take longer to heal or recover from infection. As the amount of antibody production is less, older people become more susceptible to infections and have trouble fighting them off (reinfection) so that colds and influenza develop into pneumonia. Vaccines become less effective and need to be repeated (boosted) annually.

The impact of SARS-CoV-2 (Covid-19) on the immune system depends on any underlying health issues. If the individual has a sub-optimal immune response, they are likely to develop severe Covid-19. This can trigger a 'cytokine storm' (hyper-cytokinaemia): this is an unregulated response of the inflammatory system which can overwhelm the patient leading to multi-organ collapse. Included within the cytokine storm is thrombopoietin, which is associated with abnormalities in blood clotting. Further research is needed to determine if this is responsible for the blood clotting which characterises severe Covid-19. Research (Lucas et al., 2021) has also indicated that cytokines such as eicosanoids responsible for allergic reactions (anaphylaxis) are also triggered. As these are unrelated to viral control, this was an unwelcome surprise.

Go Further 6.10

You can read more about the immune system lecture notes: www.csun. edu/~cmalone/pdf589/lect_1.pdf

---

THE MUSCULOSKELETAL SYSTEM

This system is about how locomotion is achieved through muscles moving the skeleton. Muscle tissue is comprised of long filaments (muscle cells) bundled together to form muscle fibres (see Figure 6.43), which are also bundled together to form muscles. Muscles attach to the skeleton, and this allows movement. The body has approximately 640 different skeletal muscles and most of them are bilateral (found on both sides of the body) and they comprise half of the body weight.

Skeletal muscles are voluntary (unlike cardiac or smooth muscle, which is involuntary), and have three main properties:

- Extensibility: ability to change length to lever bones
- Elasticity: ability to return to resting length after being stretched
- Contractility: ability to shorten to produce force

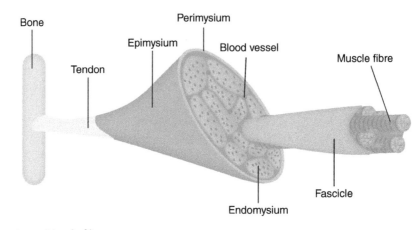

Figure 6.43   Muscle fibre

A single elongated cylindrical muscle cell is multinucleated (more than one nucleus). The cell's membrane is called the sarcolemma and its cytoplasm is called sarcoplasm. It contains contractile units called myofibrils made up of actin and myosin in repeated units called sarcomeres (see Figure 6.44).

Go Further 6.11

Research sliding filament theory; you can find this at: www.austincc.edu/apreview/PhysText/Muscle.html

And watch some YouTube animations to further your understanding.

Each cell is coated in a connective tissue called the endomysium and a bundle of cells is collectively known as a fascicle. A bundle of fascicles is surrounded by the perimysium and the whole muscle is surrounded by the epimysium. The function of skeletal muscle is to provide movement, give support to posture and a by-product is heat generation. The muscles also give the body its shape.

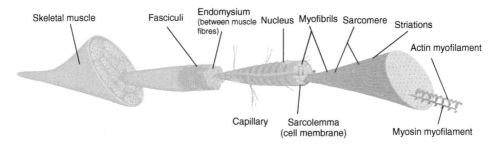

Figure 6.44   Muscle fibre showing sarcomere and myofilament

Skeletal muscles are antagonistic. This means they work in opposition to one another: when one muscle of a pair contracts, the other relaxes. For example, when one muscle in a pair contracts to bend a joint, its counterpart then contracts and pulls in the opposite direction to straighten the joint out again.

Muscle nomenclature is predominantly in Latin and there are many mnemonics (quite often rude) to help you remember them. See Table 6.10 for the rules on which the naming of muscles is predicated.

Table 6.10   The naming convention for muscles

Location (e.g. the temporalis muscle overlies the temporal bone)

Shape (e.g. the deltoid muscle group is roughly triangular or deltoid shape)

Size (minimus means small, maximus means large, brevis means short and longus means long)

Direction (rectus refers to straight, transverse or oblique means that they run on an angle)

Number of origins: biceps (2), triceps (3), quadriceps (4)

Location of origin and/or insertion (e.g. the sternocleidomastoid is named because it attaches to the sternum and the clavicle and it inserts into the mastoid process of the temporal bone)

THE SKELETAL SYSTEM

The bony framework of the body (see Figure 6.45) comprises of 206 bones (more in an infant). Its functions are complex and diverse:

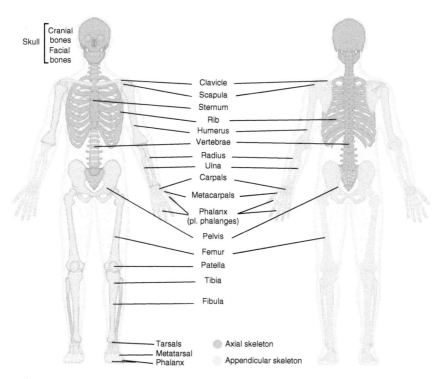

Figure 6.45   The skeleton

support, protection, movement, mineral storage and blood cell production. The naming system for bones is given in Figure 6.46 and a mnemonic in Table 6.11.

Bones are primarily made of calcium and collagen, and osteocytes are the long-lived star-shaped cells that make up bone tissue. Osteocytes do not divide but use a complex mechanism involving osteoblasts for reproduction (see Figure 6.47).

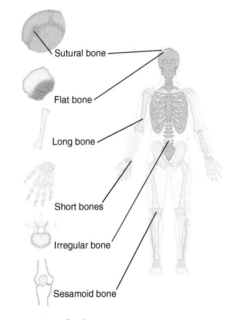

Figure 6.46   The naming convention for bones

Table 6.11   The mnemonic for naming bones: FISSSL

F = Flat	Scapula, sternum, pelvis, ribs
I = Irregular	Vertebrae, facial bones
S = Sutural	Skull bones
S = Short	Carpals and tarsals
S = Sesamoid	Patella
L = Long	Femur, tibia, fibula, humerus, radius and ulnar

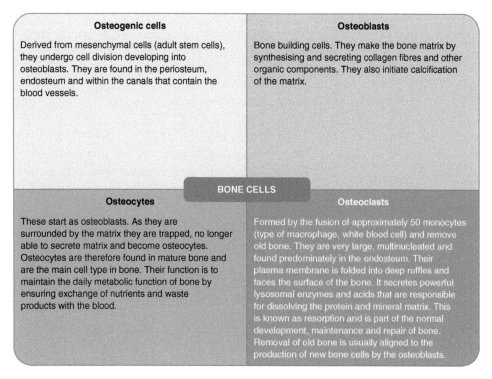

Osteogenic cells

Derived from mesenchymal cells (adult stem cells), they undergo cell division developing into osteoblasts. They are found in the periosteum, endosteum and within the canals that contain the blood vessels.

Osteoblasts

Bone building cells. They make the bone matrix by synthesising and secreting collagen fibres and other organic components. They also initiate calcification of the matrix.

BONE CELLS

Osteocytes

These start as osteoblasts. As they are surrounded by the matrix they are trapped, no longer able to secrete matrix and become osteocytes. Osteocytes are therefore found in mature bone and are the main cell type in bone. Their function is to maintain the daily metabolic function of bone by ensuring exchange of nutrients and waste products with the blood.

Osteoclasts

Formed by the fusion of approximately 50 monocytes (type of macrophage, white blood cell) and remove old bone. They are very large, multinucleated and found predominately in the endosteum. Their plasma membrane is folded into deep ruffles and faces the surface of the bone. It secretes powerful lysosomal enzymes and acids that are responsible for dissolving the protein and mineral matrix. This is known as resorption and is part of the normal development, maintenance and repair of bone. Removal of old bone is usually aligned to the production of new bone cells by the osteoblasts.

Figure 6.47   Development of bone cells

JOINTS

Joints are where bones meet and there are three types: fibrous or immovable, such as the teeth and skull; cartilaginous or slightly moveable, such as the vertebral bones and rib cage; and synovial or freely moveable joints, such as in the limbs and which are used in locomotion (the list below and Table 6.12 give more detail about the movement of bones).

Connective tissues: Remember …

- Ligament – connects bone to bone
- Tendon – connects muscle to bone
- Cartilage – cushions the joint at the end of a bone and between bones
- Bursa – fluid-filled sac that allows bones to move easily over others

Synovial joints (see Figure 6.48) allow different types of movement: **abduction** = the joint moving away from the middle of the body, and **adduction** = the joint moving towards the middle of the body. Both occur at the wrist, shoulder and hip.

Table 6.12   Synovial joint movements

Joint	Movement
Ball and socket (shoulder/hips)	Wide range of movements
Hinge (ankle/elbow)	Movement is restricted to bending and straightening only
Pivot (atlas – axis, radio – ulnar)	Movement is restricted to one bone rotating about its longitudinal axis
Condyloid (wrist/knuckles)	Allows almost as much movement as the ball and socket
Gliding (fingers/toes)	Allows a limited range of movement in all directions
Saddle (thumb)	The concave area of one bone articulates with the convex area of the adjacent bone and vice versa to allow rotation
Apophyseal (vertebrae)	Hinge-like joints that allow the flexion, extension and torsion of the spine

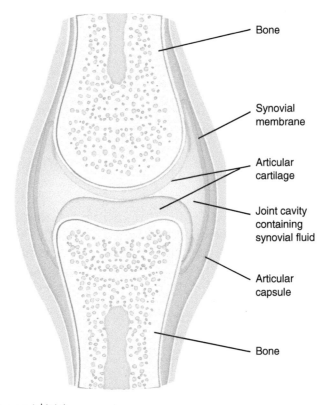

Figure 6.48   A synovial joint

THE CHILD'S MUSCULOSKELETAL SYSTEM

Babies and toddlers have more porous bone, with wider Haversian canals, which makes their bones more plastic and elastic. This means they can deform more before they break (greenstick fracture). Children's long bones grow from the ends, the epiphysis growth plate, until maturity, usually achieved about age 17. When children break a long bone, there is an excessive growth response leading to temporary limb length discrepancy, unless the break is at the epiphysis growth plate, in which case repair can take years to correct; an example of this is septic arthritis. Malnutrition can impact on bone growth, leading to stunted development; rickets leads to bow legs as the leg bones are not strong enough to take the weight of the upper body. Bone matrix deficiencies lead to many problems as does thyroid and growth hormone dysfunction. This includes osteogenesis imperfecta. Tuberculous infection in the bones can cause quite significant displacement and deformity.

Muscle mass develops during puberty and adolescence under the influence of growth hormones. The muscles and nerves (myelination) grow in tandem which allows children to improve their performance in skills that require balance, agility, strength and power; thus anything that interrupts nerve supply will also affect muscle development.

THE EFFECTS OF AGEING ON THE MUSCULOSKELETAL SYSTEM

Bones stop growing towards the end of adolescence. Nutrition has an impact on the strength of bones as a lack of calcium, protein and other nutrients during growth and development can cause bones to be small. Bones need vitamin D, which is necessary for absorption of calcium from the intestines, and vitamin C, which is necessary for collagen synthesis by osteoblasts. Levels of calcium in the blood depend upon movement of calcium into or out of bone. This is controlled by two hormones: the parathyroid hormone increases calcium, and calcitonin lowers it.

As we age, bone matrix production falls, leading to bone loss; collagen production also falls, leading to brittle bones, and for women, the rate of bone loss increases 10-fold after menopause. This leads to increased risk of fractures and can cause deformity (such as 'Dowager's hump'), loss of height (approximately 2 inches by age 80 caused by compression of vertebrae), pain, stiffness and loosening teeth.

As we age our muscles generally decrease in strength, endurance, size and weight. The muscular system ages due to loss of muscle density, lack of movement due to pain, and slower muscle–nerve interaction due to a poorer response to stimuli. Typically, we lose about 23% of our muscle mass by age 80 as both the number and size of muscle fibres decrease. These changes may be more the result of inactivity, poor nutrition and chronic illness or disease rather than the result of ageing per se and much of this decrease in muscle mass can be prevented by maintaining physical fitness.

Go Further 6.12

You can read more on the skeletal and muscular system at: www.pearson.com/content/dam/one-dot-com/one-dot-com/us/en/higher-ed/en/products-services/course-products/fremgen-6e-info/pdf/Sample_ch04_final.pdf

THE ENDOCRINE SYSTEM

This system is the collection of glands that produce the hormones that regulate metabolism, growth and development, tissue function, sexual function and reproduction (Figure 6.49). The glands are the hypothalamus, pineal gland, thymus, thyroid gland, parathyroid glands, pituitary gland, adrenal glands, pancreas, ovaries (in females) and testes (in males). Hormones circulate through the body and target their associated organs and tissues. Imbalances within the system can lead to infertility, thyroid ailments (hyper/hypothyroidism) and in the case of the pancreas, diabetes.

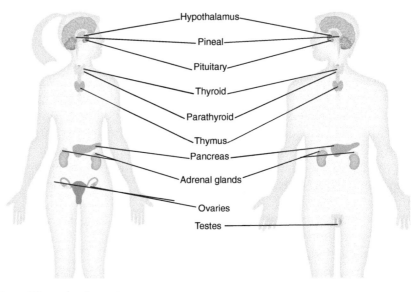

Figure 6.49   The endocrine system

Go Further 6.13

You can read more on the endocrine system at: www.lamission.edu/lifesciences/lecturenote/AliPhysio1/Endrocrine%20System.pdf

WOUND HEALING

Wound healing happens in three stages:

1. Inflammation, where pyrogens begin the process of killing invaders (see the immune system above) causing swelling, pain, heat and redness. In response to damage, the blood vessels constrict (haemostasis) and seal as the platelets are trapped in nets of fibrinogen which form a clot and stop bleeding. Bacteria and debris are phagocytosed and removed, which is characterised by the infiltration of neutrophils, macrophages and lymphocytes.
2. Proliferation, as the wound begins to heal, new healthy granulation tissue begins to grow along the wound bed. Angiogenesis is the process of growing new blood vessels within tissues made of extracellular matrix and collagen. Epithelial cells crawl across the wound bed to cover it, the wound then contracts and closes (see Figure 6.50).

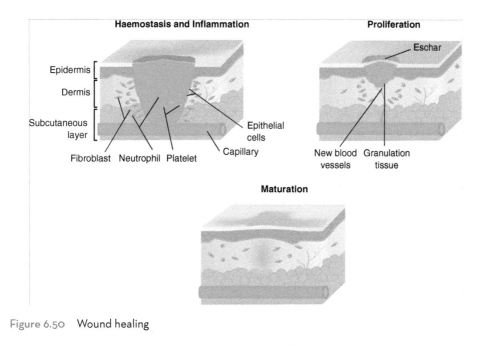

Figure 6.50   Wound healing

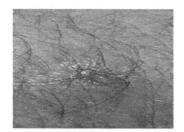

Figure 6.51   A healing burn

3. Maturation and remodelling occurs after the wound has healed over (such as image 6.51). Collagen is remodelled and realigned, dermal tissue is formed, and scar tissue reduces (this can take up to two years).

This describes an uneventful healing process; however, sometimes wounds become infected, so this process is interrupted or incomplete, and even a mature wound can suddenly burst open. Indications of infection include continuing pain, inflammation, an unpleasant smell (some infectious agents have a distinctive smell, such as *Pseudomonas* bacteria which smell sweet) and suppuration. Most chronic wounds are a result of ischaemia, vascular incompetence, diabetes and decubitus ulcers. Other factors in delayed healing are immunocompromise by iatrogenesis, age, gender and (over or under) nutrition.

Go Further 6.14

Michael Mercandetti (2021) gives a basic overview of wound healing and repair at: https://emedicine.medscape.com/article/1298129-overview#a1at

---

DEATH

Eventually, everybody dies. You need to understand that death is not an event, but a process. The dying body slowly shuts down, even bodies killed by traumatic events. Brain death may be instantaneous, but the body will take some time shutting down. It is important to remember that the last sense to close down is hearing, so we must be respectful in the things we say, even when we suspect the patient is gone. Body temperature and blood pressure drop, the pulse slows, breathing usually slows (Cheynes–Stokes). The jaw may relax due to loss of muscle control (also the bladder/bowel may void for the same reason). Breathing and heartbeat ceases – although due to the action of some drugs, heart beats may occur; an ECG might be needed to confirm that the heart has stopped. This is called clinical death and the person may be revived if resuscitation methods are used. Brain death slowly follows if no intervention takes place (biological death); when all of the systems have shut down, we consider the person to be dead. However, biochemical processes continue with rigor mortis setting in; this takes anything from 10 minutes to a few hours depending on the temperature of the body at death. Rigor mortis is caused by stiffening of the muscles and joints and lasts approximately 72 hours: it begins with smaller muscles such as those in the face first, followed by the larger muscles. Physiologically, rigor mortis is caused by depletion of ATP. Recall that

ATP separates actin-myosin bridges during muscle relaxation. Without ATP, cross-bridging locks the muscles. The onset of decomposition breaks the bridges and muscles relax. The joints are the last to unstiffen due to the action of tissue decay and leaking intercellular fluid.

CHAPTER SUMMARY

- This chapter has introduced you to basic anatomy and physiology and given details of each system as it grows, ages and dies. The chapter cannot replace a good A&P book and suggestions for further research are given throughout the chapter.
- I have included details of SARS-CoV-2 (Covid-19); however, virus research continues and, therefore, while accurate at the time of writing, further research may throw up more detailed evidence of how this virus behaves, mutates and impacts on the human body.
- Watch YouTube videos and podcasts to aid your understanding when you feel overwhelmed. I also really recommend drawing diagrams if you are a kinetic learner.
- Wound healing is a specialism in nursing (tissue viability) but it is important to understand the mechanics of both the immune system in action and the healing process to support the care of your patients.

FURTHER READING

WEBSITES

Top tip: if you type into your browser the body system you are interested in and put PDF after it, you will find whole chapters you can download.

- Test banks: https://home.pearsonvue.com/nmc/practicetests
- *Fundamentals of Anatomy and Physiology*: www.fundamentalsofanatomy.com/ (for nurses)
- Howard Hughes Medical Institute – Biointeractive: www.hhmi.org/biointeractive

VIDEOS

- Inner Body: www.innerbody.com/
- Khan Academy – Human Anatomy and Physiology: www.khanacademy.org/science/health-and-medicine/human-anatomy-and-physiology
- Anatomy and physiology crash course: www.youtube.com/watch?v=uBGl2BujkPQ

BOOKS AND ARTICLES

- British Pain Society (2014) Suggested articles and reports. Available at: www.britishpainsociety.org/about/articles-and-reports/
- Guo, S. and DiPietro, L. (2010) Factors affecting wound healing. *Journal of Dental Research*, 89(3): 219–29.
- Marieb, E. and Hoehn, K. (2018) *Human Anatomy and Physiology.* London: Pearson.
- McKissock, C. (2014) *Great Ways to Learn Anatomy and Physiology.* Basingstoke: Palgrave.
- Peate, I. and Evans, S. (eds) (2020) *Fundamentals of Anatomy and Physiology: For Nursing and Healthcare Students.* Oxford: Wiley.
- Riley, K. (2014) *Wound Care* (Nursing and Health Survival Guides). Abingdon: Routledge.
- Waugh, A. and Grant, A. (2018) *Ross and Wilson: Anatomy and Physiology in Health and Illness* (13th edn). London: Elsevier.

REFERENCES

Lucas, C., Wong, P. and Klein, J. (2021) Longitudinal analyses reveal immunological misfiring in severe COVID-19. *Nature, 584*: 463–69. https://doi.org/10.1038/s41586-020-2588-y

Molteni, E., Sudre, C., Canas, L., Bhopal, S., Hughes, R. and Antonelli, M. (2021) Illness duration and symptom profile in symptomatic UK school-aged children tested for SARS-CoV-2. doi: https://doi.org/10.1016/S2352-4642(21)00198-X

NMC (Nursing and Midwifery Council) (2018) The Code: Professional standards of practice and behaviour for nurses, midwives and nursing associates. Available at: www.nmc.org.uk/globalassets/sitedocuments/nmc-publications/nmc-code.pdf

Tang, J., Marr, L., Li, Y. and Dancer, S. (2021) Covid-19 has redefined airborne transmission. *BMJ, 373*(913). doi:10.1136/bmj.n913

7

ADVANCED HEALTH SCIENCE: GENOMICS AND PATHOPHYSIOLOGY

GILLIAN ROWE

STANDARDS OF PROFICIENCY FOR NURSING ASSOCIATES (2018)

Relevant Platforms include:

Platform 2:2.1 Understand and apply the principles of health promotion, protection and improvement and the prevention of ill health when engaging with people.

Platform 2:2.2 Promote preventative health behaviours and provide information to support people to make informed choices to improve their mental, physical behavioural health and wellbeing.

Platform 2:2.3 Describe the principles of epidemiology, demography and genomics and how these might influence health and wellbeing outcomes.

Platform 2:2.6 Understand and explain the contribution of social influences, health literacy, individual circumstances, behaviours and lifestyle choices to mental, physical and behavioural health outcomes.

Platform 2:2.7 Explain why health screening is important and identify those who are eligible for screening.

Platform 3:3.2 Demonstrate and apply knowledge of body systems and homeostasis, human anatomy and physiology, biology, genomics, pharmacology, social and behavioural sciences when delivering care.

Platform 3:3.3 Recognise and apply knowledge of commonly encountered mental, physical, behavioural and cognitive health conditions when delivering care.

Platform 3:3.19 Demonstrate an understanding of comorbidities and the demands of meeting people's holistic needs when prioritising care.

Annex A 1.1–1.13, 2.1, 2.2, 2.3.

To have striven, to have made the effort, to have been true to certain ideals – this alone is worth the struggle.

William Osler (1849–1919)

INTRODUCTION

This chapter discusses genomics and the mapping of the human genome (HGP). The mapping of all human genes is a project that began in 1990 and ended in 2003. Genomics, then, refers to all of the genes in the human genome and their interactions with each other, the environment, and other cultural and psychosocial factors. The goal of using genomics is to devise personalised medicine, using not only care planning but genomic information to allow care staff to prescribe more specific and individualised treatment and to avoid iatrogenic (adverse) treatment reactions.

This chapter then discusses the nature of the role of pathophysiology, which is the study of convergent sciences, pathology and physiology. Physiology examines the functioning of the body; pathology examines disease processes or abnormalities occurring within an organism at cellular level. Pathophysiology is studied by nurses to better understand patient diagnosis and to improve patient care by gaining the ability to explain to the patient the nature of their ailment, treatment and expected outcomes. The NMC Code (2018) states 'respect and uphold people's human rights' and 'encourage and empower people to share decisions about their treatment and care'; your knowledge of pathophysiology will help you to support your patients' care.

Pathophysiology, as a distinct science, was developed out of the need to study biomedicine – first at the Pasteur Institute (1888), then the Berlin Institute for Infectious Diseases (1891); America followed in 1901 with the Rockefeller Institute, and the UK with laboratories established at universities (various dates from 1900 on). The impetus was further driven by the 'Spanish 'flu' epidemic following the First World War (1914–18). In 1928, British pathologist Fred Griffith discovered that pneumococci could transform between antigenic types, thus alerting pathologists to the fact that bacteria contained genes. It wasn't until the electron microscope was developed in 1931 that cell organelles could be properly studied and, supported by the discovery of the shape of DNA by Watson, Crick and Franklin in 1953, cell biology emerged as a discipline. Collaborations began between biologists, pathologists, geneticists and medical scientists in determining the aetiology of disease. The future of pathogenic and epidemiological research includes epigenomics and metabolomics to determine risk factors and causal inference. For more information on this subject look at Chapter 6, Bioscience, and Chapter 8, Prevention and Control of Infection.

GENOMICS

Hereditary information is stored on the famous double helix of deoxyribonucleic acid (DNA). DNA looks like a twisted ladder, the rungs of which contain four bases, arranged in different ways and different lengths (Figure 7.1). Each section or sequence being a gene, the exact sequence of each base (adenine, cytosine, guanine, thymine) carries the information a cell needs to assemble protein and ribonucleic acid (RNA) molecules. RNA contains uracil instead of thymine.

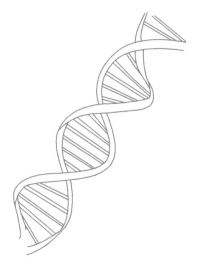

Figure 7.1   The double helix

Source: © Roo Cooper

Genes make proteins in a tightly controlled two-step process called transcription and translation, known as gene expression (Figure 7.2).

During the process of transcription, the information stored in a gene's DNA is transferred to a molecule of ribonucleic acid in the cell nucleus. Both RNA and DNA are made up of a chain of nucleotide bases but have different chemical properties. The type of RNA that contains the information for making a protein is called a messenger RNA (mRNA) because it carries the information, or message, from the DNA out of the nucleus and into the cytoplasm. Translation takes place in the cell's cytoplasm; the mRNA interacts with a ribosome which translates the code to build an amino acid. A transfer RNA (tRNA) is a non-coding RNA (ncRNA) which assembles the protein; you could imagine this as making then threading beads on a string.

Go Further 7.1

Google 'making proteins'; there are a plethora of sites and good YouTube videos available to enhance your understanding.

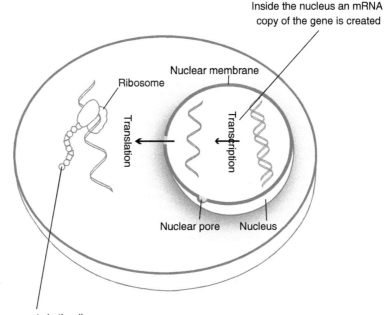

Figure 7.2   Transcription and translation

Source: Boore et al. (2017). Illustrated by Shaun Mercier, © SAGE Publications

GENETICS AND EPIGENETICS

Epigenetics, a term coined by Conrad Waddington in 1942, is the name given to chemical compounds that can affect gene expression, so they effect change in phenotype (observable characteristics) without a change in genotype (heritable genetics). They have a role in turning genes on and off and are transcribed with the gene and are also heritable. The epigenetic process is prone to making errors which can lead to abnormal gene activity (or inactivity) and can thus be responsible for genetic, metabolic and degenerative disorders. Epigenetic mutation can be impacted by environmental stressors leading to some cancers and repairing or reversing this is where current research is focused. The notion that epigenetics have some form of memory is being explored, as stress in the early years can have metabolic implications in later life.

Every human carries 46 chromosomes. When a new life is being created, each parent donates 23 chromosomes to the child, 23 chromosome pairs with a total of about 3 billion DNA base pairs. Somatic cells usually have one copy of chromosomes 1–22 from each parent, plus an X chromosome from the mother, and either an X or Y chromosome from the father, for a total of 46 chromosomes (Figure 7.3).

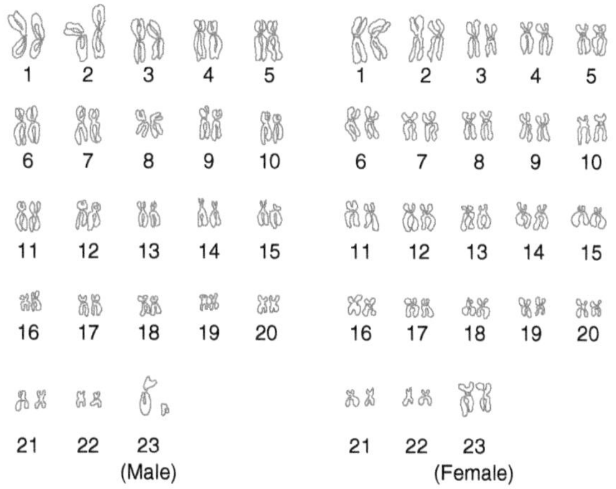

Figure 7.3   Chromosomes

Source: Boore et al. (2017). Illustrated by Shaun Mercier, © SAGE Publications

Some ailments have a distinct genetic predisposition. The first to be identified was Down syndrome in 1959. The genetic disorder Huntington's disease was located on chromosome 4 in 1983, its gene isolated in 1993. In 1990, familial breast and ovarian cancer was identified on chromosome 17 (BRCA1) and chromosome 13 (BRCA2); these are normally tumour suppressor genes, but mutations can lead to tumour formation. These mutations can lead to an increased risk of between 5 and 10 times higher than normal (NHS, 2019).

Gregor Mendel (1865) experimented with pea plant breeding and developed three principles of inheritance that described the transmission of genetic traits. He did this before anyone knew genes existed. Traits are passed down in families in different patterns; some family traits include such things as hair colour or nose shape, these are called pedigree patterns and can be seen across generations. The inheritance pattern of any such characteristic is considered dominant because it is observable in every generation. Thus, every individual who carries the genetic code for this characteristic will show evidence of the characteristic. Where a characteristic disappears for a generation, then reappears, this is called recessive.

Mendelian inheritance disorders are genetic conditions that are passed on in families in fixed proportions. They are caused by gene mutations that are present on one or both chromosomes of a pair. One gene inherited from one or both parents can cause a Mendelian disorder. These disorders are autosomal dominant (such as Huntington's disease), autosomal recessive (such as sickle cell anaemia), mitochondrial (Alpers' disease) and X-linked disorders.

Go Further 7.2

You can find good resources here: http://mitochondrialdisease.nhs.uk/patient-area/what-mitochondrial-disease/ and here: www.sciencedirect.com/topics/medicine-and-dentistry/mendelian-inheritance

---

📖 Case Study 7.1

Logan is a 11-month-old boy; his parents are concerned that he seems reluctant to crawl or walk and becomes distressed when encouraged to do so. His mother has noticed swelling and bruising on his knee and elbow joints; she thought this was due to falling when he was learning to walk, and this explained his reluctance to move. However, they became alarmed by a nosebleed (epistaxis) that wouldn't stop. Listening to their concerns, their GP referred Logan to the paediatric outpatient clinic for further investigation. Blood tests were ordered and revealed abnormalities on the blood coagulation screen (prothrombin time and activated partial thromboplastin time) and so haemophilia was suspected. Genetic analysis (FVIII assay) showed an altered haemophilia gene on his X chromosome, and he was diagnosed with haemophilia A. Logan's parents were given genetic tests to identify who carried the X mutation. Tests revealed that Logan's mother is an unknowing carrier of the haemophilia gene; this means there is a 1 in 4 chance her male children will be haemophiliac and that there is an enhanced chance any daughter she has will be a carrier of haemophilia. If Logan's mother had not carried the gene, he would not be haemophiliac as boys always inherit the X chromosome from their mothers.

Logan's condition will be managed at a specialist clinic. Treatment could include factor inhibitors, factor replacement products and adjuvant medications and management of bleeding episodes.

Haemophilia A is the most common form of haemophilia and is caused by an X-linked recessive gene, it is a bleeding disorder caused by Factor VIII deficiency. Factor VIII is created in the endoplasmic reticulum and Golgi apparatus of the endothelial cells in the liver – haemophiliacs who have a liver transplant usually find their haemophilia is cured.

Clotting factors are proteins in the blood that control bleeding. Many different clotting factors work together in a series of chemical reactions to stop bleeding, problems with Factor VIII and Factor IX are known as haemophilia A and B. **Coagulation factors** circulate in the blood in an inactive form. When a blood vessel is injured, the coagulation cascade is initiated, and each coagulation factor is activated in a specific order to lead to the formation of the blood clot. Coagulation factors are identified with Roman numerals (e.g. Factor I or FI).

Alleles are different versions of the same genes. For instance, there are two genes for eye colour: alleles for brown and blue eye colour. For any gene, a person may have the same two alleles (homozygous) or two different ones (heterozygous). The genotype is the collection of alleles that determine characteristics and can be expressed as a visible phenotype. Alleles can be dominant (typified by capital A) or recessive (typified by lower case a); therefore, dominant brown eyes are present if a person has either one or two alleles (A or AA); blue eyes are recessive and need two copies of the allele (aa).

In the case study, Logan's mother was found to carry the mutant X gene. Having a good understanding of family history is important when considering diagnosis. Genetically aware nurses take extended notes when examining and admitting patients to optimise patient outcomes by screening to identify diagnostic and therapeutic interventions, all aimed at improving individual and population health. Logan's parents could have been offered pre-pregnancy screening. Would they have chosen to have Logan had they known he would suffer from a genetic disease?

To examine the ethical and moral implications in genetic testing, the UK National Screening Committee set up the Human Genetics Commission, and the commission determined that there are 'no specific social, ethical or legal principles' against genetic pre-pregnancy screening. This type of genetic testing would examine the DNA of prospective parents before they conceive in order to assess the risk of their children inheriting a range of hereditary conditions (NHS, 2011). The commission deliberated on how to avoid discrimination and negative eugenics by the deliberate discouragement or prevention of reproduction in certain groups.

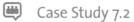 Case Study 7.2

Brenda McGrath had her first baby when she was 16 years of age; her family were ashamed of her, and she gave the baby up for adoption. In her late 20s, Brenda married and quickly became pregnant, but she did not tell her husband or her midwife about the baby given up for adoption. Blood tests revealed that Brenda was Rhesus negative (RhD-). Her midwife advised her that if she had a second child, it might be at risk of rhesus disease (haemolytic disease of the foetus and newborn) (HDFN). Brenda did not know if her previous baby was RhD positive or not and so did not know if she been previously sensitised to RhD+ blood. Brenda then disclosed her history to her midwife but begged her not to tell her husband. Brenda was given anti-D immunoglobulin injections. Had Brenda not disclosed her previous pregnancy, her baby may have needed a blood transfusion and neonatal care.

We discovered that Brenda is rhesus negative and that, should any of her blood mix with her rhesus positive baby, rhesus disease could be the outcome.

The first successful blood transfusion was carried out in 1665 by Dr Richard Lower. He used dogs as the donor and recipient. However, when they started performing transfusions on humans, they couldn't understand why the people receiving the blood kept dying. It wasn't until 1900 that Dr Karl Landsteiner discovered the ABO blood group system and realised that human patients needed to be given compatible blood. He received the Nobel Prize for his discovery. Mixing blood from two incorrectly matched individuals can lead to blood clumping or agglutination. The clumped red cells can crack and cause toxic reactions. This can have fatal consequences. Karl Landsteiner discovered that blood clumping was an immunological reaction which occurs when the receiver of a blood transfusion has antibodies against the donor blood cells.

The differences in human blood are due to the presence or absence of protein molecules called antigens and antibodies. The antigens are located on the surface of the red blood cells and the antibodies are in the blood plasma. Individuals have different types and combinations of these molecules. The blood group a person belongs to depends on parental inheritance.

Blood comes in four main groups, O, A, B and AB, and each of these can be rhesus positive or negative (Rh group). Antigens are surface markers on the red blood cells; antigens from the ABO groups are made of proteins, and antibodies are part of the immune system, floating in the blood plasma.

Box 7.1   Blood groups

- Blood group A: has A antigens on the red blood cells with anti-B antibodies in the plasma
- Blood group B: has B antigens with anti-A antibodies in the plasma
- Blood group O: has no antigens, but both anti-A and anti-B antibodies in the plasma
- Blood group AB: has both A and B antigens, but no antibodies

---

People with type O blood are universal donors, because anyone can receive a type O blood transfusion. Type O blood has no antigen on the surface that could react with antibodies in the recipient's plasma and cause a transfusion reaction.

Type AB blood is a universal recipient because this blood has no antibodies to react with donated blood.

Red blood cells have another antigen, the Rh antigen, which is a protein called RhD. This is what makes the blood positive or negative. Group O negative is safe to give to anyone in a blood transfusion. Can you work out why?

AB RhD positive (AB+)
AB RhD negative (AB−)
A RhD positive (A+)
A RhD negative (A−)
B RhD positive (B+)
B RhD negative (B−)
O RhD positive (O+)
O RhD negative (O−)

The **Kell antigen** and antibodies are the third influencing factors of blood groups. The antigens are encoded by the KEL genes and are found in association with the protein Kx on the surface of red blood cells. They are found elsewhere in the body, for example, in the liver and bone marrow, and Kell is located on chromosome 7 and has 31 alleles which are dominant (K1 and K2 or K and k). K1 is an immunogen and antibodies generated against antigens in the Kell system can cause transfusion reactions. Kell occurs in approximately 90% of the global population.

Other antigenic glycoprotein blood types include Duffy, which plays a role in inflammation and malaria, Kidd, Lewis, Lutheran and I and P.

Go Further 7.3

The Nobel Prize organisation have devised a game to help nurses understand blood groups and how they interact. Have a go and try not to kill the patient!

https://educationalgames.nobelprize.org/educational/medicine/bloodtyping-game/

MULTIFACTORIAL INHERITANCE

Multifactorial inheritance involves the combined contribution of multiple genes and environmental factors as the cause of a particular disease or trait. Environmental factors would include exposure to pollutants or toxins and lifestyle factors such as poor diet, and risk-taking activities such as smoking, excessive alcohol intake and illegal drugs. Other multifactorial diseases are complex disorders such as diabetes, heart disease and obesity. These may or may not cluster in families, but they do not have the same dominant or recessive pattern of other inherited disorders.

Nursing associates need to collect family history going back three generations (if possible) to identify if someone is at genetic risk; the nursing associate would then be able to offer advice and guidance if a risk factor presents itself. There is now genetic testing for more than 1600 genetic disorders, ranging from single-gene disorders, such as cystic fibrosis, to complex disorders, such as diabetes; however, some of these are only available commercially or not accessible due to NICE regulations.

Many companies engage in direct marketing of genetic testing kits to the public, and the danger here is that, without education, individual consumers may be misled or misinformed or misinterpret the information given to them. Most predisposition genetic tests are not sensitive or specific enough to allow prediction with any degree of certainty that a disorder will occur, nor will a negative test result rule out any likelihood of disease occurring in the future (NHS, 2018). The actor Angelina Jolie had a bilateral mastectomy when she discovered she was carrying the BRCA1 gene. When she publicised this, women in the USA, Australia and Western Europe responded by demanding genetic testing. But research carried out by Desai and Jena (2016) revealed that while celebrity endorsement increased awareness of breast cancer, it did not target the populations most at risk; so the tests failed to increase breast cancer diagnoses.

Screening is available for genetic predisposition among some ethnic groupings, such as sickle cell anaemia which is predominant in the West African and Afro-Caribbean population, or Tay–Sacks which is predominant in Ashkenazi Jewish populations.

Go Further 7.4

The Genomics Education Programme (GEP) provides online resources for NHS staff, accessible through the training portal. It includes 'Introduction to Genomics' and 'Introduction to Bioinformatics': www.genomicseducation.hee.nhs.uk/

Medical pharmacology is an evolving field. **Pharmacogenetics** deals with the unpredictability of individuals' responses to medications due to genetic variation and considers a patient's genetic information regarding how drugs are transported and metabolised in their body and their specific drug receptors. Some individuals are prone to side effects with some drugs due to their genetic predisposition. Drug efficacy may also vary with genetic makeup. There is more detail on this in Chapter 9, Essential Skills for Care. For instance, research by Budnitz et al. (2007) evidenced that 17% of people over age 65 had an adverse reaction to warfarin requiring emergency treatment. Individual genetic markers are among the factors that contribute to the determination of warfarin dose requirements: research by Lea et al. (2008) has indicated the genes CYP2C9 and VKORC1 and their ability to affect the metabolism of warfarin. The genetically competent nursing associate would recommend gene testing prior to warfarin prescription to reduce the incidence of haemorrhage or thrombosis because of individual responses regulated by genetic makeup.

The American National Cancer Institute has researched drug combinations and colonic cancers, discovering that some gene combinations mitigate against the efficacy of chemotherapy and cetuximab. The current focus of pharmacological companies is to design products for the individual against their genetic makeup.

PATHOPHYSIOLOGY

When someone is developing an ailment, they develop clinical manifestations known as signs and symptoms. These are objective and can be measured: for instance, temperature, blood pressure, pulse, etc. Some signs are focal such as a pain or swelling and some are systemic such as a fever or a rash all over the body. The prodromal or insidious phase describes vague symptoms such as lethargy, aches, loss of appetite until more specific symptoms reveal themselves and a diagnosis can be made. Pathophysiology looks at what is happening to tissues and cells as they respond to infectious agents or trauma.

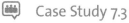 Case Study 7.3

Paula Kellow is a 52-year-old woman of Afro-Caribbean descent. She has two adult children and works full-time; she is mildly obese and smokes 10 cigarettes a day. She has a sedentary day job but is physically active at weekends as she takes her grandchildren swimming and horse riding. Paula has been feeling tired lately but puts this down to stress at work. Late one Sunday evening, she experiences pain in her jaw, shoulders and back and feels nauseous; she suspects 'flu and goes to bed. Later she wakes with severe pain in her left arm. She rings the out of hours service, who suggests she visit A&E, where she is given an ECG which indicates a heart attack.

Cardiovascular disease (CVD) and cardiac events are of major public health importance: 34% of all UK deaths were due to CVD in 2018 (NICE, 2018) – this is 159,000 deaths, of which 30% were under age 70 and considered premature and avoidable. The British Heart Foundation estimates over 4 million people in the UK are living with CVD and that there are 96,000 new cases of angina annually. This comes with a £32 billion cost to the NHS. CVD affects a greater proportion of people in lower socioeconomic groups, especially those living in areas of deprivation, and helps to explain their lower life expectancy (–8.2 years). The blame for this is laid at modifiable risks, smoking, excess alcohol, poor diet, lack of exercise, high blood pressure, high cholesterol, diabetes and psychological stress (NICE, 2018).

Paula was fortunate in having a responder who recognised her symptoms. Heart attack is often misdiagnosed in women, and it would seem that women might experience heart disease differently to men. There is also evidence that historical bias may have a role: heart disease was explained by the Canadian physician Sir William Osler (1849–1919) as something experienced by keen and ambitious men (Cushing, 1925). Research into heart disease was mainly conducted with male patients: the 1982 Multiple Risk Factor Intervention Trial, one of the first to establish a link between cholesterol and heart disease, involved 12,866 men and no women, and this is not the only example. Women tend to have atypical symptoms, such as pain in the jaw, shoulders or back and have nausea and vomiting due to stomach pain as opposed to crushing pain in the chest.

Myocardial infarction (MI) occurs when the blood supply to the coronary arteries ceases, usually due to **thrombosis** (clot) or atheroma embolism or both (Burke, 2015), causing tissue death (**infarction**) in the cardiac muscle (**myocardium**). Most MIs are caused by **coronary artery disease** (CAD) accelerated by insulin resistance, smoking and hypertension (Lilly, 2011). Blockage of a coronary artery is often caused by atheroma plaque rupture (see Figure 7.5), and the severity of the MI depends on the site of the blockage. It should be noted that an MI is not a cardiac arrest (ventricular fibrillation) but can cause this.

Diagnosis is confirmed by ECG, blood tests (elevated troponin levels) and angiography. The ECG will confirm an elevated ST segment (STEMI), in which case percutaneous coronary intervention (PCI) will be performed, which is a procedure that uses a catheter to insert a stent to open up a blood vessel. A non-ST elevation myocardial infarction (NSTEMI) is managed with heparin, or if severe, a PCI. Where blockages are revealed in multiple coronary arteries, a coronary artery bypass (CABG) may be performed rather than angioplasty, which is a procedure used to widen blocked or narrowed coronary arteries.

Cardiac activity is monitored using an ECG. This shows the electrical activity drawn in waves and recorded on specific graph paper. Three, five, or 10 electrodes are attached to the body, and each gives a reading. Usually the three- or five-lead readings are carried out continuously (such as during an operation or in an ambulance) whereas the 10-lead will be printed on paper.

An ECG is the best way to measure and diagnose abnormal rhythms of the heart, particularly abnormal rhythms caused by damage to the conductive tissue that carries electrical signals, or abnormal rhythms caused by electrolyte imbalances.

So what is happening inside Paula's body?

SYSTEMIC RESPONSE TO CARDIAC FAILURE

When cardiac output fails for whatever reason, the body responds systemically.

1. The sympathetic nervous system reacts to decreased blood pressure, thus the feedback system forces increased myocardial contraction while causing vasoconstriction of arterioles. This will keep the patient alive but will increase the afterload by vasoconstriction.
2. The renin-angiotensin-aldosterone (RAA) system attempts to maintain blood pressure and fluid volumes by decreasing tissue perfusion; this releases renin from the kidney which forms angiotensin I from angiotensinogen. Angiotensin II is formed by an enzyme reaction which cascades reactions, as shown in Figure 7.4. The RAA system supports life but adds to the fluid burden on the heart.

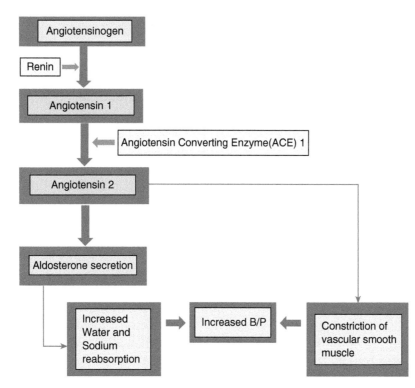

Figure 7.4   Renin-angiotensin-aldosterone system

Source: © Gillian Rowe

3. Energy production metabolic systems move to anaerobic production of ATP. This is less effective than aerobic systems and generates lactic acid; however, lactic acidosis acts to inhibit myocardial contractions, inducing failure.

4. Myocardial hypertrophy and dilation will increase oxygen demand by the myocardium, thus increasing stress.
5. Pulmonary stress occurs when the pulmonary system (from either side of the heart) is congested with blood that cannot be transported through the heart, called pulmonary oedema. Fluid fills the interstitial tissues and alveoli impairing gaseous exchange. This results in the patient experiencing dyspnoea and later orthopnoea, also cardiac asthma.
6. The patient may also have pitting oedema, hepatic splenomegaly, and distension of the neck veins. This is especially visible in right side heart failure where the right ventricle cannot fully pump stroke volume and thus increases pressure in the systemic venous system.

WHAT HAD LED TO PAULA DEVELOPING A HEART CONDITION?

Paula has a sedentary job but is active at weekends, she is of Afro-Caribbean descent, mildly obese and smokes cigarettes. How had her lifestyle contributed to health?

A good diet is health promoting, the problem is knowing what a good diet consists of. Advice changes like the wind and many diets are fads promoted by people with little nutritional knowledge. The NHS offers the 'eatwell plate', which indicates portion sizes of the various food groups. Cardiologists such as Dr Aseem Malhotra argue that sugar and processed food have a greater implication in heart disease than dietary fats. Malhotra is co-author of The Pioppi Diet, which recommends a daily intake of olive oil, which as an HDL (high density lipoprotein) has a role in reverse cholesterol transport (Berrougui et al., 2015), the process whereby cholesterol is transported back to the liver for excretion. However, the jury is still out, and the NHS suggests that a diet rich in vegetables and legumes is equally health protective.

Cholesterol is a required lipid used for cell membranes, the production of hormones such as oestrogen, progesterone and testosterone, and, essentially, for vitamin D metabolism. The debate about cholesterol levels has been raging since the 1950s when Ancel Keys determined that saturated fat consumption has a strong predictive relationship with cardiovascular disease. He extended his work to a seven-country survey (Greece, Italy, Spain, South Africa, Japan, USA and Finland) of men aged 49–59 and followed up at 5-year intervals. This reinforced his findings. Populations with saturated fatty acid intake of less than 10% of daily energy needs have low coronary heart disease or thrombotic stroke rates, despite widely varying total fat intake or usual levels of blood pressure or rates of tobacco use.

Clinical examination looks at total cholesterol levels, and **HDL** (high density lipoprotein) (also known as good) and **LDL** (low density lipoprotein) (also known as bad). HDL and LDL are not cholesterol, they are **lipoproteins**, molecules that transport cholesterol around the body.

Dyslipidaemias are abnormal amounts of fat (cholesterol and triglycerides); prolonged elevation of insulin can also cause dyslipidaemia suggesting dietary causes. This can lead to the build up of **atherosclerosis**, which are fatty plaques that narrow arteries.

LDL comes in small dense particles that are able to pass through artery walls. As they are more readily oxidised, it is currently thought these might drive heart disease as atherosclerosis begins within the wall of the artery (subendothelial) in association with LDL particles and this may be a trigger for the inflammatory process, as the major constituents of atherosclerosis are macrophages, monocytes and basophils. Figure 7.5 shows this process.

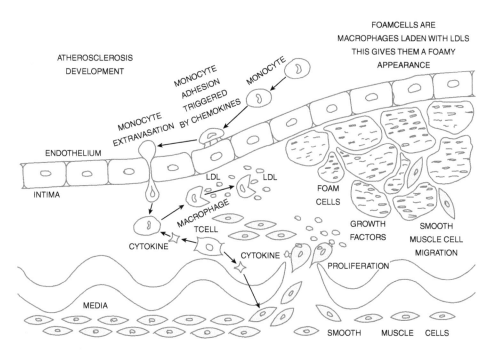

Figure 7.5   Atherosclerosis

Source: © Gillian Rowe

LDL also comes in larger particles which do not pass through the artery wall and here studies become conflicting, as some research indicates that saturated fat changes small dense LDL into large LDL (Dreon et al., 1998; Nichols et al., 1976; Siri-Tarino et al., 2010) and that some saturated fat could, in fact, be health protective. A Cochrane review performed a meta-analysis of extant data evidence and found that reducing saturated fat has no effect on death or death from heart disease. However, researchers found that replacing saturated fats with unsaturated fats reduced the risk of cardiac events by 14% (Hooper et al., 2011). This is especially true for those who have familial hypercholesterolaemia or the gene variant ApoE4, which is part of chromosome 19. This gene has a strong relationship with the development of Alzheimer's disease in those with high serum total cholesterol and high blood pressure.

However, what these studies collaboratively did show is that consuming highly processed carbohydrates, sugars and processed trans fats was a strong indicator of risk of CVD and that a lower carbohydrate diet is health protective.

Fruit in the diet is another contentious issue; back in your grandparent's day, fruit was an occasional treat that provided vitamin C and in the case of bananas, potassium. After the Second World War and based on no empirical evidence, the American National Cancer Institute and the Fruit and Vegetable Growers Association of America decided that eating 'five a day' would be health protective from cancer. This article of faith was comprehensively debunked after 30 years of research, the latest from the UK EPIC4 study (Key, 2011).

Modern fruit has been specially bred to be sweeter than ancestral fruit (Nookaraju et al., 2010) and contains not just fructose (which does not invoke an insulin reaction) but glucose, which provokes a pancreatic response and thus is stored as glycogen. Modern fruit is fattening. Leafy green vegetables such as spinach, kale and broccoli are vitamin and mineral rich and these should be promoted along with limited amounts of tree nuts such as walnuts, almonds, brazil nuts and pecans.

Paula lives a sedentary life, with bursts of activity at weekends, people who have had heart problems are reluctant to engage in exercise for fear of provoking a further cardiac event, especially those who have not been particularly active prior to their illness. The cardiac aware nurse will be able to explain the concept of **ischaemic preconditioning**. When patients begin to exercise, they feel breathless or an angina type pain, so they stop. However, if they walk a little further or engage in light stretching and then carry on, they are being heart protective. 'Warm-up angina' is a well-known phenomenon when building up to moderate exercise. Exercise makes the heart more resilient by developing muscle and building strength, thus is life prolonging and reduces mortality rates. However, *and this is particularly important*, all cardiac rehabilitation done in the first 12 weeks after a cardiac event should be supervised and assessed.

Cardiac rehabilitation requires a range of interventions including psychological support (Heran et al., 2011), especially for those suffering from anxiety and depression. People with type A behavioural patterns seem particularly susceptible to MIs as they live 'stressful, fast paced lives with multiple responsibilities leading to an inability to cope' (Mierzynska et al., 2010). Mierzynska's research shows that depression has more of an impact on rehabilitation than previously considered, as it impacts on social anchoring (limited socialisation, development of agoraphobia). She determined that having a close supportive family is health protective, as they can offer encouragement to make life changes (smoking cessation, diet and exercise) in preparation for returning to work. Developing optimism after a cardiac event is also health protective and cognitive behavioural therapy (CBT) has been shown to support recovery (Ronaldson et al., 2015).

Paula's smoking habit is contributing to her poor health. The number of people smoking in the UK began to fall significantly after the smoking in public places ban (Health Act 2006) was introduced in 2007 (22% of population, now 18%). This kickstarted a cultural shift to 'denormalise' smoking. There was concern that people would start drinking and smoking at home and put children at greater risk of second-hand smoke, but evidence does not bear this out (Cheeseman et al., 2017). It is also illegal to smoke in a vehicle carrying anyone under the age of 18. This law is mostly self-enforced, with the Chartered Institute of Environmental Health reporting high levels of compliance, and it is widely expected that smoking will be banned in all cars in the future (ASH, 2019).

There has been a slight increase in the number of hospital admissions related to smoking. This may be related to the ageing demographic, who have the highest historic levels of smoking over their lifespan, and therefore will have a higher level of smoking-related ailments. In 2017, 22% of all admissions for respiratory diseases, 15% of all admissions for circulatory diseases and 9% of all admissions for cancers were estimated to be attributable to smoking. People in the industrial northwest and northeast have the highest smoking attributable admission rates (NHS Digital, 2019).

Besides being a risk factor for CVD, smoking has a multiplicative interaction with diabetes and high blood pressure (hypertension). Smoking enhances lipid mobilisation due to nicotine-induced lipolysis leading to increased hepatic LDL secretion (Hellerstein et al., 1994), thus leading to high cholesterol levels. Smoking also has a demonstrable and significant role in insulin resistance – this also increasing the risk of CVD. Facchini et al. (1992) evidenced that chronic cigarette smokers are insulin resistant, hyperinsulinaemic and dyslipidaemic.

Smoking in older people promotes **macular degeneration** in the eyes, for which there is no available treatment; it also has an impact on **bone density**. Women's bones are protected by oestrogen until menopause; as women age, the body makes less dense bone and they become fragile. At 52, Paula is likely to be menopausal. The exact mechanism of smoking impact to bone density is poorly understood but a meta-analysis conducted by Law and Hackshaw (1997) showed that postmenopausal women who smoked had a 19% increased risk of fracture over non-smoking postmenopausal women.

Some of the chemicals in tobacco smoke promote coagulation with increased risk of deep venous thrombosis (DVT) and MI; they also produce irritants (especially nitric oxide) which promote an inflammatory response and thus have a role in atherosclerosis plaque formation. It is noted that smokers have a higher preponderance of **peripheral arterial disease** in the lower extremities (Solberg and Strong, 1983). Smoke chemicals also inhibit bronchial cilia, disrupting the mucus escalator, which is why smokers cough to remove mucus and debris, and this has a role in repeated chest infections. Recent research is focusing on the impact of tobacco smoke on the blood brain barrier (BBB) and the implications of small vessel ischaemic disease and resultant cerebral infarction.

If Paula can be persuaded to stop smoking, she will reduce her death rate probability of dying from CVD and cerebrovascular disease significantly after 6 months' cessation, and after 5 years' abstinence, will have a similar rate to non-smokers.

As Paula is of Afro-Caribbean descent, she might carry the sickle cell anaemia (SCA) gene. Therefore, cultural assessment, knowledge and skills are needed for effective nursing and to improve patient and family health outcomes.

The sickle cell trait comes from one parent being heterozygous for the abnormal haemoglobin gene HbS; the carrier would not have any symptoms of the disease but might have some sickle erythrocytes. However, if two parents carry the gene there is a 50% chance any offspring will carry the trait, and a 25% chance they will have SCA, as this is an autosomal recessive gene disease. The trait offers protection from *Plasmodium falciparum* malaria.

Current thinking considers sickle cell to be an evolutionary development in high malarial areas. Malaria is a leading cause of disability and death in Africa, and WHO states there are 219 million people globally suffering from malaria and in 2018 435,000 people died from the disease (WHO, 2022). People of African heritage are more likely to carry the trait – incidentally thalassaemia and other blood cell dyscrasias are also thought to provide anti-malarial protection.

Sickle cells are red blood cells shaped like a sickle with haemoglobin that forms long, stiff fibres that distort red blood. The sickle cell allele codes for a modified haemoglobin protein. This haemoglobin carries reduced amounts of oxygen, and in low oxygen conditions the cells become sticky. The condition becomes relevant when someone flies at over 10,000 feet in an unpressurised aircraft or on long haul flights and is significant when a patient with sickle cell undergoes procedures under anaesthetic (dental or surgical).

The life cycle of *Plasmodium* transmission via the *Anopheles* mosquito is as follows. The *Anopheles* mosquito feeds by sucking blood from a human host, while injecting either *Plasmodium malariae, P. falciparum, P. vivax* or *P. ovale* sporozoites from its salivary glands into the bloodstream. The sporozoites are passed through the liver via the hepatic portal system, where they damage liver cells by forming schizonts and the parasites mutate into merozoites. Some sporozoites seem to hibernate (hypnozoites) for many years before activating (especially *P. viva* and *P. ovale*). The schizont bursts releasing merozoites to infect erythrocytes, where they again mutate becoming trophozoites which are the *Plasmodium* gametes, which is how a mosquito in turn becomes infected when it sucks blood from the human host.

The clinical signs of the disease become apparent when the infected red blood cell lyses and releases the merozoites, hemozoin pigment and other toxic factors. This stimulates macrophage and cytokine reactions which provoke fever and rigour. The patient suffers from fever, chills, sweats, nausea, body ache and malaise, known collectively as **malarial crisis**. Medical examination may reveal enlarged liver and spleen, jaundice and increased respiration rate. Microscopy would reveal parasitic infestation, thrombocytopenia, and elevation of bilirubin and aminotransferases.

Pregnancy decreases any malarial protection the mother may have gained, and babies of malarial mothers are either delivered prematurely or with low birth weight, with consequently decreased chances of survival during the early months of life. Children of parents with SCA are at greater risk of stroke, especially between the ages of 2 and 16, and so children of African descent parents are tested at birth by heel prick.

The main symptoms of sickle cell disorder are anaemia and episodes of severe pain. The pain occurs when erythrocytes (red blood cells) change shape (conformation) when squeezing through small capillaries. The sickle shape prevents red cell deformation and thus blood flow, causing blockages in the capillaries. Long-term and chronic conditions include blindness, elevated stroke risk, and damage to the liver, spleen, kidneys, heart and lungs.

📖 Case Study 7.4

Robert is a 17-year-old male, he developed **Crohn's disease** in early childhood and aged 10 had surgical interventions, bowel resection, stoma and anastomosis. Robert has been given corticosteroids, immunomodulators and primary nutrition therapy with limited success. He has had quite severe bouts of abdominal pain leading to hospital admission for management. Robert has developed fistula and has scored over 300 on the Crohn's Disease Activity Index and would have a Harvey–Bradshaw score of over 9. Robert has been prescribed a biologic drug (infliximab), which he has tolerated well and has a maintenance dose every 8 weeks. Patients taking infliximab need an annual review to ensure the drug is effective, but at review Robert has blood tests which show some worrying results. Robert is referred to a gastroenterologist and visits the endoscopy department for bowel scope screening colonoscopy and chromoscopy. Polyps are located and a biopsy performed for histological proof for diagnosis.

Crohn's disease (CD) is somewhat similar to ulcerative colitis (UC) in that they are both inflammatory bowel diseases and share symptomatology including abdominal pain, bloating, rectal bleeding, fever, diarrhoea and weight loss. Crohn's can affect any part of the gastrointestinal tract (GIT). Complications of this disease can be local or systemic – Box 7.2 gives details.

Box 7.2

Local: Abscess, bile salt diarrhoea (especially in the ilium), fissure, fistula, strictures, small intestinal bacterial overgrowth (SIBO)

Systemic: Malabsorption and malnutrition, axial and peripheral arthritis, more rarely ankylosing spondylitis, erythema nodosum, pyoderma gangrenosum, bone loss due to steroidal therapy, episcleritis of the eyes, kidney stones, uric acid stones, hydronephrosis, gallstones, hepatitis, pancreatitis, growth delays in young children

---

Crohn's disease has always been thought of as an autoimmune reaction but recent research questions this, and suggests it results from a complex interplay between genetics, the environment and the immune system. The genetic component is that 20% of CD sufferers have a familial relationship. Globally rare, it is a disease more usually experienced in industrial nations, and more prevalent in white populations, especially Ashkenazi Jews. The UK has one of the highest rates of incidence in the world, which has increased since industrialisation (Logan, 1998). Peak incidence is in teenage years and early adulthood.

The role of the intestine is to host the enzymes that break down food into cellular products and absorb the products for protein catabolism and anabolism and energy use. Absorption is via villi and micro villi. The villus, a finger-like projection, is comprised of four differentiated cells, made from stem cells seated in the Crypt of Lieberkühn. These are absorptive cells (enterocytes) and secretory cells (goblet cells, tuft cells and Paneth cells) (see Figure 7.6). These cells migrate to the tip of the villi and then are shed into the lumen in a process that takes approximately a week.

As the intestines are exposed to environmental insults, the epithelial layer is capable of rapid regeneration. However, defective regeneration in response to inflammation and disease will disrupt normal intestinal homeostasis and can lead to tumours developing (tumorigenesis). The epithelium is protected by a pre-epithelial layer comprised of mucus glycoproteins, trefoil peptides, IgA and antimicrobial peptides (AMPs). Just below the epithelial layer, dendritic cells, which are part of the innate immune system, are continuously sampling luminal antigens and directing other immune cells such as neutrophils towards mounting a response. The dendritic cells do this via activation of signalling pathways such as the Toll-like receptors and NOD2 receptors (nucleotide-binding domain 2). These proteins are produced by intestinal epithelial cells and detect peptidoglycan from the gut microflora, triggering a protective inflammatory response which maintains intestinal homeostasis. However, if a NOD2 mutation occurs, the protective inflammatory process is lost and leads to intestinal barrier dysfunction as these signalling pathways fail to modulate the immune response in Crohn's disease, and the dendritic cells are then unable to induce tolerance to normal gut commensal micro-organisms.

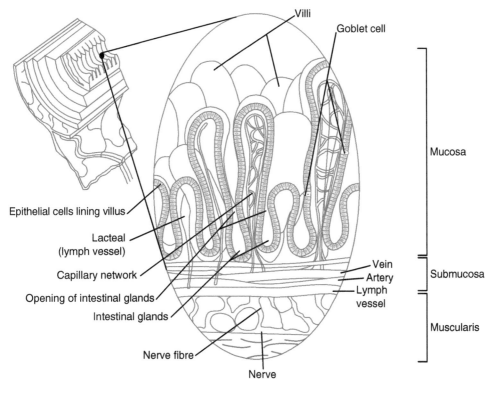

Figure 7.6   Villus

Source: Boore et al. (2017). Illustrated by Shaun Mercier, © SAGE Publications.

The mucus layer has a strong relationship with the innate immune system. Goblet cells secrete mucus which should be devoid of pathogens; however, patients with CD have a compromised mucus layer rendering it available to bacterial colonisation. Paneth cells have an antimicrobial role and defects increase a susceptibility to inflammation. Once inflammation has been initiated at the mucosal surface, it is maintained by an excess of inflammatory cytokines such as TNF-alpha (TNF-α), IFN-gamma (IFN-γ) and IL-17.

When the epithelial layer is exposed to pathogens or disease processes, the turnover rate shifts into a higher gear, and if this process is not tightly controlled or the control system fails, unrestrained regeneration may foster tumour growth. **Colonic cancer** has a strong relationship with persistent inflammation and is a response to ongoing regenerative repair leading to polyp formation. Genetic studies have associated CD with several transcription factors involved in epithelial regeneration, such as HNF4A and NKX2-3 (Darsigny et al., 2009).

Autophagy is the process by which cells degrade and recycle their components, and it has a role in infection control and inflammation reduction. The gene ATG16L1 is essential for all forms of autophagy, and the coding mutation T300A is associated with increased risk of Crohn's disease. Experiments with mice show that an absence of ATG16L1 always leads to CD or UC (Cooney et al., 2010).

Genome-wide association studies (GWAS) have evidenced similarity in CD and UC suggesting comparable contributory genetic predispositions and pathophysiological pathways (Khor et al., 2011). Although currently poorly understood, genetic relationships are undergoing significant research, especially to understand signalling pathways and genetic mutations on B- and T-cells. The CARD15 gene was one of the first genes to be associated with the development of Crohn's disease, and amongst other things, encodes NOD2.

As to why CD develops during the teenage years, current thinking associates this with **Peyer's patches**, which are aggregated lymphoid nodules in the mucosal layer and classed as 'gut-associated lymphoid tissue' (GALT). These are located only in the small bowel and particularly in the distal ileum. They are populated with immune cells (Bs and Ts) whose role is monitoring intestinal bacteria populations and preventing the growth of pathogenic bacteria in the intestines. The brush border is partially interrupted where it meets Peyer's patches. The surface epithelium of Peyer's patches is overlaid with specialised cells called microfold cells (M-cells) that detect pathogenic antigens. When antigens are present, the M-cell uses endocytosis to transport the antigen to a mucosal pocket for phagocytosis by dendritic cells, some of which become antigen-presenting cells. Adolescent iliums have the highest number of Peyer's patches, which decrease after age 30, and are thus implicated in Crohn's.

BIOLOGIC DRUGS

The first biologic drugs were vaccines, blood transfusions and insulin since biologic drugs are derived from living organisms. Biologic drugs are complex protein-based medications that control the actions of other proteins and cellular processes; they might also be cells that secrete hormones or neurotransmitters to suppress or activate components of the immune system. Their role is to trick directed cells to manufacture desired proteins using biotechnology. Each gene codes for one protein; after the gene has undergone genetic modification, it needs to be inserted into a host cell, then reproduced in order to create a useable drug. This is an incredibly complex challenge using molecular biology, recombinant biotechnology and cell culture techniques. The host cells currently in use are yeasts, *E. coli* and a Chinese hamster cell called CHO (O for ovary). This is a biological, not chemical, process and the cells are grown in large vats called bioreactors.

Treatments using biologic drugs include those developed for Crohn's disease, ulcerative colitis, rheumatoid arthritis and various other autoimmune diseases. Some biologic drugs have revolutionised cancer treatment, delayed or reversed the course of immune related conditions, and changed the lives of people with rare diseases. As biologic drugs are inactivated by the digestive system, they are given by injection or infusion.

As with all other medications, they have unwanted off-target interactions leading to side effects, especially those that suppress the immune system; opportunist micro-organisms can become invasive and harmless commensals can become incursive.

Making biologic drugs is an incredibly expensive process: few are recommended by NICE purely on the basis of cost and each has to be clinically justified. Once a drug comes off patent, generic biosimilar drugs can be produced at reduced cost offering wider access. An estimate of costs for Robert is given in Box 7.3. The drug cost crisis came to a head with the cost of antiretroviral drugs for AIDS treatment, which in America were prohibitive even with health insurance. Activists all over the world campaigned for cheaper drugs, which led to the Doha Declaration in 2001, stating that countries could override a protected 20-year patent in the interests of public health.

Box 7.3

Infliximab works by blocking a cytokine activity called tumour necrosis factor alpha (TNF-α); this does not cure Crohn's disease but makes the symptoms more manageable.

Robert has been taking infliximab every 8 weeks for a year.

100 mg vial of infliximab is £419.62 (2021) plus VAT at 20% (£83.80) (hospitals pay VAT on drugs) equalling £503.42.

However, the dose is adjusted for weight, 5 mg/kg. At 8 stone (50.8 kg) he would receive 250 mg infused over two hours costing £1258. 55.

The medical administration cost is approximately £258.00 per infusion; therefore, the cost of each dose is £1516.55 approximately. Times this by 6 to total £9099.30 per year (figures from NICE, 2019b). Robert's clinicians could offer Robert biosimilar drugs (Inflectra and Remsima) as these have been proven effective and cost £377.66 per 100 mg, generating a saving of £41.96 per 100 mg (mims. co.uk, 2021).

NUTRITIONAL STATUS

Protecting nutritional status is health affirming for CD sufferers as they frequently experience **malabsorption**, which can have serious consequences. Therefore, measurement of ferritin, vitamin B12 and folate can help determine nutritional status as B12 is absorbed in the terminal ileum, which is the area most commonly affected in Crohn's disease. Iron deficiency is due to blood loss.

Blood tests might include C-reactive protein (CRP) and erythrocyte sedimentation rate (ESR) as they might be raised. Liver and renal function results may be poor due to the chronic nature of the ailment. Patients taking glucocorticosteroids should be offered periodic dual energy X-ray absorptiometry (DEXA) scans for bone density.

CD sufferers might need nutritional support in addition to folate, iron and vitamin B12. Calcium and vitamin D should be recommended when a patient is taking glucocorticosteroids. Certain foods can trigger an episode, so a food diary should be kept and, once identified, these foods should be excluded from the diet. This is personal to the patient as no two patients will have the same triggers. There is no recommended diet, it is purely trial and error.

PSYCHOLOGICAL SUPPORT

Patients with Crohn's disease are often young, and this makes psychological adjustment difficult for some patients, especially if they are managing a stoma. They are known to have an increased risk of developing mental health disorders such as depression and anxiety (Silva et al., 2017) and so will often benefit from counselling, cognitive behavioural therapy and the informal support network of close family and friends. School SENCOs should be given advice and information to support young people in educational settings.

COLONIC CANCER

The result of Robert's colonoscopy and chromoscopy evidence abnormal adenomatous tissue in the terminal ilium. The symptoms of small bowel cancer are the same as Crohn's disease, abdominal pain, occult blood loss, diarrhoea and abdominal mass so symptoms might be misconstrued. Robert had previous surgery to remove a 25 cm segment of bowel with multiple fibrous strictures with no evidence of malignancy, the bowel was resected, rested by use of a stoma, then anastomosed (re-joined). The average age for bowel cancer is approximately 64 years old, and the average age for cancer with Crohn's disease is approximately 48 (Balaji et al., 2017) so Robert is a non-traditional candidate. The risk of malignant transformation from CD/UC to cancer is particularly high, with one study finding that

CD/UC patients are up to 30 times more likely to develop colonic cancer and three times more likely to die from colonic cancer than the general population (Katsanos et al., 2007). Chromosome 18 may offer some clues as to why this should be. An area of this chromosome called 18q21 contains DCC, a tumour suppressor gene. Reduction in DCC expression levels is associated with tumour progression and metastasis. Also, the tumour suppressor genes SMAD2 and SMAD4 are within this region. SMAD2 has been hypothesised to play a role in the development of colonic cancer in inflammatory bowel disease (IBD) patients (Terdiman et al., 2006). The full genetic analysis has yet to be elucidated and although there currently is no known genetic relationship between CD and Lynch syndrome (an autosomal dominant genetic condition that is associated with a high risk of colonic cancer) occasionally the two coexist. Future investigation into inflammatory states will probably hold the key.

THE SEARCH FOR AN EFFECTIVE COVID-19 VACCINATION

Once SARs-CoV-2 (Covid-19) became a pandemic, the search was on internationally to find a preventative vaccine. The RNA virus needs a host cell to reproduce, which it does by hijacking the cell's reproductive system (see Chapter 6). As of 2022, the duration of immunity both from natural immunity (surviving the disease) and vaccination is uncertain. Many factors impact on immune system response (age, weight, pre-existing conditions) to exposure to the disease, although there is some evidence that those who survive serious illness have a longer lasting protection.

Covid-19 is a respiratory infection but goes beyond severe acute respiratory distress syndrome (ARDS). It can cause multiple blood clots anywhere in the cardiovascular system as a result of triggering an exacerbated inflammatory response leading to a cytokine storm. Many people who have had the disease experience 'long Covid', a type of post-viral syndrome. Symptoms include breathing difficulties/breathlessness, fatigue/malaise, chest/throat pain, headache, abdominal symptoms, myalgia, other pain, cognitive symptoms and anxiety/depression. Long Covid is described as symptoms that last between 3 and 6 months. Only time will tell if it lasts longer and has the same profile as other post-viral syndromes such as myalgic encephalomyelitis/chronic fatigue syndrome (ME/CFS).

The SARS-CoV-2 genome encodes four structural proteins: the spike, envelope, membrane and nucleocapsid. The spike protein is further divided into two subunits, S1 and S2: these facilitate host cell attachment and infiltration. By binding at the receptor, S1 attaches to angiotensin converting enzyme 2 (ACE2) (see Chapter 6 for more detail) on the host cell; this then begins a conformational change in S2 that results in virus–host cell membrane fusion and viral entry by endocytosis.

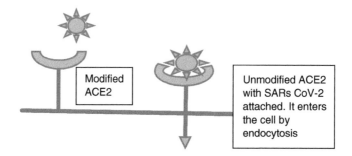

Figure 7.7   Modified ACE2 and SARS-CoV-2

The ACE2 receptor is most populous in epithelial cells which make up the tissues of the cardio, respiratory and intestinal systems. Therefore, research scientists have looked for ways to prevent or reduce the seriousness of infection. In the UK, the Oxford-AstraZeneca vaccine uses an unrelated harmless virus viral vector that delivers SARS-CoV-2 genetic material to prompt an immune system response. Unfortunately, it is not yet clear how long the immune system retains the information to produce memory B-cells and boosters are needed. The Moderna and Pfizer-BioNTech vaccines contain a segment of genetic material of the SARS-CoV-2 virus again to trigger an immune response and B-cell memory. Other types of vaccines are in testing (such as an attenuated vaccine) but are not as yet proven and licensed.

Researchers have taken monoclonal antibodies (mAb) cells from people who have recovered from Covid-19 and reproduced them using hamster or mouse ovary cells. The antibodies that these cells manufacture are extracted and purified. Once infused, therapeutic neutralising monoclonal antibodies (nMAB) can bind to the spike protein and thus reduce the viral load. Higuchi et al. (2021) have engineered modified ACE2 receptors (see Figure 7.7), which has also proved promising as the research has evidenced resistance to escape mutations of virus.

📖   Case Study 7.5

Samantha Taylor is a 48-year-old woman with type 2 diabetes (previously known as non-insulin dependent diabetes or NIDD). She was diagnosed aged 30. She has a direct family member who is also diabetic and there may be a genetic component to her diagnosis. She has successfully reduced her weight but is still mildly obese and has ophthalmic complications associated with the disease.

Glucose is the end product of the metabolic breakdown of carbohydrates. Glucoregulation is a negative feedback system that maintains homeostasis, which keeps a constant internal environment for cellular activity in the body. The glucoregulatory hormones are insulin, glucagon, amylin, GLP-1, glucose-dependent insulinotropic peptide (GIP), epinephrine, cortisol and growth hormone. Of these, insulin and amylin are derived from the β-cells (beta), glucagon from the α-cells (alpha) of the pancreas, and GLP-1 and GIP from the L-cells in the intestine. Within the pancreas are the Islets of Langerhans (Figure 7.8): these were discovered by the German pathological anatomist Paul Langerhans in 1869 and are islands of endocrine cells scattered throughout the parenchyma of the pancreas. Human islets consist of about 30% glucagon-producing α-cells, about 60% insulin producing β-cells, with the remaining 10% being pancreatic polypeptide-producing, and ε-cells (ghrelin-producing cells).

Elevated blood glucose concentration will stimulate the release of insulin, which then acts on cells throughout the body to stimulate uptake and storage of glucose. Insulin facilitates entry of glucose into muscle, adipose and other cells by way of facilitated diffusion through GLUT-4 hexose transporters. The brain uses GLUT-1 transport to move glucose across the blood brain barrier; the liver however does not use GLUTs: this is because insulin activates enzymes which promote the liver to store glucose in the form of glycogen in the hepatocytes. The net effect of storage is to reduce blood glucose concentration, so as concentration falls, insulin production ceases. As neurons need a constant supply of glucose, most of the stored glycogen is provided from this reserve.

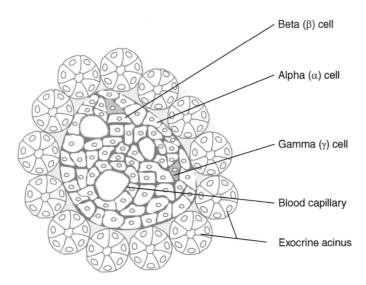

Figure 7.8   Islets of Langerhans

Source: Boore et al. (2017). Illustrated by Shaun Mercier, © SAGE Publications

When insulin levels fall, cells cannot access glucose and fall back on fatty acids for energy (ketosis). Falling insulin levels stimulate production of glucagon, which in turn breaks down glycogen to glucose and returns blood glucose to normal levels. However, when the hepatocytes in the liver are saturated with glucose, they pass through metabolic pathways and are converted to fatty acids. Glucose is a six-carbon sugar molecule. It is first converted into two three-carbon pyruvate molecules through the process of glycolysis and then into acetyl CoA in the cells' mitochondria; this is then exported from the liver as lipoproteins, which pass through the circulatory system and enter cells as free fatty acids and are stored in adipocytes which make up adipose tissue. Insulin also progresses the accumulation of fat in the adipocytes. As insulin promotes glucose uptake within the cell, it has a role in the synthesis of glycerol, which, along with the fatty acids, creates triglycerides – these are discussed in Box 7.4 showing the lipid profile values.

Box 7.4

Excess sugar is turned into fat and stored as triglycerides; hypertriglyceridemia is an excess of fat which contributes to arteriosclerosis leading to diseases of the cardiovascular system (see previous pages).

Lipid profile values

Normal – Less than 150 milligrams per decilitre (mg/dL), or less than 1.7 millimoles per litre (mmol/L)

Borderline high – 150–199 mg/dL (1.8–2.2 mmol/L)

High – 200–499 mg/dL (2.3–5.6 mmol/L)

Very high – 500 mg/dL or above (5.7 mmol/L or above)

Samantha was diagnosed with diabetes in her early 30s, which fits with an emerging pattern of younger people developing what used to be known as maturity onset diabetes. A 2012 study undertaken by Imperatore et al. for the American Diabetic Society projected a likely quadrupling of young people (aged 10–18) diagnosed with type 2 diabetes. Diabetes develops as a result of insulin resistance or reduced insulin production (beta dysfunction). However, while the mechanisms controlling the interplay of these two impairments are unclear, it seems the target cells fail to respond, and disease symptoms are revealed. These include tiredness, excessive thirst (polydipsia) and concomitant need to urinate (polyuria), reduced wound healing, invasive commensals such as *Candida albicans* (thrush in women/ balanitis in men), blurred vision, and unplanned weight loss. A more contentious symptom is polyphagia, the inability to control eating.

Samantha is overweight, which is a feature of the majority of T2 sufferers. Abdominal adipose clearly has a crucial role within the adipose endocrine organ hypothesis, but also ectopic fat storage syndrome, triglyceride fats stored in muscle and the liver, is under investigation as a possible explanation. Another is Taylor's (2013) 'twin cycle' hypothesis, which suggests that insulin resistance increases liver lipogenesis, that increased liver fat will cause a relative resistance to insulin suppression of hepatic glucose production and that, over time, this cycle becomes established. However, Taylor asserts that a low calorie diet can reverse this process and re-establish euglycemia. Other research by Busko (2019) determined that a low carbohydrate diet with intermittent fasting is effective for rapid weight loss and participants measured reduced low density lipoprotein cholesterol.

There is no doubt we live in an **obesogenic environment**, with access to energy dense, low nutritional value foods. The pace of life and a lack of work–life balance mean that people have less energy to prepare and cook meals from scratch. The knowledgeable nursing associate should be aware that any recommended diet should be within the patient's financial reach and cultural milieu. Muslim patients required to fast for Ramadan should monitor their blood sugar closely and seek religious and medical advice if complications arise.

Whilst you cannot outrun a poor diet, moderate exercise can delay the progression of diabetes by using up excess calories. A randomised control trial conducted by Church et al. (2010) indicated that a combination of aerobic and resistance training was effective in the lowering of HbA1c levels, blood pressure and waist measurement, and reduced circulating triglycerides.

Samantha has a close relative with diabetes. Genome-Wide Association Studies (GWAS) have identified over 40 genetic variants that are associated with β-cell function and insulin resistance. For instance, research by Chiefari et al. (2011) indicated the A1 (HMGA1) protein is a key regulator of the insulin receptor gene (INSR) and that functional variants of the HMGA1 gene are associated with an increased risk of diabetes.

Diabetes affects many of the body systems and Box 7.5 gives some of the more common effects. Haffner et al. (1999) developed the 'ticking clock' hypothesis of complications, asserting that the clock starts ticking for microvascular risk at the onset of hyperglycaemia.

Box 7.5

1. The CV system is affected due to elevated levels of small, dense low density lipoprotein (LDL) cholesterol particles.

2. Patients with diabetes are more likely to suffer cognitive declines, exhibiting the type of symptoms seen in early Alzheimer's disease and they are also more likely to report depression.

(Continued)

3. Diabetic retinopathy is caused by damage to the blood vessels of the retina at the back of the eye and can lead to blindness.

4. Diabetes is a major contributor to end-stage renal disease which requires dialysis or transplant.

5. Diabetic neuropathy and vasculopathy is the leading cause of non-traumatic lower limb amputations.

6. Diabetics have a higher risk of postoperative pneumonia.

Samantha has ophthalmic complications. Diabetes can affect the lens, vitreous and retina, causing visual distortions, and glycaemic control is essential to reversing retinopathy, although advanced or long-term retinopathy may not show signs of improvement, especially for those with hypertension (high blood pressure). Laser photocoagulation is a possible early intervention remedy but cannot restore lost sight.

Metformin is the medication of choice; it is an established drug for reducing plasma glucose as it improves insulin sensitivity and reduces hepatic glucose production. Metformin can be prescribed for pre-diabetes as a preventative measure. As with all drugs, there are off-target side effects, including muscle weakness and pain, diarrhoea or constipation, bloating and flatulence, low levels of vitamin B12, hypoglycaemia, nausea, and a liability to chest infections. While not listed as a side effect, many patients complain that metformin appears to promote weight gain. This can lead to mistrust between both the patient and nurse, therefore when discussing weight loss, tact should be used.

Metformin is contraindicated in the elderly due to increased renal dysfunction and should not be prescribed to the over-80s unless tests evidence normal renal function. If metformin does not alleviate the symptoms, a second complementary drug is usually offered, such as glitazones or sulphonylureas, which stimulate insulin release. Alpha-glucosidase inhibitors, which delay glucose absorption, are another option, and there are many other drugs available for the research orientated nurse to investigate.

Insulin remains an option when clinically indicated. This is a biologic drug with a short storage liability. Insulin can be rapid acting or retarded. Rapid-acting insulin analogues take between 5 and 15 minutes to take effect and, dose and brand dependent, last between 2 and 5 hours. Regular human insulin is retarded, taking between 30 minutes and an hour to take effect but lasts (dose dependent) up to 8 hours. NPH human insulin is an intermediate insulin, taking over an hour to be effective, and lasting 4–6 hours. There are some very long-acting insulins, which can be used overnight or by people undertaking a fast, and which, depending on dose and brand, can last 24 hours.

Insulin is delivered via a pen or pump depending on need. The pens include an insulin cartridge, a dial to measure dosage and a disposable needle, and can be disposable or reusable; however, a new disposable needle must be used every time insulin is injected. The drawbacks of this delivery system are that not all insulins can be used, and insulin cannot be mixed, necessitating two or more pens. Patients need to be taught the correct storage and administration of the drug. Patients with cognitive deficits who are unable to use the pens for self-administration would need a different delivery system.

Type 1 diabetics are treated with insulin, and it is now becoming more common for long-term or medication-resistant type 2 diabetics to receive insulin support. Figure 7.9 shows two typical insulin pens.

As with all type diabetics, Samantha should conduct blood sugar testing to ensure good management, while weight loss is first line management. Good glucose control requires a haemoglobin A1c (HbA1c) count of less than 6.4%. There are many makes of blood monitoring machines, most require a finger prick and a drop of blood applied to a small plastic strip, which is then read by the machine. Pre-meal readings (fasting) should be within the 4–7 mmol/L range, post-meal (post-prandial) readings taken 90 minutes after eating should be under 8.5 mmol/L (NICE guidelines, 2019a). New types of blood sugar reading machines are less invasive, and from September 2022, all type 1 diabetics and type 2 diabetics with a learning disability will be offered a Dexcom flash monitor (NHS England, 2022) which is a wearable device which sends readings to a reader or smartphone (Figure 7.10). The flash device measures the amount of sugar in the interstitial fluid so finger prick measurements will still be needed for accuracy. There are also continuous glucose monitoring (CGM) devices which the NHS offers for certain conditions such as hypoglycaemic events without warning.

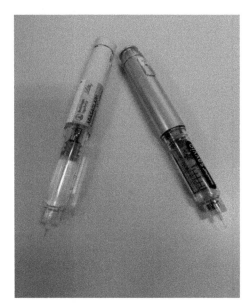

Figure 7.9   Insulin pens

Source: © Gillian Rowe

Good management should ensure hypoglycaemia does not occur, and nurses and patients should remember the admonishment 'under 4, on the floor'. Patients are advised to carry a prepared drink or sweet as a preventative. The NHS recommends Lucozade, but reformulation of the product has changed the recommended intake: 100 ml used to deliver 20 g of sugar but with the advent of the sugar tax, this has been reduced to 8.9 g/100 ml, and so 170–225 ml (15–20 g sugar) is the current recommended dose for the new formulation (Harrold, 2017).

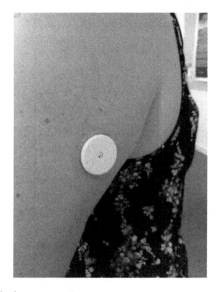

Figure 7.10   Diabetes flash glucose monitor

Diabetic neuropathy is insidious and has consequences. There are four main types of neuropathies, which are detailed in Box 7.6. Peripheral neuropathy can lead to amputation of the lower limb, and it is not uncommon for progressive amputations to occur.

Box 7.6

- **Peripheral neuropathy** is the most common type of diabetic neuropathy: it affects the toes, feet and legs first then progresses to hands and arms. Symptoms include various types of pain sensations (burning, tingling, cramp), muscle weakness, loss of reflex, loss of balance and coordination.
- **Autonomic neuropathy**: as the autonomic nervous system controls the heart, bladder, stomach, intestines, sex organs and eyes, any of these can be affected leading to loss of function.
- **Radiculoplexus neuropathy** (also known as femoral neuropathy) affects nerves in the thighs, hips, buttocks and legs leading to pain on locomotion.

- **Mononeuropathy** (also known as focal neuropathy) affects a specific nerve, the pain is intense but fortuitously, spontaneously goes into remission. It can paralyse one side of the face leading to Bell's palsy or cause loss of vision in one eye.

Good foot care is required. Nerve damage leads to loss of sensation and inadvertent damage which goes unnoticed, therefore daily foot inspection is essential, and water temperature should be checked before bathing. Foot ulcers and Charcot foot can result in amputation if ulceration is full thickness of the dermis (Wagner/Seattle system). Although cleaning the wound by debridement and hydrogel dressing has been found to be effective (Hunt, 2009), therapeutic footwear is considered a helpful preventative intervention. It has to be said that many NHS Trusts, under resource pressure, are failing to comply with NICE guidelines on foot care provision (Jeffcoate, 2019) and that nurse and nursing associate education clearly has a role here in amputation prevention.

CHAPTER SUMMARY

This chapter has introduced you to the history of pathophysiology and genetics. You will have read through case studies to enhance your understanding of genomics and pathophysiology, and this will allow you to engage in further and wider reading to deepen your knowledge of disease processes and pathophysiology. This chapter has been updated to introduce some of the foundational research searching for successful treatments for Covid-19. The future of medication is in personalised medicine and genetic testing; however, there remain ethical questions to be answered to ensure access for all in a cost-conscious world.

📖 FURTHER READING

VIDEOS

- What is Pathophysiology: www.youtube.com/watch?v=SY_829wmRo8
- Pathophysiology Ch 1 Introduction to Pathophysiology: www.youtube.com/watch?v=-2BUEjuhD-Y
- Introducing Genomics in Healthcare: www.youtube.com/watch?v=KiQgrK3tge8
- Nursing in the Genomic Era: www.youtube.com/watch?v=LaHSMJGUco8

REFERENCES

ASH (Action on Smoking and Health) (2019) 12 years on from England going smoke-free, support for the Government to do more to tackle smoking is continuing to grow. Available at: http://ash.org.uk/media-and-news/press-releases-media-and-news/12-years-on-from-england-going-smokefree-support-for-the-government-to-do-more-to-tackle-smoking-is-continuing-to-grow/

Balaji, K., Vijayaraghavan, S., Diao, L., Tong, P., Fan, Y., Carey, J.P., Bui, T.N., Warner, S., Heymach, J.V., Hunt, K.K., Wang, J., Byers, L.A. and Keyomarsi, K. (2017) AXL inhibition suppresses the DNA damage response and sensitizes cells to PARP inhibition in multiple cancers. *Molecular Cancer Research*, 15: 45–58.

Berrougui, H., Ikhlef, S. and Khalil, A. (2015) Extra virgin olive oil polyphenols promote cholesterol efflux and improve HDL functionality. *Journal of Evidenced Based Complementary Medicine*. Available at: www.ncbi.nlm.nih.gov/pmc/articles/PMC4606102/

Budnitz, D.S., Shehab, N., Kegler, S.R. and Richards, C.L. (2007) Medication use leading to emergency department visits for adverse drug events in older adults. *Annals of Internal Medicine*, 147: 755–65.

Burke, A.P. (2015) Pathology of acute myocardial infarction. *Medscape*. Available at: https://emedicine.medscape.com/article/1960472-overview#a3

Busko, M. (2019) Intermittent fasting plus lower-calorie diet may be best. *Medscape*. Available at: www.medscape.com/viewarticle/908041

Cheeseman, H., Anderson, W. and Butterworth, G. (2017) Political priorities and public health services in English local authorities: the case of tobacco control and smoking cessation services. *Journal of Public Health*, 40: e269–e274.

Chiefari, E., Tanyolac, S., Paonessa, F., Pullinger, C.R., Capula, C., Iiritano, S., et al. (2011) Functional variants of the HMGA1 gene and type 2 diabetes mellitus. *Journal of the American Medical Association*, 305(9): 903–12.

Church, T.S., Blair, S.N., Cocreham, S., Johannsen, N., Johnson, W., Kramer, K., et al. (2010) Effects of aerobic and resistance training on haemoglobin A1c levels in patients with type 2 diabetes: a randomized controlled trial. *Journal of the American Medical Association*, 304(20): 2253–62.

Cooney, R., Baker, J., Brain, O., Danis, B., Pichulik, T., Allan, P., Ferguson, D.J., Campbell, B.J., Jewell, D. and Simmons, A. (2010) NOD2 stimulation induces autophagy in dendritic cells influencing bacterial handling and antigen presentation. *Nature Medicine*, 16(1): 90–7.

Cushing, H. (1925) *The Life of Sir William Osler*. Oxford: Clarendon Press

Darsigny, M., Babeu, J.-P., Dupuis, A.-A., Furth, E.E., Seidman, E.G., Lévy, É., et al. (2009) Loss of hepatocyte-nuclear-factor-4α affects colonic ion transport and causes chronic inflammation resembling inflammatory bowel disease in mice. *PLoS ONE*, 4(10): e7609. https://doi.org/10.1371/journal.pone.0007609

Desai, S. and Jena, A. (2016) Do celebrity endorsements matter? Observational study of BRCA gene testing and mastectomy rates after Angelina Jolie's New York Times editorial. *British Medical Journal*, 355: i6357.

Dreon, D.M., Fernstrom, H.A., Campos, H., Blanche, P., Williams, P.T. and Krauss, R.M. (1998) Change in dietary saturated fat intake is correlated with change in mass of large low-density-lipoprotein particles in men. *American Journal of Clinical Nutrition*; 67(5): 828–36.

Facchini, F.S., Hollenbeck, C.B., Jeppesen, J., Chen, Y.D. and Reaven, G.M. (1992) Insulin resistance and cigarette smoking. *Lancet, 339*(8802): 1128–30.

Haffner, S.M., D'Agostino, R. Jr, Mykkänen, L., Tracy, R., Howard, B., Rewers, M., Selby, J., Savage, P.J. and Saad, M.F. (1999) Insulin sensitivity in subjects with type 2 diabetes. Relationship to cardiovascular risk factors: the Insulin Resistance Atherosclerosis Study. *Diabetes Care, 22*(4): 562–8.

Harrold, A. (2017) Diabetic patients should be warned about changes to Lucozade glucose content. *Nursing in Practice*. Available at: www.nursinginpractice.com/article/diabetic-patients-should-be-warned-about-changes-lucozade-glucose-content

Hellerstein, M.K., Benowitz, N.L. and Neese, R.A. (1994) Effects of cigarette smoking and its cessation on lipid metabolism and energy expenditure in heavy smokers. *Journal of Clinical Investigation, 93*: 265–72.

Heran, B.S., Chen, J.M. and Ebrahim, S. (2011) Exercise-based cardiac rehabilitation for coronary heart disease. *Cochrane Database of Systematic Reviews, 7*: CD001800. doi:10.1002/14651858.CD001800.pub2

Higuchi, Y., Suzuki, T. and Arimori, T. (2021) Engineered ACE2 receptor therapy overcomes mutational escape of SARS-CoV-2. *Nature Communications, 12*: 3802. https://doi.org/10.1038/s41467-021-24013-y

Hooper, L., Summerbell, C., Thompson, R., Sills, D., Roberts, F., Moore, H. and Smith, G.D. (2011) Reduced or modified dietary fat for preventing cardiovascular disease. *Cochrane Systematic Review – Intervention Version* DOI: 10.1002/14651858.CD002137.pub2

Hunt, D. (2009) Diabetes: foot ulcers and amputations. *BMJ Clinical Evidence*, 0602.

Imperatore, G., Boyle, J.P., Thompson, T.J., Case, D., Dabelea, D., Hamman, R.F., Lawrence, J.M., Liese, A.D., Liu, L.L., Mayer-Davis, E.J., Rodriguez, B.L. and Standiford, D. (2012) Projections of type 1 and type 2 diabetes burden in the U.S. population aged <20 years through 2050. *Diabetes Care, 35*(12): 2515–20.

Jeffcoate, W. (2019) Is diabetic footcare in the UK still a 'Cinderella' service? *Medscape*. Available at: www.medscape.com/viewarticle/909936?src=WNL_exclus_uk_190315_MSCPEDIT&uac=318414EV&impID=1909125&faf=1#vp_2

Katsanos, K.H., Vermeire, S., Christodoulou, D.K., Riis, L., Wolters, F., Odes, S., Freitas, J., Hoie, O., Beltrami, M. and Fornaciari, G. (2007) Dysplasia and cancer in inflammatory bowel disease 10 years after diagnosis: results of a population-based European collaborative follow-up study. *Digestion, 75*: 113–21.

Key, T.J. (2011) Fruit and vegetables and cancer risk. *British Journal of Cancer, 104*: 6–11.

Khor, B., Gardet, A. and Xavier, R.J. (2011) Genetics and pathogenesis of inflammatory bowel disease. *Nature, 474*(7351): 307–17.

Law, M. and Hackshaw, A. (1997) A meta-analysis of cigarette smoking, bone mineral density and risk of hip fracture: recognition of a major effect. *British Medical Journal, 315*: 841–6.

Lea, D.H., Feero, G. and Jenkins, J.F. (2008) Warfarin therapy and pharmacogenomics: a step towards personalized medicine. *American Nurse Today, 3*(5): 12–13.

Lilly, L. (2011) *Pathophysiology of Heart Disease: A Collaborative Project of Medical Students and Faculty*. Baltimore: Lippincott Williams & Wilkins.

Logan, R.F.A. (1998) Inflammatory bowel disease incidence: up, down or unchanged? *Gut, 42*(3): 309–11.

Mierzynska, A., Kowalska, M., Stepnowska, M. and Ryszard, P. (2010) Psychological support for patients following myocardial infarction. *Cardiology Journal, 17*(3):

319–24. Available at https://journals.viamedica.pl/cardiology_journal/article/download/21380/16984

MIMS (2021) Available at: www.mims.co.uk/remsima-inflectra-new-infliximab-biosimilars/dermatology/article/1333839

NHS (2011) Genetic testing is 'ethically sound'. Available at: www.nicswell.co.uk/health-news/genetic-testing-is-ethically-sound

NHS (2018) Predictive genetic tests for cancer risk genes. Available at: www.nhs.uk/conditions/predictive-genetic-tests-cancer/

NHS (2019) Genetic inheritance. Available at: www.nhs.uk/conditions/genetic-and-genomic-testing/

NHS Digital (2019) Statistics on smoking – England, 2018 [PAS]. Available at: https://digital.nhs.uk/data-and-information/publications/statistical/statistics-on-smoking/statistics-on-smoking-england-2018/part-1-smoking-related-ill-health-and-mortality

NHS England (2022) NHS to roll out life-changing glucose monitors to all type 1 diabetes patients. Available at: www.england.nhs.uk/2022/08/nhs-to-roll-out-life-changing-glucose-monitors-to-all-type-1-diabetes-patients/

NICE (National Institute for Health and Care Excellence) (2018) Cardiovascular disease: risk assessment and reduction, including lipid modification. Available at: www.nice.org.uk/guidance/cg181

NICE (National Institute for Health and Care Excellence) (2019a) Diabetes. Available at: www.nice.org.uk/guidance/conditions-and-diseases/diabetes-and-other-endocrinal--nutritional-and-metabolic-conditions/diabetes

NICE (National Institute for Health and Care Excellence) (2019b) Crohn's disease: management. Available at: www.nice.org.uk/guidance/ng129

NICE (National Institute for Health and Care Excellence) (2010, 2019) Infliximab and adalimumab for the treatment of Crohn's disease. Available at: www.nice.org.uk/guidance/ta187/chapter/3-The-technologies

Nichols, A.B., Ravenscroft, C., Lamphiear, D.E. and Ostrander, L.D. Jr (1976) Daily nutritional intake and serum lipid levels: the Tecumseh study. *American Journal of Clinical Nutrition*, *29*(12): 1384–92.

Nookaraju, A., Upadhyaya, P.C., Pandey, S.K., Young, K.E., Hong, S.J., Park, S.K. and Park, S.W. (2010) Molecular approaches for enhancing sweetness in fruits and vegetables. *Scientia Horticulturae*, *127*: 1–15.

Ronaldson, A., Molloy, G.J., Wikman, A., Poole, L., Kaski, J.C. and Steptoe, A. (2015) Optimism and recovery after acute coronary syndrome: a clinical cohort study. *Psychosomatic Medicine*, *77*(3): 311–18.

Silva, N.M., Santos, M.A.D., Rosado, S.R., Galvão, C.M. and Sonobe, H.M. (2017) Psychological aspects of patients with intestinal stoma: integrative review. *Review of Latin American Nursing 25*: e2950. doi:10.1590/1518-8345.2231.2950

Siri-Tarino, P.W.I., Sun, Q., Hu, F.B. and Krauss, R.M. (2010) Saturated fat, carbohydrate, and cardiovascular disease. *American Journal of Clinical Nutrition*, *91*(3): 502–9.

Solberg, L.A. and Strong, J.P. (1983) Risk factors and atherosclerotic lesions: a review of autopsy studies. *Arteriosclerosis*, *3*(3): 187–98.

Taylor, R. (2013) Type 2 diabetes: aetiology and reversibility. *Medscape*. Available at: www.medscape.com/viewarticle/781719_1

Terdiman, J.P., Aust, D.E. and Chang, C.G. (2006) High resolution analysis of chromosome 18 alterations in ulcerative colitis-related colorectal cancer. *Cancer Genetics* and *Cytogenetics*, *136*: 129–37.

WHO (World Health Organization) (2022) Sickle cell disease. Available at: www.afro.who.int/health-topics/sickle-cell-disease

8

PREVENTION AND CONTROL OF INFECTION

DEBORAH GEE

STANDARDS OF PROFICIENCY FOR NURSING ASSOCIATES (2018)

Relevant Platforms include:

Platform 2:2.9 Protect health through understanding and applying the principles of infection prevention and control, including communicable disease surveillance and antimicrobial stewardship and resistance.

Platform 4:4.3 Understand and apply the principle of human factors and environmental factors when working in teams.

Platform 5:5.1 Understand and apply the principles of health and safety legislation and regulations and maintain safe work and care environments.

Platform 5:5.4 Respond to and escalate potential hazards that may affect the safety of people.

Annex B Monitor wounds and undertake wound care using appropriate evidence-based techniques 3.6.

Annex B Infection control 8.1–8.8.

Prevention and management of infection is the responsibility of all staff working in health and social care.

Sunley et al. (2017)

This chapter will introduce you to the importance of infection control within health and social care settings. It covers the core principles in managing the spread of infection through institutions and the preventative measures available. It also examines the legislation that supports infection control. This chapter links with bioscience, which is the focus of Chapter 6, and will remind you of the body's immune system functions. This chapter will also give you essential details about sepsis, spotting and treating it.

Glossary

- **CQC** Care Quality Commission
- **Evidence-based practice** Ways of working that have been proved to be effective
- **Healthcare-associated Infection (HCAI)** Infection as a result of receiving healthcare in hospital or community settings
- **HSE** The Health and Safety Executive
- **PPE** Personal protective equipment
- **RCN** The Royal College of Nursing
- **RIDDOR** Reporting of Injuries, Diseases and Dangerous Occurrences Regulations 2013

INTRODUCTION

All nursing associates, healthcare practitioners, nurses and midwives have a professional and ethical responsibility to ensure their knowledge and skills are up-to-date and that they are able to practise safely and competently at all times. The Code for Professional Standards of Practice and Behaviour for Nurses, Midwives and Nursing Associates states specifically that nurses must 'keep to and promote recommended practice in relation to controlling and preventing infection' and 'take all reasonable personal precautions necessary to avoid any potential health risks to colleagues, people receiving care and the public' (19.3+4, NMC Code, 2018). With over 4 million people across Europe developing a Healthcare-associated Infection (HCAI) each year, managing the spread of infection within practice is a constant challenge (PHE, 2016). Infection prevention and control is a practical, evidence-based approach which prevents patients and healthcare workers from being harmed by avoidable infections.

HCAIs bring increased morbidity and mortality to the patients, with Public Health England reporting that approximately 37,000 people die each year from HCAI (PHE, 2016). Patients with infection are likely to experience increased pain and discomfort, not forgetting the financial burden prolonged treatments can bring to both the care provider and the patient themselves.

Using an evidence-based approach, this chapter will provide those working in health and social care settings with the knowledge and skills to practise safe infection prevention and control when working with patients. It will also introduce some of the health and safety legislation linked to safety and will offer suggested areas for critical reflection and further reading.

THE IMPORTANCE OF INFECTION CONTROL IN HEALTHCARE PRACTICE

Within healthcare practice over the past two decades there has been a plethora of government initiatives to address the increasing numbers of healthcare associated infections.

With the number of infections rising, the subsequent extensive use of available antibiotics to treat these infections has resulted in an increased number of infections such as MRSA (methicillin-resistant *Staphylococcus aureus*), VRE (vancomycin-resistant enterococci), *Clostridium difficile* (*C. difficile*), *Escherichia coli* (*E. coli*) and ESBL (extended-spectrum beta-lactamases), all of which are increasingly resistant to many of the current antibiotics available, and this brings increased challenges for the health and social care profession.

The World Health Organization (WHO) states that antimicrobial resistance is one of the top 10 global public health threats facing humanity, warning of the need for global changes to how antibiotics are prescribed and used within society. Antibiotic resistance is a definite risk to individuals, making our ability to successfully treat common infectious diseases increasingly more difficult. WHO also note that changes in the way in which antibiotics are prescribed and used alone will not be sufficient to manage the threat to individuals; they suggest additional behaviour changes should also include actions to reduce the spread of infections through measures such as effective handwashing and vaccination (WHO, 2020).

CORONAVIRUS

In December 2019 a wider public health threat to the population emerged: a novel coronavirus was identified in China. Although coronaviruses were first discovered in domestic poultry in the 1930s it was not until the 1960s that they were identified in humans.

There are seven strains that cause an immediate threat of disease to humans (NCIRD, 2020) (see Table 8.1). Four of the seven are more related to milder symptoms such as the common cold. The other three include two types of Severe Acute Respiratory Syndrome (SARS-CoV; SARS-CoV-2) and Middle East Respiratory Syndrome coronavirus (MERS-CoV), causing more severe symptom presentation in humans, with increased risk of serious respiratory infections that regularly require hospital care for recovery; however, these can and sometimes do lead to death. SARS is noted by the World Health Organization as one of the first severe transmissible diseases of the twenty-first century; it is an airborne virus and can be spread in a similar way to colds and influenza. SARS may also be spread indirectly, from hard surfaces for example (WHO, 2021).

CORONAVIRUS PREVENTION AND TREATMENT

There is no cure for SARS or MERS; treatments should be supportive and focused around the patients presenting symptoms. Controlling outbreaks relies upon behavioural measures to help contain and prevent the spread of the virus. The personal preventative measures include frequent hand-washing using soap or alcohol-based disinfectants. Those working in areas where they are at a greater risk of contracting the virus should be wearing appropriate personal protective equipment (PPE).

Scientists have made significant progress with the development of antiviral treatments and specific vaccines to tackle the novel coronovirus SARS-CoV-2 known as Covid-19; several companies are known to be working on antiviral drugs and vaccines have been developed and approved. Access to safe and effective vaccines across the world is critical but it is the actions taken by those working within healthcare practice to ensure that people in society are fully vaccinated that is key to ending the Covid-19 pandemic.

Table 8.1   Human coronavirus types

Type	Impact upon humans
1. 229E (alpha coronavirus) 2. NL63 (alpha coronavirus) 3. OC43 (beta coronavirus) 4. HKU1 (beta coronavirus)	Rhinorroea, nasal congestion, sneezing, sore throat and cough with a potential fever. Symptoms usually peak on day 3–4 of the illness.
5. SARS-CoV (beta coronavirus)	A high temperature >38°C, headache malaise and muscle pain. At the onset some have mild respiratory symptoms. After 3–7 days there can be a dry cough, shortness of breath and low blood oxygen levels. Incubation is 2–7 days but can be as long as 10 days.
6. MERS-CoV (beta coronavirus)	MERS-CoV symptoms can range from a person being asymptomatic to having mild or severe symptoms. These include a fever, cough and shortness of breath. Pneumonia is commonly noted. Gastrointestinal problems such as diarrhoea have also been reported. The virus seems to cause more problems in older people and those with chronic diseases such as renal disease, cancer, chronic lung disease and diabetes.
7. SARS-CoV-2 (novel coronavirus)	Common symptoms: a high temperature >38°C, a new continuous cough, a loss of or changes in sense of taste or smell and fatigue. Serious symptoms: shortness of breath, loss of speech or mobility, confusion and chest pain. On average it takes 5–6 days from when someone is infected with the virus for the symptoms to show, however it can take longer, up to 14 days.

Case Study   8.1   Mr Neville Jones

Mr Jones was brought into the hospital emergency department after his neighbour called an ambulance on noticing he was short of breath and not quite his usual cheery self. On arrival at the emergency department Mr Jones has a temperature of 38.2, pulse of 91 bpm and his respirations are 22 bpm. His blood pressure is 140/95. Saturations 94% in room air.

Mr Jones is 69 years old, 5 ft 8 in (172 cms) and weighs 12 stone (78 kg). Mr Jones is an ex-smoker. He wears spectacles and uses a hearing aid. He always refuses his annual influenza vaccine stating that 'it gives him the flu'.

He was widowed more than 5 years ago and is an active member of the church committee. Mr Jones does not drink regularly, describing himself as an occasional drinker; he is usually quite active and enjoys looking after his garden.

Activity 8.1   Critical thinking

As a nursing associate working within the emergency department, using the Case Study 8.1 what would your initial thoughts and feelings be about Mr Jones and his presenting condition? Considering the risks associated with coronavirus infections, what personal and professional challenges do you think you will be faced with when caring for Mr Jones?

An outline answer is given at the end of this chapter.

Go Further 8.1

In 2021 Public Health England launched the 'Supporting Excellence in Infection Prevention and Control Behaviours Toolkit' to support practitioners. The 'Every Action Counts' resources have been developed to support NHS organisations to communicate with and apply compliance interventions to staff, patient and visitor groups. You can access more information on this toolkit via this link: www.england. nhs.uk/coronavirus/publication/every-action-counts/

THE BODY'S DEFENCE SYSTEMS

Individuals in healthcare settings such as hospitals are vulnerable to the risk of infection for several reasons, including their reduced immunity, the presence of invasive devices and the fact that they have increased risk of being in contact with other patients who are suffering from infection.

Infections themselves are generally caused by micro-organisms and the term 'infectious agent' is frequently used to describe these. The body, however, has its own natural defences and has several specific ways of protecting itself from infection. You can find more discussion of the immune system in Chapter 6, Bioscience.

The body's defence mechanisms are divided into two categories: non-specific defence mechanisms and specific defence mechanisms. Let's look at non-specific mechanisms first. These are effective against any invader.

NON-SPECIFIC DEFENCE

The skin protects most of the body surface, but there are also other protective features, for example, sticky mucus, which traps microbes and other foreign materials and prevents tissues from drying out, and body fluids that can contain antimicrobial substances, for example, gastric juices contain hydrochloric acids. Saliva, which washes the surface of the teeth, also contains lysozomes and enzymes that can break down bacteria. These are classed as the first lines of non-specific defence (Figure 8.1). They prevent entry and minimise further passage of microbes and other foreign material into the body. Good oral hygiene prevents dental and gum infections which can compromise the beneficial effects of saliva.

Healthy, intact skin and mucus membrane provide an effective barrier. The sebum and sweat excreted provide a good defence to pathogens as they both contain antibacterial and antifungal substances.

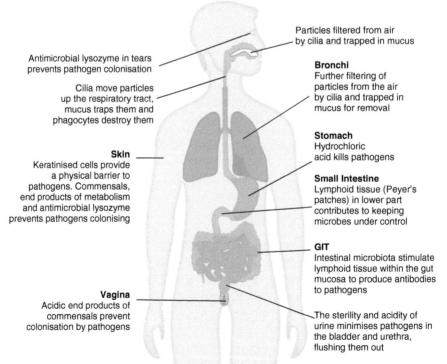

Figure 8.1 Non-specific defence

Epithelial membranes lining body cavities like the respiratory, urinary and digestive tracts, although delicate, are also well defended by antibacterial secretions. The epithelia produce more secretions, often acidic, containing antibodies and enzymes as well as sticky mucus for trapping passing microbes. Table 8.2 lists natural antimicrobial substances.

Another of the non-specific defence mechanisms is phagocytosis. This is known as 'cell eating'. The phagocytic defence cells such as macrophages and neutrophils are the body's first line of cellular defence. These cells naturally migrate to the site of inflammation and infection and engulf the targets. They indiscriminately digest and destroy foreign cells.

Table 8.2   Natural antimicrobial substances

Hydrochloric acid	Kills most ingested microbes
Lysozyme	Antibacterial enzyme. Destroys bacterial cell walls but does not affect viruses or other pathogens. Found in tears, mucus, saliva, sweat, milk, cervical mucus, leucocytes and kidney tissue
Antibodies	Protective proteins found coating membranes and body fluids and inactive bacteria
Saliva	Secreted into mouth and washes away debris, preventing bacteria and tooth decay
Interferons	Chemicals produced by T-lymphocytes and macrophages. They prevent viral replication in cells
Complement	System of approximately 20 proteins found in blood and tissues (see also Chapter 6)

The inflammatory response is the physical response to tissue damage. Its purpose is protective: to isolate, inactivate and remove both the cause and the damaged tissues.

Another defence mechanism is immunological surveillance. A population of lymphocytes called NK (natural killer) cells patrol the body looking for abnormal cells. Once a cell is detected the NK cells destroy it.

SPECIFIC DEFENCE

Specific defence is when the body generates a specific response against any substance it identifies as foreign. These substances are known as antigens and include:

- Pollen from flowers and plants
- Bacteria and other microbes
- Cancer cells or transplanted tissue cells

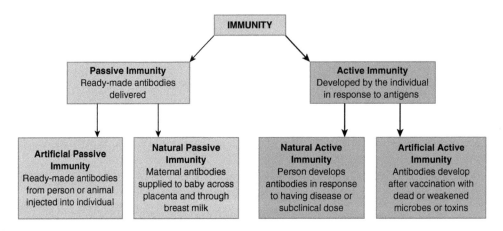

Figure 8.2   Specific defence

These antigens then induce the immune system to produce antibodies and a specific immune response (see Figure 8.2).

If the body's first line of non-specific defences is overwhelmed, then there is an activation of the powerful immune system. Immunity has three key attributes:

1. Specificity – immune response directed at a specific antigen.
2. Memory – the response usually forms a memory and therefore if the body is faced with the same challenge again, it will act faster.
3. Tolerance – the cells of the immune system can be aggressive and destructive. Healthy 'self' cells display marker proteins that tell the immune cells that they are 'OK'. Issues can happen when 'non-self' cells are present, such as transplanted cells and cancer cells.

TYPES OF IMMUNITY

1. CELLULAR IMMUNITY

- Carried out by T-cells. When the T-cell encounters an antigen for the first time, it becomes sensitised to it.
- Antigen-presenting cell (macrophage). Macrophages are like Pac-Man, they chase down and eat (by phagocytosis) invading bacteria; they then mature into antigen-presenting cells to attract T-cells and to produce cytokines (antibodies).
- Infected cells are killed by cytotoxic T-cells.

2. ANTIBODY OR HUMORAL IMMUNITY

- Carried out by B-cells.
- Antibodies are produced and remain in the bloodstream.
- Antibodies bind to antigens and deactivate them.

3. NATURAL AND ACQUIRED IMMUNITY

- Some of the activated T- and B-cells become memory cells. The next time an individual meets up with the same antigen the immune system can respond and destroy it. Depending upon the route of entry into the body and the amount and type of antigen produced, the immunity can be strong or weak, short-lived or long-lasting.
- Immunity can also be influenced by inherited genes.
- An immune response can be sparked not only by infection but also by immunisation with vaccines. Vaccines contain specially treated micro-organisms. Once administered, they provoke an immune response to the specific disease.
- Immunity can also be transferred from one individual to another. The immunological responses of a baby are generally weak, however prior to birth the mother will transfer additional antibodies to the baby to boost its immune system. This protection can be further enhanced by mothers who breastfeed their babies; however, this passive immunity typically lasts only a few weeks or months (NHS Choices, 2017).

WHEN INFECTION OCCURS

Despite the body's specific and non-specific defences against infection there are occasions when infections do occur. However, certain conditions need to be met for a micro-organism or infectious disease to be spread from person to person. This process is referred to as the 'chain of infection' (see Figure 8.3).

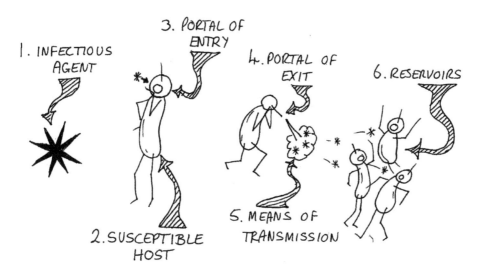

Figure 8.3   The chain of infection

THE CHAIN OF INFECTION

THE INFECTIOUS AGENT

Germs (the infectious agent) are generally all around us and play an important part in helping us remain healthy. There are also many germs that are not helpful to our health and can cause disease. The challenge arises when a germ leaves its usual 'healthy' place of residence and travels elsewhere in the body.

THE RESERVOIR

This 'place' where germs can live and multiply is called a reservoir. This can be a person, who may be either a service user or a member of staff. BUT … it can also be any part of the surrounding area of a health or social care setting, such as fixtures and fittings, including soft furnishings, in addition to any equipment used for patient care.

THE PORTAL OF EXIT FROM THE RESERVOIR

The portal of exit can vary depending upon the type of infection. There are both human and non-human means by which the germs can escape.

- **Human** – a healthcare worker touches a used commode, and some of the germs move onto that person's hands. Their hands are now the 'portal of exit' – how the germs are able to move from the commode to another place.
- **Non-human** portals include items of equipment that have not been properly cleaned, such as commodes, bed mattresses, pillows and reusable equipment, which would become the infectious agent (portal of infection).

MODES/MEANS OF TRANSMISSION

Awareness of the methods by which a disease is transmitted is important in infection control; it also highlights the importance of effective handwashing in controlling the spread of infection.

The most common modes of transmission that occur in the care environment are:

- Contact
- Droplet
- Airborne

CONTACT SPREAD

In contact spread, the susceptible person has either direct or indirect contact with the infected source or reservoir.

Direct (patient) contact occurs when there is actual physical contact between the source and the susceptible person. It is necessary for the source and the susceptible person to be exposed to skin and body secretions via close contact. Remember that organisms can also be transmitted from one part of a person's body, such as their skin, to another part of their own body or to another person, for example through touching a wound.

Indirect (contaminated object) transmission usually occurs when a piece of equipment is used on more than one person and has not been properly cleaned in between uses.

DROPLET TRANSMISSION

Droplet particles cannot be transmitted beyond a radius of a few feet of the source. The large particles generally expelled from respiratory secretions by coughing, sneezing or talking rapidly settle on horizontal surfaces or are deposited on the susceptible person's conjunctivae, nasal membranes or mouth. For instance, viral influenza pathogens are transmitted this way.

AIRBORNE SPREAD

Airborne particles are disseminated by having a true airborne phase; this is usually a distance of several feet or more between the source and the susceptible person. Pathogens that are transmitted this way include varicella and tuberculosis.

PORTALS OF ENTRY

Microbes can enter the body through four sites:

- Respiratory tract
- Gastrointestinal tract
- Urogenital tract
- Breaks in the skin surface

The portals of entry in healthcare practice are listed in Table 8.3.

Table 8.3 Portals of entry in healthcare practice

An opening to the skin
Catheter being placed into the bladder (suprapubic or urinary)
Enteral feeding
Central venous catheterisation
Injections/used needles

A SUSCEPTIBLE HOST

The development of an infection from any transferred pathogens is dependent upon the ability of the organism to cause disease and the body's ability to resist it. As we have seen in this chapter, the ability of the body to defend itself is called immunity, and previous exposure and immune response will also play a role. Healthy people are generally able to 'fight off' infection; however, some (both apparently well and unwell) people are unable to fight infection, making them susceptible hosts when their bodies are invaded.

In 2016, the Royal College of Nursing (RCN) provided practitioners with a toolkit with an overarching framework to help meet the challenge of reducing and sustaining the reduction in HCAIs. However, the reduction of HCAIs remains high on the government's safety and quality agenda and in the general public's expectations for quality of care. The *Code of Practice on the Prevention and Control of Infections* (Department of Health, 2015) applies to all registered providers of healthcare and adult social care in England. The Code of Practice (Part 2) sets out the 10 criteria against which the Care Quality Commission (CQC) will judge a registered provider on how it complies with the infection prevention requirements set out in regulations.

> ⚙ Activity 8.2   Critical thinking
>
> Hospitals and care providers have for many years recognised the significance of infection prevention and control and employ specialist infection control staff. Are you able to identify nominated person(s) in your workplace?

CORE PRINCIPLES IN INFECTION PREVENTION AND CONTROL

The prevention and control of infection is the responsibility of all staff working within health and social care settings, and all have a duty to ensure that those they care for are not at risk from poor practice.

The acquisition of an HCAI has potential implications for:

- Patients
- Visitors
- Staff
- Workers such as electricians and plumbers working in buildings
- The employing organisation, e.g. healthcare trust, care home, hospice
- The National Health Service (NHS)

The effective implementation of basic core principles is the first step in managing the control and spread of infection because poor practice related to hygiene increases the risk of hospital-acquired infections, and this in turn can lead to pain, distress, unwanted exposure to medication (and negative side effects), lengthened hospital stays, long-term complications and even death for your patient. We must also consider the impact upon the NHS and other healthcare providers of such things as increased costs, reduced public confidence and reduced staff morale.

The core principles of infection prevention and control are:

- Effective handwashing
- Protective clothing
- Barrier or isolation nursing
- Laundry and waste management
- Cleanliness of the environment
- Decontamination of equipment

Activity 8.3   Evidence-based practice and research

Consider what the potential implications are when a patient has acquired an HCAI.

ASEPTIC NON-TOUCH TECHNIQUE (ANTT)

ANTT could also be used as a mnemonic:

Always decontaminate hands effectively

Never contaminate key parts or sites

Touch non key parts with confidence

Take appropriate infection control precautions

Nurses need to assess the precautions for infection risk when required to maintain asepsis; you should be trained and assessed as competent before using ANTT. Previously, sterile procedures required full sterile protection; now called the aseptic field, only certain parts of the procedure (micro critical aseptic fields) are judged to require sterility. Key sites for ANTT are urinary catheterisation, open wounds, sites of invasive procedures, and central and peripheral line management. High impact assessment tools should be used for data gathering for the insertion phase and during ongoing care while any insert remains in situ.

The activity should be strictly controlled using the five steps to ANTT:

1. The work environment should be disinfected to convention
2. Hands should be cleaned and dried (see below for hand cleaning guidance) before the activity commences (such as drawing up drugs for line delivery); PPE worn

3. Critical aseptic fields: key parts protected (critical management states only sterilised or aseptic equipment such as sterile gloves and drapes should come into contact with a critical aseptic field)
4. Non-touch technique
5. Decontamination/disposal to prevent cross-infection

Go Further 8.2

You can find more information about ANTT at: www.gwh.nhs.uk/media/y03bms4s/aseptic-non-touch-technique-policy.pdf

---

Recent research has voiced concern about reusable tourniquets used in venepuncture, as evidence reveals these are seldom cleaned and often contaminated, with the potential for dissemination of micro-organisms. Osorio et al.'s (2019) research states that single-use disposable tourniquets would be cost effective in infection control and reducing HCAIs.

HAND HYGIENE

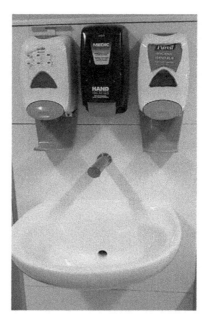

Figure 8.4   Hand hygiene

One of the most effective and non-invasive ways of preventing HCAIs is through good hand hygiene (see Figure 8.4). Hands carry two different types of micro-organisms: transient and resident. Infection can occur when micro-organisms are transferred from one patient to another, either from equipment or the environment between patients and staff, resulting in a disruption to a patient's 'normal bacterial flora'.

Transient micro-organisms are found on the skin surface. These are readily acquired from contact with other body sites, people and the environment, and are easily transferred to others. The disruption to the normal body flora can predispose the individual to infection if the bacteria are being transferred from one part of the body to another where they are not normally resident; for example, if faecal bacteria from the groin are transferred to the face during washing or performing mouth care without the healthcare worker undertaking effective hand hygiene or changing their gloves.

Resident micro-organisms are part of our normal skin flora and are found in deeper skin layers, hair follicles and sweat glands, and they are more difficult to remove than transient micro-organisms.

It is essential for all healthcare workers to ensure they clean their hands at the right times and in the right way.

HOW SHOULD WE WASH OUR HANDS?

Despite awareness of the importance of effective handwashing, studies repeatedly show that effective handwashing is dependent upon many factors, including the selection of the appropriate cleansing product in addition to the technique used (WHO, 2009). Figure 8.5 shows commonly missed areas as a result of poor technique.

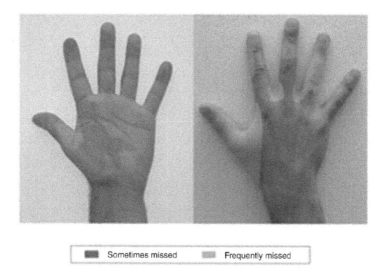

Sometimes missed   Frequently missed

Figure 8.5   Commonly missed areas

In practice, there are generally three different ways hands are cleaned:

1. Soap and water – effective in removing dirt and soiling and transient micro-organisms
2. Antimicrobial detergent – effective in removing dirt and soiling and more effective in removing resident micro-organisms
3. Alcohol-based hand rubs – effective on non-soiled hands, quick and effective way of destroying transient bacteria. Note: not effective with *C. difficile* infections (WHO, 2009)

What is the correct technique? Effective handwashing involves three stages: *preparation, washing* and *rinsing,* and *drying.*

*   **Preparation**: Wet hands under tepid running water before applying the recommended amount of liquid soap or an antimicrobial preparation.
*   **Washing**: Hands should be washed and rinsed thoroughly. The hand-wash solution must come into contact with all of the surfaces of the hand and the hands should be rubbed together for 10–15 seconds (Loveday, 2014).

Within healthcare practice the consensus across the literature would appear to be that the six-step approach first provided by Ayliffe et al. in the late 1970s is the most effective method (see Figure 8.6):

1. Rub hands palm to palm.
2. Rub right palm over the back of the other hand with interlaced fingers and vice versa.
3. Rub palm to palm with the fingers interlaced.
4. Rub the backs of fingers to opposing palms with fingers interlocked.
5. Use rotational rubbing of the left thumb clasped in the right palm and vice versa.
6. Use rotational rubbing, backwards and forwards with clasped fingers of the right hand in the left palm and vice versa (Ayliffe et al., 1978).

*   **Drying**: In healthcare practice always use good-quality paper towels to dry the hands thoroughly (Loveday, 2014).

Go Further 8.3

You might read the original research by Ayliffe, Babb and Quoraishi. You can find it at: http://jcp.bmj.com/content/jclinpath/31/10/923.full.pdf. It is an interesting read, as due to poor handwashing, several research participants became very unwell.

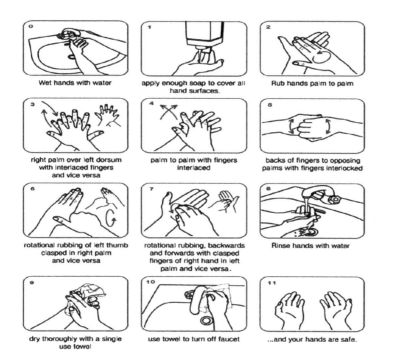

Figure 8.6   Effective hand cleaning

Source: Reproduced with the permission of WHO (www.who.int/infection-prevention/en/)

⚙ Activity 8.4   Test your knowledge

Answer as many of the following questions as you can without referring back to the literature.

1. What does the acronym HCAI stand for?
2. What does MRSA stand for?
3. How many steps are there to effective handwashing using the Ayliffe technique?
4. According to the Health and Safety at Work Act 1974 what must employers provide where there is a risk of infection?
5. HCAIs are only acquired in the hospital setting. True or False?
6. How is MRSA spread?
7. *Clostridium difficile* usually causes what kind of infection in humans?
8. How many coronavirus infections are known to affect humans?
9. In 2002 COSHH were introduced, what does COSHH stand for?
10. The COSHH legislation ensures that all healthcare workers wear protective clothing when caring for infected patients. True or False?

Answers are available at the end of the chapter.

The World Health Organization (WHO, 2006) advocates five key moments for hand hygiene (see Figure 8.7):

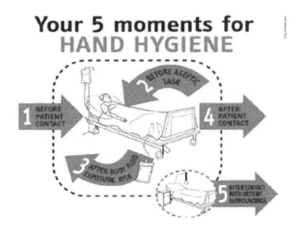

Figure 8.7   Hand hygiene at the point of care

Source: Reproduced with the permission of WHO (www.who.int/infection-prevention/en/)

1. **Before patient contact**: The need to decontaminate our hands prior to contact with a patient, and this includes arrival on duty.
2. **Before aseptic task**: The aseptic technique is used in practice to reduce the risk of infection occurring as a result of a procedure taking place. This usually follows a set of specific actions. Staff expected to perform aseptic procedures will receive appropriate training and will be deemed as competent before performing this independently. Practice examples where the need for aseptic technique is required are when changing a patient's wound dressings or when dealing with intravenous fluid administration.
3. **After body fluid exposure risk**: Relates to fluids such as blood, faeces, vomit and urine. This includes after protective gloves have been removed as it is important to consider that:

   - gloves may become damaged in use (the damage may be visible or microscopic)
   - hands may also be contaminated accidentally when gloves are being removed
   - the environment inside the glove may promote microbial growth on the user's hands
   - handwashing after taking off gloves may also remove particles of the material that the gloves are made of, e.g. latex, and so reduce the risk of developing an allergy.

4. **After patient contact:** For example, when undertaking moving and handling tasks.
5. **After contact with patient surroundings:** As micro-organisms live on both hard surfaces and soft furnishings (Figure 8.8).

PERSONAL PROTECTIVE EQUIPMENT

When working in the health or social care setting, health and safety regulations (HSE, 1992) state that in order to protect you from any risk to your health and safety your employer must undertake appropriate risk assessments and provide you with the personal protective equipment (PPE) necessary to reduce the risks. All employees must be provided with information, instruction and training on the PPE available for use.

Some of the most common pieces of PPE are: disposable gloves, disposable plastic aprons, and masks, visors and eye protection.

DISPOSABLE GLOVES

These are essential in the prevention and control of infection within healthcare practice. However, it is important to wear gloves only when necessary as unnecessary use can arguably undermine the current hand hygiene initiatives. There is also the potential health risk to the healthcare worker, as wearing gloves when they are not necessary can lead to other problems such as contact dermatitis or exacerbation of other skin problems.

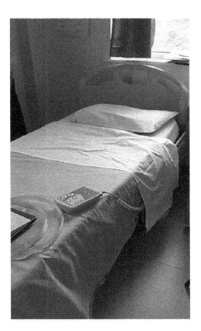

Figure 8.8   Ward bed

There are many different types of disposable gloves available to choose from and health workers need to ensure that they use the correct gloves and that the ones chosen are fit for purpose.

Powdered latex and natural rubber latex gloves should not generally be used as they increase the risk of allergic reaction in patients and staff with existing allergies. Latex can also lead to allergic contact dermatitis and occupational asthma in sensitised individuals. If latex gloves are to be used, they must only be used following a thorough risk assessment for suitability and safety. If they are selected for use, they must be low protein and single use (HSE, 2011).

In addition to latex, other chemicals known as accelerators can present a risk of work-related dermatitis. The Health and Safety Executive states that health surveillance checks should be carried out on those exposed to hazardous substances.

Under the Reporting of Injuries, Diseases and Dangerous Occurrences Regulations (RIDDOR, 2013) there is a legal requirement to report occupational asthma or dermatitis related to normal rubber latex to the Health and Safety Executive (HSE).

1. Neoprene and nitrile gloves are good alternatives to natural rubber latex. These are a synthetic glove and have been shown in clinical studies to be comparable in use to the rubber latex ones.
2. Vinyl gloves can be used for many tasks in the healthcare setting but may not be appropriate when handling bloodstained products, cytotoxic drugs or other high-risk substances.
3. Polythene gloves are not suitable for use in healthcare practice.

DISPOSABLE PLASTIC APRONS

These provide a physical barrier between clothing/skin and prevent contamination and wetting of uniforms/clothing during bathing or washing or equipment cleaning.

Aprons should be worn whenever there is a risk of contamination with blood or bodily fluids and when the patient has a suspected or known infection.

✷ Activity 8.5   Critical thinking

Employers provide different coloured plastic aprons for use in the clinical area – how many can you identify in your area? What is the rationale for this?

MASKS, VISORS AND EYE PROTECTION

These items should be worn when it is likely that blood or bodily fluids may splash into the eyes, face or mouth. They should be worn when there is likelihood of exposure to bodily fluids, such as in childbirth, trauma or operation theatre environments.

Masks may also be necessary if infection can be spread by an airborne route. All staff should be trained in how to fit a mask safely. If we are at risk in our environment, then the employer has a legal obligation to provide this protection under the Health and Safety at Work Act 1974 (Section 9).

BARRIER OR ISOLATION NURSING

Within healthcare practice, there are times when patients need to be barrier nursed or cared for in isolation. This is sometimes necessary to reduce the risk of spreading infection, including to those resistant to antibiotic treatment, and to protect patients who are more susceptible to infection, for example those who may have a compromised immune system because of their illness or the medications they are taking.

Barrier nursing involves the healthcare practitioner taking extra precautions to prevent the spread of the germs. Isolation nursing usually involves the patient being in a side room. The infection prevention control professional from your practice area will be able to offer specific advice regarding this.

SAFE HANDLING AND DISPOSAL OF WASTE

Any healthcare worker who produces waste as a part of their job is classified as a waste producer. Within health and social care practice waste is produced from those providing such care to patients, either in their own homes or within a healthcare organisation. There are three categories of waste: clinical, hazardous and offensive (RCN, 2014).

Waste reduction, segregation and disposal are all crucial to sustaining a healthy environment and reducing costs. As healthcare waste can include human waste and bodily fluids in addition to sharps (needles, scalpels, glass vials, etc.) and other biohazardous materials that may be infectious, it is essential that all waste products are disposed of correctly (Figure 8.9).

All health and social care organisations should have their own policy which will specify how an organisation manages its waste and identifies who is responsible for this within the organisation. This policy should provide employees with guidance and procedures to ensure that they dispose of waste safely and in compliance with all relevant legislation (Department of Health, 2013a, 2013b).

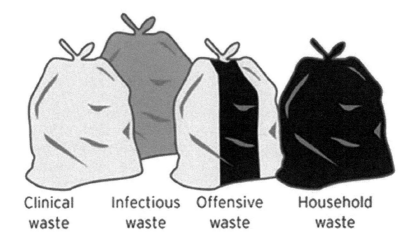

Clinical   Infectious   Offensive   Household
waste   waste   waste   waste

Figure 8.9   Waste bags

📷   Case Study 8.2   Wilfred, Annie and Daisy

At 4 pm you are advised that there has been an outbreak of diarrhoea and vomiting within the care home where you work. There are three residents severely affected, with Wilfred, Annie and Daisy all presenting with severe diarrhoea and vomiting within the last 2 hours.

⚙️   Activity 8.6   Evidence-based practice

Consider the information in Case Study 8.2 Wilfred, Annie and Daisy. As a member of the nursing team what things would you need to establish in order to manage the situation properly?

As a member of the nursing team how are you going to protect yourself and reduce the risk that you might spread infection to other service users?

Sample answers are offered at the end of the chapter.

The safe disposal of waste from health and social care is dependent upon the healthcare worker being able to classify the category of waste and use the correct waste container. The RCN (2014) highlights that effective segregation is not only essential for compliance with waste regulations, it is essential to promote good health and safety at work. The *Health Care Waste Management Manual* (Department of Health, 2013b) suggests use of an appropriate classification framework to support healthcare workers in this process. The RCN (2014) also provides further information on how to appropriately classify waste and points out that 'This may be a bag for soft wastes or more rigid container for sharps or medicinal wastes'.

The *Health Care Waste Management Manual* (Department of Health, 2013b: Section 3.2) provides suggested colours for waste containers which can be used to quickly identify the types of waste that should be disposed of within them. Colour coding for waste containers is important as it makes clear the end disposal/treatment route of the waste. Whichever colour is used, the waste producer is subject to their duty of care (a legal requirement) and should ensure any container is clearly labelled in a manner that makes the subsequent holder aware of its contents.

SAFE HANDLING OF SHARPS

Sharps are items (or parts of items) that could cause cuts or puncture wounds, including needles, the needle part of a syringe, scalpels and other blades, broken glass ampoules and the patient end of an infusion set (cannula/Venflon, etc.).

The use of sharps within a procedure can increase the risk of injuries, and therefore to ensure that those working with sharps reduce their risk of injury and infection it is essential that sharps are used and disposed of appropriately (Health and Safety at Work Act 1974).

In May 2013, the European Sharps Directive came into force in the UK. This states that the use of sharps should be eliminated where possible, and employers should consider the use of safety engineered sharps devices where elimination is not possible.

Table 8.4 summarises sharps best practice.

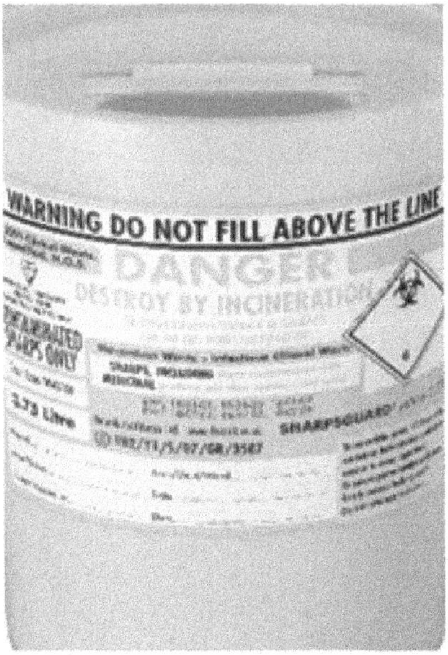

Figure 8.10   Sharps box

Table 8.4   Sharps best practice points

Ensure syringes and needles are placed as complete items straight into a sharps container (see Figure 8.10) following use
Needles should never be re-sheathed or re-capped
All sharps containers should conform to UN standard 3291 and British Standard 7320
Sharps containers should not be overfilled
Staff should attend training on the safe use of sharps, including safety engineered devices
Staff should report sharps injuries in line with local reporting procedures

Source: RCN (2012)

CLEANLINESS OF THE ENVIRONMENT

All healthcare providers must make sure that the care they provide is safe for service users. They must ensure that they take appropriate measures to prevent and control the spread of infection, ensuring that the premises and any equipment used are safe, and where applicable available in sufficient quantities (Department of Health, 2015).

A dirty clinical environment is one of the factors that may contribute towards infection rates. Effective cleaning to remove contaminants such as dust, faeces, blood and bodily fluids will help reduce the risk of cross-infection.

There are several different methods for cleaning: traditional methods such as detergent with water and microfibre cloths, the use of appropriate cleaning wipes for some items, and the specialist technologies such as hydrogen peroxide vapour cleaning (RCN, 2012).

Local policies should be consulted with regard to the cleaning regime and all healthcare workers have a duty to ensure that standards of cleanliness are maintained, reporting any concerns as per employer policy.

Spillages of all blood and bodily fluids should be dealt with quickly following your workplace written policy for managing these incidents. You should understand these *before* such incidents happen. This policy should include details of the chemicals staff should use to deal with the incident properly, for example there will be differences if the spillage is on a hard surface or a carpeted floor either in a care setting or in a patient's home.

DECONTAMINATION OF EQUIPMENT

Within healthcare practice there are several specific types of equipment available for use (see Table 8.5).

Table 8.5 Permissible use of different types of equipment

Type of equipment	Used more than once?	Examples
Single use	No	Needles, syringes, thermometer covers
Single patient use	Yes, for the same patient but still needs to be cleaned in between use	Pulse oximeter probes, nebulisers
Re-useable multi-patient use	Yes, but needs decontamination in between use	Beds, commodes, shower chairs, blood pressure cuffs

Decontamination of equipment is a term used for the removal of microbial contamination to make an item safe. All multi-patient use equipment needs to be cleaned and decontaminated in between patients. The process can involve cleaning, disinfection and sterilisation.

Cleaning is the most effective way of reducing the risk of infection from equipment and is essential in the process of disinfection and sterilisation.

Disinfection is used to decontaminate the micro-organisms from the environment, and multi-use equipment such as beds, commodes, bath chairs and blood pressure cuffs.

Sterilisation is the process involving the removal of all types of micro-organisms; however, it is impossible to ensure that every micro-organism is destroyed, and therefore effective, thorough cleaning is essential in the process to optimise the results.

All health and social care staff must be aware of the implications of ineffective decontamination of equipment, and employing organisations need to ensure that all staff are trained and competent to ensure they keep themselves and patients/service users safe.

📖 Case Study 8.3   Donna Davies

Donna is 33 years old and has moderate learning disabilities. She lives at home with her parents, who are her main carers. Donna eats well although often prefers to eat sweet foods rather than savoury. She is approximately 157 cms (5 ft 2) in and weighs 84 kg (12 stone 9lbs).

Donna is admitted to the hospital ward for a minor surgical procedure; she is currently in a bay with five other female patients all recovering from surgery. She will be required to stay in hospital for 2–3 days following her procedure.

Upon admission Donna was routinely screened for MRSA as per Hospital Trust policy.

⚙ Activity 8.7   Evidence-based practice

You have received a telephone call from the Infection Control and Prevention Team within the hospital. Your patient Donna Davies (Case Study 8.3) has tested positive for MRSA.

What would be the immediate priorities required when caring for Donna knowing she is now positive for MRSA?

What things would you consider when preparing to inform Donna that she is MRSA positive?

What are the risks to Donna, other patients and staff?

What things would need to be considered when preparing to send Donna to theatre?

Donna will be discharged home in 2–3 days. What would need to be considered when discharging Donna home?

See end of chapter for model answers.

IMPLICATIONS FOR PRACTICE: SEPSIS

Sepsis is a common and potentially life-threatening condition triggered by the body's own response to infection. Sepsis most commonly occurs in response to bacterial infections of the lungs, urinary tract, abdominal organs or skin and soft tissues. If left untreated, this infection that can lead to shock, organ failure or death.

The Sepsis Trust estimates that in the UK sepsis claims at least 46,000 lives each year, with suggestions this figure may even be as high as 67,000. Sepsis is reported to cost the NHS somewhere between £1.5 billion and £2 billion each year, with further financial implications for the wider economy estimated to be as high as £15.6 billion (Sepsis Trust, 2017). In 2016 the National Institute for Health Care and Excellence produced Guideline NG51 for healthcare professionals which covers the recognition, diagnosis and early management of sepsis for all populations (NICE, 2016). Sepsis is a condition that can affect any patient presenting to any area of healthcare. Spotting signs of sepsis is not always easy: sometimes the patient can present with symptoms that look like influenza, gastroenteritis or a chest infection.

SPOTTING SEPSIS

All healthcare professionals should be aware of their own role in spotting and treating sepsis to ensure lives are saved. Sepsis should be considered if the patient:

- Presents with any signs of infection
- Triggers an early warning score
- Looks ill to a health professional or a relative

(Sepsis Trust, 2017)

TREATING SEPSIS

In 2002, following international collaboration, the Surviving Sepsis Campaign developed the 'Sepsis Six' guidance to support those caring for patients at risk of sepsis (Figure 8.11). The campaign has continued worldwide with the commitment to reducing mortality from severe sepsis and septic shock. This involves six elements: three treatments and three tests (within the first hour).

Tests:

- Taking blood cultures to identify the type of bacteria causing sepsis
- Taking a blood sample to assess the severity of sepsis
- Monitoring urine output to assess kidney function

Treatments:

- Giving antibiotics
- Giving fluids intravenously
- Giving oxygen if levels are low (<90%)

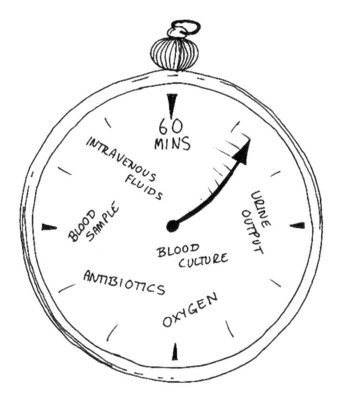

Figure 8.11   Sepsis Six guidance

CHAPTER SUMMARY

- The topic of control and prevention of infection is complex.
- For those working within health and social care practice, it is essential that you not only have the skills to practise safely, but also that you understand the implications poor practice can have on the patient/service user, yourself, your employer and the wider community.
- In the ongoing fight against infection, it is essential that all those working within health and social care, wherever the setting, work safely as prevention and management of infection is everyone's responsibility.

⚙ Activity model answers

Activity 8.1 Critical thinking

Based upon the Case Study 8.1 Mr Neville Jones.

Your immediate thoughts should be with the patient and providing fundamental nursing care. Mr Jones is presenting as clinically unwell and there are concerns relating to his temperature, pulse, respiration and blood pressure. The use of the appropriate monitoring in line with your employing organisation's protocols would be appropriate.

Considering the presenting symptoms of Mr Jones, there are concerns or a potential need for PPE to be worn. It is undetermined if Mr Jones has coronavirus although he is presenting with many of the atypical symptoms. It would be an appropriate case for testing and management.

Mr Jones is self-declaring that he has not been immunised against influenza and there is no mention of any uptake of vaccine for coronavirus. As healthcare professionals it is important that we make every contact count with our patients and service users and therefore this would be an opportunity to promote the vaccine uptake with Mr Jones once he recovers from this episode of illness.

Activity 8.4 Test your knowledge

1. Healthcare Associated Infections
2. Methicillin-resistant *Staphylococcus aureus*
3. Six
4. Clothing, gloves, aprons and gowns.
5. False, these are most likely to occur in hospital but can also occur in GP surgeries, care homes, mental health trusts, ambulances and in people's own homes.
6. Via hands, equipment and environment.
7. Gastrointestinal infections, however it can be part of normal gut flora and live in the body without causing harm. Certain antibiotics can cause the bacteria to produce toxins that cause diarrhoea.
8. Seven.
9. Control of Substances Hazardous to Health
10. False. The role of this legislation is to ensure that all hazardous substances used in healthcare settings are identified, labelled and stored safely.

Activity 8.6 Evidence-based practice

Wilfred, Annie and Daisy

- As a member of the nursing team what actions would you need to take in order to manage the situation properly?

Your priority would be to provide immediate care for Wilfred, Annie and Daisy.

You may consider asking if the symptoms are persisting.

Consider if there are any non-infectious reasons for the symptoms, for example medications.

Establish if any staff are affected; if so you may need to consider sending them home.

Consider contacting the doctor to examine the affected residents, initiate appropriate investigations and to offer provisional diagnosis.

Look up the outbreak plan, have isolation measures been started, do they reflect the guidance in the organisation's policies?

Do the affected residents have dedicated toilets or commodes?

Contact the Infection Prevention and Control Team for advice.

- As a member of the nursing team how are you going to protect yourself and reduce the risk that you might spread infection to other service users?

Follow standard precautions.

Wash hands regularly following the Ayliffe technique.

Wear protective clothing when dealing with affected residents.

Deal with any spillages/waste appropriately.

Ensure high-risk areas such as toilets are regularly inspected and cleaned.

Follow the infected laundry policy.

Ensure that there are supplies of PPE.

Allow only essential staff /resident movement.

Activity 8.7 Evidence-based practice

- What would be the immediate priorities required when caring for Donna knowing she is now positive for MRSA?

Consideration should be given to the position Donna occupies on the ward. If there is the ability to nurse her in a separate room this would be appropriate.

All nursing staff should be alerted and nursing care should be undertaken with the appropriate use of PPE.

(Continued)

- What things would you consider when preparing to inform Donna that she is MRSA positive?

Donna has mild learning difficulties, there is a need to consider the appropriate communication style and use of appropriate literature to inform Donna of her diagnosis. Consider if Donna's parents need to be present during the discussion with consent from Donna.

- What are the risks to Donna, other patients and staff?

MRSA is a transmissible infection, any vulnerable patients on the ward are at increased risk. The ward is a surgical ward and therefore patients are likely to have wounds, which increases the risk of infection.

- What things would need to be considered when preparing to send Donna to theatre?

Donna should be offered appropriate treatment for MRSA as per hospital protocol; the theatre team including the surgeon will need to be informed and there may be a potential need for the theatre slot to be changed to the last on the list followed up by the need for a deep clean. Alternatively Donna's minor procedure may be postponed until she is no longer MRSA positive.

- Donna will be discharged home in 2–3 days. What would need to be considered when discharging Donna home?

Following your organisation's protocol Donna may need to be discharged with a treatment regime and if there is a need for any community nursing follow-up there should be notification of the MRSA positive test.

FURTHER READING

WEBSITES

Researching these websites will enhance your understanding and deepen your knowledge of the prevention and control of infection:

- Sepsis: recognition, diagnosis and early management: www.nice.org.uk/guidance/ng51
- Healthcare-associated infections: www.nice.org.uk/guidance/cg139/chapter/key-priorities-for-implementation
- About the Surviving Sepsis Campaign: www.sccm.org/SurvivingSepsisCampaign/Home
- NHS Improvement: www.gov.uk/government/organisations/monitor/about

- Health and Social Care Act: www.gov.uk/government/uploads/system/ uploads/attachment_data/file/449049/Code_of_practice_280715_acc. pdf
- Care Quality Commission: www.cqc.org.uk/content/what-we-do
- NHS England Regional Teams: www.england.nhs.uk/about/regional-area-teams/
- Public Health England: www.england.nhs.uk/coronavirus/wp-content/ uploads/sites/52/2021/03/C1116-supporting-excellence-in-ipc-behaviours-imp-toolkit.pdf
- World Health Organization: www.who.int/

VIDEOS

- Infection Control (Handwashing): www.youtube.com/watch?v=0skgEnZzE5I
- Infection Prevention and Control Best Practice: www.youtube.com/ watch?v=0p-kJuRaBpY

Sepsis Six – six interventions for patients who are suffering severe sepsis: www.youtube.com/watch?v=NKtiC0HRrqc

BOOKS

- Tilmouth, T., Davies, E. and Williams, B. (2011) *Foundation Degree in Health and Social Care.* London: Hodder Education.
- Waugh, A. and Grant, A. (2014) *Anatomy and Physiology in Health and Illness* (12th edn). London: Churchill Livingstone.

REFERENCES

Ayliffe, G.A.J., Babb, J.R. and Quoraishi, H. (1978) A test for 'hygienic' hand disinfection. *Journal of Clinical Pathology*, 31: 923–8.

Department of Health (2013a) *Managing Regulated Medical Waste.* Available at: www.health.ny.gov/facilities/waste/

Department of Health (2013b) *Health Care Waste Management Manual.* Available at: www.doh.gov.ph/sites/default/files/publications/Health_Care_Waste_ Management_Manual.pdf

Department of Health (2015) *The Health and Social Care Act 2008: Code of Practice on the Prevention and Control of Infections and Related Guidance.* Available at: www. gov.uk/government/uploads/system/uploads/attachment_data/file/449049/ Code_of_practice_280715_acc.pdf

HSE (Health and Safety Executive) (1992) *Personal Protective Equipment (PPE).* Available at: www.hse.gov.uk/toolbox/ppe.htm

HSE (Health and Safety Executive) (2011) *Latex Allergies in Health and Social Care.* Available at: www.hse.gov.uk/healthservices/latex/

Loveday, H.P. (2014) Epic 3: national evidence-based guidelines for preventing healthcare associated infections in NHS hospitals in England. *Journal of Hospital Infection*, 86S1: S1–S70.

NCIRD (National Centre for Immunization and Respiratory Diseases) (2020) Human coronavirus types. Available at: www.cdc.gov/coronavirus/types.html

NHS Choices (2017) Benefits of breastfeeding. Available at: www.nhs.uk/condi tions/pregnancy-and-baby/Pages/benefits-breastfeeding.aspx

NICE (National Institute for Health and Care Excellence) (2016) Sepsis: Recognition, diagnosis and early management. Guideline NG51. Available at: www.nice.org. uk/guidance/NG51

NMC (Nursing and Midwifery Council) (2018) *The Code: Professional Standards of Practice and Behaviour for Nurses, Midwives and Nursing Associates*. Available at: www.nmc.org.uk/standards/code/

Osorio, N. Oliveira, A. Oliveira, V. Costa, P. Gama, F. (2019) Tourniquets used in peripheral venepuncture as a potential vehicle for transmission of microorgan-isms: scoping review. *Portuguese Journal of Infection* DOI:10.22354/in.v24i2.839

PHE (Public Health England) (2016) *Healthcare Associated Infections (HAI): Point Prevalence Survey, England*. Available at: www.gov.uk/government/publications/ healthcare-associated-infections-hcai-point-prevalence-survey-england

RCN (Royal College of Nursing) (2012) Sharpes Safety. Available at: www.rcn.org. uk/professional-development/publications/pub-004135

RCN (Royal College of Nursing) (2014) *The Management of Waste from Health, Social and Personal Care*. London: RCN.

RCN (Royal College of Nursing) and Infection Prevention Society (IPS) (2016) *Infection Prevention and Control Commissioning Toolkit*. Available at: www.rcn.org. uk/professional-development/publications/pub-005375#detailTab

RIDDOR (Reporting of Injuries, Diseases and Dangerous Occurrences Regulations) (2013) Available at: www.hse.gov.uk/pubns/indg453.htm

Sepsis Trust (2017) Available at: http://sepsistrust.org/

Sunley, K., Gallagher, R., Reidy, P. and Dunn, H. (2017) Essential practice for infection prevention and control. Available at: www.rcn.org.uk/Professional-Development/publications/pub-005940

WHO (World Health Organization) (2006) Five moments for hand hygiene. Available at: www.who.int/campaigns/world-hand-hygiene-day

WHO (World Health Organization) (2009) *First Global Patient Safety Challenge Clean Care is Safe Care*. World Health Organization Guidelines on Hand Hygiene in Healthcare. Geneva: WHO.

WHO (World Health Organization) (2020) Antibiotic resistance. Available at: www. who.int/news-room/fact-sheets/detail/antibiotic-resistance

WHO (World Health Organization) (2021) Severe Acute Respiratory Syndrome (SARS). Available at: www.who.int/health-topics/severe-acute-respiratory-syndrome#tab=tab_1

9

ESSENTIAL SKILLS FOR CARE

GILLIAN ROWE

STANDARDS OF PROFICIENCY FOR NURSING ASSOCIATES (2018)

Relevant Platforms include:

Platform 1:1.14 Demonstrate the ability to keep complete, clear, accurate and timely records.

Platform 3:3.4 Demonstrate the knowledge, communication and relationship management skills required to provide people, families and carers with accurate information that meets their needs before, during and after a range of interventions.

Platform 3:3.6 Demonstrate the knowledge, skills and ability to perform a range of nursing procedures and manage devices, to meet people's need for safe effective and person-centred care.

Platform 3:3.7 Demonstrate and apply an understanding of how and when to escalate to the appropriate professional for expert help and advice.

Platform 3:3.8 Demonstrate and apply an understanding of how people's needs for safety, dignity, privacy, comfort and sleep can be met.

Platform 3:3.9 Demonstrate the knowledge, skills and ability required to meet people's needs in terms of nutrition, hydration, and bladder and bowel health.

Platform 3:3.10 Demonstrate the knowledge, skills and ability to act as required to meet people's needs related to mobility, hygiene, oral care, wound care and skin integrity.

Platform 3:3.11 Demonstrate the ability to recognise when a person's condition has improved or deteriorated by undertaking health monitoring. Interpret, promptly respond, share findings and escalate as needed.

Platform 3:3.12 Demonstrate the knowledge and skills required to support people with commonly encountered symptoms including anxiety, confusion, discomfort and pain.

(Continued)

Platform 4:4.4 Demonstrate the ability to effectively and responsibly access, input and apply information and data using a range of methods including digital technologies, and share appropriately within interdisciplinary teams.

Platform 5:5.1 Understand and apply the principles of health and safety legislation and regulations and maintain safe work and care environments.

Platform 5:5.3 Accurately undertake risk assessments, using contemporary assessment tools.

Platform 5:5.4 Respond to and escalate potential hazards that may affect the safety of people.

Annex A 1.1–1.13, 2.4–2.9, 4.1–4.4.

Annex B 1.1, 1.2, 1.4, 1.5, 1.8, 2.1–2.6, 3.1–3.5, 4.1–4.4, 5.1–5.4, 6.1–6.4, 7.2, 7.4, 9.1–9.3, 10–10.10.

I'm not telling you it's going to be easy; I'm telling you it's going to be worth it.

Art Williams

This chapter will introduce you to the skills you need to become an effective nursing associate or healthcare practitioner. Whilst it is beyond the scope of this handbook to cover all of the clinical investigations you are likely to undertake (such as ECG or venepuncture), I have considered the most common activities that you will engage in. As you work through the chapter, you will develop an understanding of the risks and hazards of clinical care and how to prepare both yourself and your patient for clinical observations. You will examine the importance of accurate record keeping and widen your knowledge of interpreting physiological measurements.

You will have a Practice Assessment Document (PAD), which details your skills development and is an ongoing record of your achievements. The NA PAD has been developed to ensure that student nursing associates are prepared to successfully meet the Standards of proficiency for nursing associates (NMC Code, 2018). Figure 9.1 is a table of expected achievements in order to complete your qualification.

This document will contain details of your placement initial, mid point and final interviews and record your working and learning activities (episodes of care and medicines management), you may also have an Ongoing Achievement Record (OAR) if you are training through a university. This chapter will support your confidence in performing your skills.

Criteria for Assessment in Practice – Overall Framework Years 1 & 2

Guided participation in care and performing with increasing knowledge, skills and confidence.

Year 1

Practising independently with minimal supervision, provides and monitors care, demonstrating increasing knowledge skills and confidence.

Year 2

Guided participation in care and performing with increasing knowledge, skills and confidence.

Year 1

Practising independently with minimal supervision, provides and monitors care, demonstrating increasing knowledge, skills and confidence.

Year 2

PAD 1: Guided participation in Care

'Achieved' must be obtained in all three criteria by the student by the end of the year.

Achieved	Knowledge	Skills	Attitude and values
YES	Is able to identify the appropriate knowledge base required to deliver safe, person-centred care under some guidance.	In commonly encountered situations is able to utilise appropriate skills in the delivery of person-centred care with some guidance.	Is able to demonstrate a professional attitude in delivering person-centred care. Demonstrates positive engagement with own learing.
NO	Is not able to demonstrate an adequate knowledge base and has significant gaps in understanding, leading to poor practice.	Under direct supervision is not able to demonstrate safe practice in delivering care despite repeated guidance and prompting in familiar taks.	Inconsistent professional attitude towards others and lacks self-awareness. Is not asking questions nor engaging with own learning needs.

PAD 2: Provides and monitors care with minimal guidance and increasing confidence.

'Achieved' must be obtained in all three criteria by the student by the end of the year.

Achieved	Knowledge	Skills	Attitude and Values
YES	Has a sound knowledge base to support safe and effective practice and provide the rationale to support decision making.	Utilises a range of skills to provide and monitor safe, person-centred and evidence-based care with increased confidence and in range of contexts.	Demonstrates an understanding of professional roles and responsibilities within the multidisciplinary team. Maximises opportunities to extend own knowledge.
NO	Has a superficial knowledge base and is unable to provide a rationale for care, demonstrating unsafe practice.	With supervision is not able to provide safe care and is unable to perform the activity and/or follow instructions despite repeated guidance.	Demonstrates lack of self-awareness and understanding of professional role and responsibilities. Is not asking appropriate questions nor engaged with their own learning.

Figure 9.1   Criteria for assessment in practice

Glossary

- **Clinical waste** This includes 'sharps', such as needles, bodily fluids and used dressings, and used PPE
- **Consent and the patient's rights** The patient's agreement to receive care, interventions and procedures
- **Fluid balance** The measurement of fluids going into the body and fluids being excreted from the body
- **Health and Safety at Work Act 1974 (HASWA)** This legislation applies to the safety of yourself, your colleagues and the people you support
- **Indication** The use of that drug for treating a particular disease
- **Observations and physiological monitoring** Measuring vital signs
- **Stress and resilience** The ability to deal with the pressure of working and studying

INTRODUCTION

This chapter is about the essential skills you will need in your day-to-day work: such as assessing risks and judging hazards with an eye on legislation and promoting good practice. All work for health and care takes place within a framework of legislation; this chapter discusses health and safety legislation applied to health and social care. This is to ensure you and your patients are kept safe when undertaking monitoring activities. You will learn how to take physiological measurements to monitor your patient's health and to aid diagnosis. These skills need to be practised under supervision until you have been assessed competent to practise. Developing clinical skills is hard work, but as Art Williams (quoted above) states, it is worth the effort. The more confident you are in your skills, the more effective you will be in your practice. The NMC Code asks you to treat people as individuals and uphold their dignity, you should:

1.1 Treat people with kindness, respect and compassion

1.2 Make sure you deliver the fundamentals of care effectively

1.3 Avoid making assumptions and recognise diversity and individual choice

1.4 Make sure that any treatment, assistance or care for which you are responsible is delivered without undue delay

1.5 Respect and uphold people's human rights

The Code continues, 'The fundamentals of care include, but are not limited to, nutrition, hydration, bladder and bowel care, physical handling and making sure that those receiving care are kept in clean and hygienic conditions. It includes making sure that those receiving care have adequate access to nutrition and hydration and making sure that you provide help to those who are not able to feed themselves or drink fluid unaided.'

Part 2 of the Code considers that the patient is a partner in their care (2.1) and should be consulted and empowered (2.3) to make healthy choices, but that you should accept that patients have the right to refuse care if they so choose (2.5).

HEALTH AND SAFETY AT WORK

What is a risk and what is a hazard?

A hazard is an object that can potentially do harm, and risk is the likelihood of harm occurring. Healthcare work is classed as a hazardous occupation due to the nature of the work. The potential for infection is high. The latest figures available from the Health and Safety Executive (HSE) cite 'infection rates of about 30 per 100,000 workers per year amongst nurses and about 100 per 100,000 per year amongst care workers in residential homes' (HSE, 2016, 2021a). There were about 5 million lost working days (1.78 days per worker) due to work-related illness and injury in the health and social care sector (pre Covid). This is one of the highest levels in any employment sector. Chapter 8, Prevention and Control of Infection, gives greater detail on self-protection. Although, statistically, the infection rates have not changed over the last few years, work-related health issues such as stress and anxiety have significantly increased (HSE, 2021b).

In the time of Covid, work-related stress has been an almost intolerable burden and workers need to manage their stress to avoid burnout.

Employers and employees must abide by the Health and Safety at Work Act 1974 (HASWA) and its many amendments and regulations by providing you with a safe working environment, protective equipment and health and safety training. Employers or their designated persons must carry out risk assessments and put control measures in place to reduce risks to all people who use, visit or work in their setting. You, as an employee, are obligated to take reasonable care of yourself and others, and not put yourself or others at risk by your actions or inactions, and you must cooperate with your employer on health and safety matters.

Your employer should risk assess procedures and produce guidance for you to follow. You should understand these protocols are there to protect you and your patients. However, you too should risk assess each activity to ensure you are engaging in safe working practice and are monitoring the risk and modifying the process if it is needed.

LEGISLATION

Control of risk from biohazardous agents rests with the employer but each employee is bound by the Control of Substances Hazardous to Health 2002 (COSHH) legislation. Patients are at risk from care workers through healthcare-associated infections (HCAIs) (see Chapter 8), especially now that so many infectious agents are becoming resistant to antibiotics.

Staff are at great risk of needlestick injuries and attention needs to be paid when drawing up, giving and removing needles. It is easy to be distracted and then accidents happen. Safe disposal of used needles and syringes should be in accordance with infection control protocols; they are usually put into a sharps box. The risk from non safety needles is highest overall and the people most likely to receive a sharps injury are the cleaning staff, when sharps are not properly disposed of (Unison, 2018). The most common risks of sharps contamination are hepatitis B (HBV), hepatitis C (HCV) and human immunodeficiency virus (HIV). Workplace vaccination is mandatory to protect healthcare workers.

Any workplace accidents need to be recorded and reported under the Reporting of Injuries, Diseases and Dangerous Occurrences Regulations 2013 (RIDDOR). The forms used are provided by the HSE and this is a legal document which is submissible in a court of law.

Staff are also at risk when moving and handling patients. You should receive special training to prevent damage both to yourself and your patients (Manual Handling Operations Regulations 1992). Legislation in the form of the Provision and Use of Work Equipment Regulations 1998 (PUWER) and the Lifting Operations and Lifting Equipment Regulations 1998 (LOLER) are regulations to support safe working practice. You should never undertake the use of mechanical lifting equipment until you have received training on each piece of equipment and, if relevant, how to use and check slings. You will also need training for safe manual handling and the use of such aids as transfer belts and sliding sheets. Your trainer should provide you with a certificate of competence when you have been assessed and this should be renewed annually.

Patients at risk of falls should be assessed using the 'timed up and go test' or 'turn 180° test'. Timed up and go times how long it takes an individual to get up and walk 3 metres: if it takes them longer than 15 seconds, they are at risk of falls. The turn 180° test asks the patient to turn around by 180 degrees: if it takes more than four steps, they are at risk of falls. Frail patients should be assessed using the Electronic Frailty Index (eFI): this is cumulative deficit model for patients over age 65, using information gathered from the patient's primary care records. Information such as clinical signs and symptoms, diseases, disability and vulnerability are entered into the e-system to predict likelihood of falls.

In 2020, 30% of all non-fatal accidents in health and social care settings were musculoskeletal injuries (HSE, 2021c). Read Scenario 9.1 and think about how correct attention to health and safety could have prevented this incident.

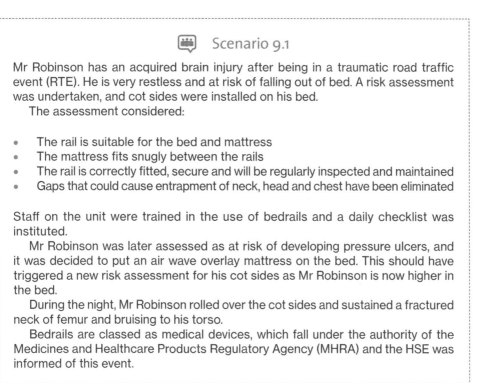

Scenario 9.1

Mr Robinson has an acquired brain injury after being in a traumatic road traffic event (RTE). He is very restless and at risk of falling out of bed. A risk assessment was undertaken, and cot sides were installed on his bed.
The assessment considered:

- The rail is suitable for the bed and mattress
- The mattress fits snugly between the rails
- The rail is correctly fitted, secure and will be regularly inspected and maintained
- Gaps that could cause entrapment of neck, head and chest have been eliminated

Staff on the unit were trained in the use of bedrails and a daily checklist was instituted.
Mr Robinson was later assessed as at risk of developing pressure ulcers, and it was decided to put an air wave overlay mattress on the bed. This should have triggered a new risk assessment for his cot sides as Mr Robinson is now higher in the bed.
During the night, Mr Robinson rolled over the cot sides and sustained a fractured neck of femur and bruising to his torso.
Bedrails are classed as medical devices, which fall under the authority of the Medicines and Healthcare Products Regulatory Agency (MHRA) and the HSE was informed of this event.

Go Further 9.1

Type 'bedrail assessment' into a search engine and you will find free resources which are useful in ensuring that you understand safe practice with bedrails. If your patients use bedrails in your setting, ask for training to assess the bedrails and ensure that you have a recording method in place for monitoring their safety.

COMMUNICATION

Ensure that before engaging in an activity, you explain the purpose to the patient. Use clear concise language, do not use acronyms of technical terms. The NMC Code (2018) explains that you should 'take reasonable steps to meet people's language and communication needs, providing, wherever possible, assistance to those who need help to communicate their own or other people's needs' (7.2) and you should also 'use a range of verbal and non-verbal communication methods, and consider cultural sensitivities, to better understand and respond to people's personal and health needs' (7.3). The Code then states you should 'check people's understanding from time to time to keep misunderstanding or mistakes to a minimum' (7.4). Thus, the patient is more likely to consent to an activity if they understand why it is taking place, and you can reassure any anxiety they may experience: 'recognise when people are anxious or in distress and respond compassionately and politely' (2.6).

PATIENTS' RIGHTS

Before you undertake any activity with your patient, you must receive consent. Patients have fundamental legal and ethical rights to determine what happens to their own bodies; also, seeking consent is a matter of common courtesy. Discuss what you are going to do and say why you need to do it. Explain carefully, using language the patient understands. The NMC Code requires you to 'use terms that people in your care, colleagues and the public can understand' (7.1). Remember that consent must be voluntary and informed. If the activity is going to be uncomfortable, say so, don't lie, or imply the patient is being difficult if they complain they are uncomfortable. If patients are properly prepared, they are more likely to give valid consent. The NMC Code states: 'make sure that you get properly informed consent and document it before carrying out any action' (4.2). Documenting consent is essential in case anything untoward occurs during or after the procedure, or if a complaint arises.

When taking repeated observations or measurements, ask for consent each time, do not assume that agreeing to the procedure once is an implicit consent for continued observations or measurements. The same applies to any activity you do for or with the patient. For example, good oral hygiene promotes good health and supports the immune system; consent should be sought when supporting a patient with oral hygiene, rather than assuming the patients is happy for you to remove or replace dentures.

If the patient is incapable of giving consent, remember that any activities should be in their 'best interests', and you should seek permission (in writing and recorded) from a family member or mental capacity advocate. Table 9.1 tells you who can give consent.

Table 9.1   What is consent and who can give it

The parents of a child under the age of 14

A child of 14 or over who is assessed as 'Gillick competent'

Any adult over the age of 18 has a right under common law to grant or withhold consent to examination/investigation or treatment, except in certain special circumstances, such as those with a community treatment order (CTO) under the Mental Health Act 2007 (amended 2008)

Competent adults also have a right to refuse procedures or treatment for reasons that are 'rational, irrational or for no reason'

Consent must not be induced by force or fraud, neither must the withholding or withdrawing of consent during an examination, investigation or treatment affect the quality of care the patient receives

Those of you who have supported many clients and patients with personal hygiene will understand that bodies come in many shapes, sizes and colours and that 'normal' is an indefinite term. However, knowing what the range of 'normal' looks like will help you to recognise 'abnormal' when you see it. Supporting patients with personal care (bed bathing, etc.) is an opportunity to check for anything that might have been missed, such as signs of abuse or other non-diagnosed ailments and is therefore a learning opportunity to be embraced.

MAKING CLINICAL OBSERVATIONS AND MONITORING VITAL SIGNS

WEIGHT AND NUTRITION

It is important to monitor your patients' weight (see below) but you should also monitor what they are eating and record their daily consumption. For this you could use a Malnutrition Universal Screening Tool (MUST). Quite often, obese or underweight adults are suffering from malnutrition either because they are not eating enough or because they are eating cheap energy-dense foods that lack vital nutrients. Poor quality foods can affect the patient's immune system, which can impair wound healing and delay recovery (see Chapter 6, Bioscience, for more detail). Excess weight can promote type 2 diabetes and add to the risk of developing heart disease; being overweight can also lead to depression and poor self-image which can lead to self-neglect. Activity 9.1 shows you how to calculate someone's BMI using different methods.

Nutritional support may be needed if the patient has issues with swallowing. This can include thickening agents, soft diet, or artificial feeding systems such as enteral or parenteral nutrition.

⚙️ Activity 9.1

To calculate a BMI:

- First: divide weight in kilograms (kg) by height in metres (m)
- Then: divide the answer by height again to get the BMI

$$BMI = \frac{Weight\ (Kg)}{Height\ (m)^2}$$

A BMI in the 20–25 range is desirable, below 18 is underweight and over 30 is very obese.

For example, Mrs Brown is 5 foot 2 inches tall and weighs 12 stone. What is her BMI?

(Continued)

Change her weight and height into metric:

Height: 5 ft 2 in = 1.58 metres

Weight: 12 stone = 168 lbs = 76.2 kg

Therefore: 76.2 ÷ 1.58 = 48.2

48.2 ÷ 1.58 = 30.5 therefore her BMI is 30.5

If the patient does not know their height or weight, or is unable to communicate, you can estimate their BMI by taking a measurement of their mid-arm circumference. If it is greater than 32 cm they are likely to be overweight, if it is under 23 cm, they are likely to be underweight.

LIMITATIONS OF BMI

Measuring BMI is a good indicator, but it does have its limitations, especially with athletes and for the elderly. For athletes, a BMI may overestimate the amount of fat and for the elderly it may underestimate the amount of fat due to muscle loss. Measuring waist circumference helps screen for possible health risks that come with obesity, therefore measuring waist and hips can give a better indication of health risk: a waist size that is greater than 35 inches for women or greater than 40 inches for men can indicate a risk of type 2 diabetes and heart disease.

PREPARING FOR OBSERVATION

When you first see your patient, employ what has been called 'the medical gaze' (Foucault, 1963). This is looking for 'telling signs' and reading your patient's body language. Look at their demeanour (sad, tired, happy, in pain, tearful), the way they sit or lie, their skin colour (pallor, flushed, sweaty).

Recent weight loss or gain can be judged by looking at the patient's clothing: is it loose or tight? Look at the patient's hands, are rings loose or tight?

They may have been neglecting themselves: do they look clean and well cared for or do their clothes look unkempt? Do they smell unpleasantly, is their hair clean and brushed?

What about their breath? Have they cleaned their teeth or dentures? Breath smelling of acetone (smells like they have been sucking pear drops) can indicate diabetes.

Are their eyes red rimmed and rheumy, are the whites of their eyes red? They may have an eye infection.

When you speak to the patient, ask how they are, does their response match your summation of their condition? Quite often people will try to put on a brave face, they don't like to be a bother, or feel embarrassed if they need pain relief or need help with an activity they can normally do themselves.

PREPARING THE ENVIRONMENT

Ensure the area is private to maintain the patient's dignity, quiet, free from draughts, is well lit and that the patient is comfortable. Also, check the area is free from risks or hazards to you and the patient. You have responsibilities under the Health and Safety at Work Act 1974. Table 9.2 tells you what some of these are.

Table 9.2   Health and Safety at Work Act 1974 (HASWA)

Take reasonable care for your own health and safety and for others who may be affected by what you do or do not do
Cooperate with your employer on health and safety
Correctly use work items provided by your employer, including personal protective equipment, in accordance with training or instructions
Do not interfere with or misuse anything provided for your health and safety or welfare

Source: www.hse.gov.uk (2017, 2021)

PREPARING YOURSELF

Physical contact with patients carries risk of contamination and therefore you need to be wearing personal protective equipment (PPE) (see also Chapter 8). Your employer is legally obliged provide such things as single use vinyl gloves and aprons. Some organisations still use latex gloves, but these are being phased out due to the number of allergies they provoke in staff. In order to reduce cross-infection and contamination, it is vital that you use PPE and change it every time you move on to another patient. You may need to wear a face mask and gown if the patient is infectious and, in some cases, white boots need to be worn too. Depending on the patient's condition, these may be kept inside their room if you are 'barrier nursing' (protecting yourself from the patient) or outside their room if you are 'reverse barrier' nursing (protecting the patient from you).

TO GLOVE OR NOT TO GLOVE

Overuse of gloves can put you at risk of work-related contact dermatitis, therefore current advice (RCN, 2019) is to risk assess the activity to decide if glove use is appropriate. If you develop dermatitis, you should inform your line manager who might move you to a non-clinical area while your hands are treated. The RCN considers that glove use is 'often unnecessary' and could instead lead to poor hand hygiene, thus increasing the risk of infection. Its guidance does state that gloves should be worn if there is a risk of coming into contact with blood/body fluid, non-intact skin, or mucus and mucus membranes, and when using certain chemicals such as disinfectants, preserving agents or cytotoxic drugs (RCN, 2019).

ASEPTIC NON-TOUCH TECHNIQUE

ANTT is the use of aseptic technique without wearing sterile gloves. ANTT should be considered for invasive clinical procedures, such as inserting or accessing intravenous (IV) devices, phlebotomy, urinary catheterisation, wound dressings, minor surgical procedures and biopsies.

The main principles are:

A: Always ensure hands are decontaminated effectively prior to the procedure

N: Never contaminate key parts of sterile equipment

T: Touch non-key parts with confidence

T: Take appropriate infection prevention and control (IPC) precautions at all times

For ANTT procedures, the immediate environment needs to be considered, such as using a clinical room; if the procedure takes place by the bedside, ensure that a sterile field is created, and hand decontamination takes place before and after the procedure. Further in-depth details of ANTT procedures can be found in Chapter 8.

HANDWASHING

Handwashing is the most significant procedure in preventing cross-infection, this prevents cross-contamination between patients and between staff and patients.

Handwashing is critical to infection control. Chapter 8, Prevention and Control of Infection, goes into this in greater detail and describes the correct 12-step procedure (see Figure 8.6 in Chapter 8). It also discusses the use of cleansing gels, but remember they are not a substitute for handwashing, but complementary to washing. Wash your hands before and after any patient contact (Table 9.3). During the time of Covid, many healthcare workers suffered from chapped sore hands which carried the risk of contamination (to themselves and others); invest in a good quality unperfumed hand cream and use it as often as possible.

Table 9.3   Handwashing: Remember ...

Before doing anything... Wash your hands (Figure 9.2)
After doing anything... Wash your hands
And wear PPE

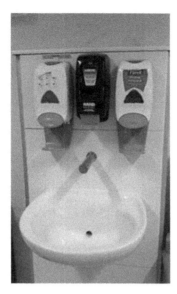

Figure 9.2   Washing your hands

Your employer should provide 'clinical hazard' bags (usually bright yellow) for you to place used PPE in. These bags need to be collected by a specialist company who are licensed by the local authority to dispose of the contents safely. The bags therefore need to be stored safely until collection.

Ensure that you have a nurse's fob watch (cheap from online sources and some organisations give them away free). Some watches can be removed from the rubber or plastic case so that the case can be cleaned to reduce the risk of cross-infection. Please do not use your mobile phone as a timing device as it will become a source of contamination and you will put yourself and anyone else who uses your phone at risk.

PREPARING THE EQUIPMENT

Make sure you have enough space and the right resources to undertake the measurement and that any electrical equipment you are using has been recently PAT tested (PAT = Portable Appliance Testing) and is functioning. If it is battery powered, ensure you have spare batteries in case of malfunction, or that it has been properly charged and has been stored in a safe place. Any broken or faulty equipment must be reported as soon as possible, and a faulty sign appended to it to warn others.

PREPARING THE PATIENT

Prior to your measuring their vital signs, the patient should have the opportunity to sit for approximately 5 minutes to calm them down, especially if you have asked the patient to walk from one area to another. This will allow their blood pressure to resolve while they are resting and give an accurate resting pulse. If you leave the patient to rest, ensure that you come back within 10 minutes at the most. Any longer than that and the patient may become anxious as they will think they have been forgotten, which could give misleading high blood pressure results.

The patient should be asked to, or assisted to, loosen clothing or remove arm coverings (cardigans/jumpers) ready for you to take their blood pressure. Also, if you are taking the patient's blood pressure, ensure they visit the toilet first, as a full bladder increases blood pressure and can give a false reading. The patient should be sitting comfortably and not on the edge of a bed if there is a risk of falling. Ensure that you remember the four Rs when taking the observations:

- **Respect** the patient's dignity and privacy
- **Reassure** the patient in a manner that minimises fears or concerns
- **Record** the results
- **Report** any concerns

MEASURING VITAL SIGNS

Physiological measurements are an important part of your caring role because they allow the patient's condition to be monitored and ensure prompt detection of adverse events, deteriorating or developing conditions. These are essential skills, included in your PAD 1 and 2 (Professional Values P1–8), and referenced in both the NMC standards and the AP standards of care.

WHAT IS NORMAL?

Biomarker measurement ranges are arrived at by taking mass measurements and arriving at a median. For instance: normal temperature (98.4°F/36°C) was determined by Carl Wunderlich (in the early nineteenth century) by taking the temperature of 25,000 patients. He also noted that normal temperature varies through the circadian cycle and is consistently lower in older individuals – something that is not always acknowledged when considering fever in the elderly.

PAIN

Pain is not a normal daily event and is always an indicator that something is not right, therefore any pain is abnormal and is an indicator of the presence of an ailment. Patients should be assessed for the presence of pain, and it should be treated promptly and effectively. It can adversely affect measurement accuracy in the same way that anxiety can, possibly leading to a misdiagnosis. You should have an understanding of the factors that may influence a patient's experience and expression of pain (this can be culturally mediated); it can also be age mediated, as older people can experience multiple or concurrent causes of pain and yet are less likely to report it. Pain assessment tools are many and varied, which tool is used will depend on your organisation; it should be used and applied consistently, and the results documented. Acute pain should be reported and escalated.

Chronic persistent pain is pain that lasts more than three months. NICE (2021b) recently updated their guidelines on the management of primary pain: this is when the cause of the pain is unclear (secondary pain is the type of chronic pain caused by underlying conditions such as osteoarthritis, rheumatoid arthritis, ulcerative colitis). Rather than paracetamol or non-steroidal anti-inflammatory (NSAID) drugs, benzodiazepines or opioids, NICE recommend exercise programmes, psychological therapies such as cognitive behavioural therapy (CBT) and acceptance and commitment therapy (ACT). Acupuncture is also considered as an option.

Pain can prevent the patient from getting a restorative night's sleep. Support patients with suitable pain relief to minimise insomnia.

WEIGHT

Patients should be weighed when they enter your setting, and in residential care settings, they should be weighed each month to monitor their overall health. Weight loss or gain can be indicative of an underlying health issue which can be psychological and/or physical. Unplanned weight loss is an acute risk factor and may indicate an underlying health condition such as diabetes.

MEASUREMENT OF PHYSIOLOGICAL PARAMETERS

The NEWS2 (National Early Warning Score, updated in 2017) chart (Table 9.4) has replaced previous recording charts as it is more dynamic in assisting diagnosis. It is traffic light colour coded showing warning (amber) and danger (red) areas which should alert you to a patient's condition. This gives an aggregated score showing areas of risk. A downloadable version of the NEWS2 chart can be found at www.rcplondon.ac.uk/projects/outputs/national-early-warning-score-news. All Trusts have been obliged to use this scoring system since March 2019 and training can be found at www.e-lfh.org.uk/recognising-and-managing-deterioration-elearning-a-free-programme-for-all-health-and-social-care-professionals/. This system has been improved to aid early diagnosis of septicaemia.

Table 9.4   National Early Warning Scores (NEWS2)

The physiological parameters which form the basis of the scoring system are:

1. Respiratory rate
2. Oxygen saturations
3. Temperature
4. Systolic blood pressure
5. Pulse rate
6. Level of consciousness

Source: Royal College of Physicians. National Early Warning Score (NEWS) 2: Standardising the assessment of acute-illness severity in the NHS. Updated report of a working party. London: RCP, 2017.

TEMPERATURE

The normal body temperature of a person varies depending on gender, recent activity, food and fluid consumption, time of day, and for women, the stage of the menstrual cycle. Older people or people with disabilities that restrict movement have a lower 'normal or usual' temperature. It also changes depending on the site in the body where the reading is taken. A rectal reading will be higher than one taken in the axilla (armpit). Therefore, when taking a reading it is important to be consistent in the chosen site (oral, aural, rectal, axillary). Aural thermometers quite often have single use plastic covers to prevent cross-infection and these are to be preferred where possible. Tempa-dot thermometers are single use and need to be disposed of safely and to organisational convention.

It is also important to use the same device to ensure accuracy, whether it is a digital or chemical tool, as the reading will differ by as much as 1 degree. Some settings use liquid crystal scan strips which are placed on the forehead; while these are safer than glass thermometers, they are not known for their accuracy, whereas the Tempa-dot chemical thermometers are more accurate than the strips, but not as accurate as an aural or rectal thermometer.

It is important that you understand what temperature is. Body temperature is generated by heat produced through movement and metabolic activity; it is regulated in the hypothalamus area of the brain and the brain is informed by thermoreceptors in muscles and the liver and sensory receptors in the peripheral nervous system. Thermoregulation is a negative feedback system and is one of the functions of homeostasis.

When preparing to take the temperature, do not do it after the patient has just had a hot or chilled drink, smoked a cigarette, had a hot bath/shower or engaged in moderate/vigorous exercise as this will give a false high or low reading, which can lead to an incorrect diagnosis and inappropriate treatment. An inaccurate reading will also be given if you do not leave the thermometer in place for long enough, or in the case of a tympanic thermometer, not insert it correctly. Look at Table 9.5 to see what normal and abnormal temperature is.

Table 9.5   Temperature gradients for children and adults

Normal temperature	36–37.5°C
Hypothermia	<35°C
Low grade pyrexia	38–39.5°C
Moderate to high pyrexia	38–40°C
Hyperpyrexia	40+°C

PULSE

The pulse is the pressure wave of blood moving through pliable arteries, and a reading can be taken at pulse points where an artery passes over a bone. This is a fairly accurate way to assess the condition of the heart and circulatory system. The reading will indicate the number of heart beats and can also be used to examine the strength of the beat (full and bounding/ weak and thready) and the regularity of the beat. Various machines can count the pulse, but they cannot give this additional information, so it is always useful to do a manual pulse check as well as a digital reading.

Compress the chosen artery with two fingers, ease off the pressure slightly as you do not want to cut off the blood flow, and using a watch, time your count for a full 60 seconds. This will give you the resting heart rate. Table 9.6 gives the range of pulse rates.

The pulse rate changes often and rapidly. It is affected by caffeine, smoking, exercise, stress, anxiety, fever, weight and medication.

Table 9.6   Pulse rates

	Beats per minutes
Babies	100–160
Young children	60–140
Adolescents and adults	60–80
Athletes	40–60
Bradycardia	Less than 60
Tachycardia	More than 100

RESPIRATION

Breathing is the act of inhaling oxygen-rich air and exhaling carbon-dioxide-rich air. Oxygen is attached to red blood cells in the alveoli of the lungs for transportation around the body and is then used in cellular respiration. Pulse and respiration are related because the heart and lungs work together. Normally, an increase or decrease in one causes the same effect on the other.

Observing someone breathing can lead to them breathing more rapidly, so try to be surreptitious about it. There isn't a machine that can do this, so you must practise breathing observation and counting breaths over a minute by watching the patient's chest rise and fall. Note that *one breath = breathing in and out.*

Respiration rates may increase with fever; also note whether a person has any difficulty breathing such as dyspnoea, stridor, stertor (while sleeping), wheezing, rasping, or chest noises that could indicate a chest infection, asthma, bronchitis or COPD (chronic obstructive pulmonary disease – emphysema). Patients with bronchial ailments such as asthma may have inhalers to take medication; these are usually classed as preventers and relievers, although there are combination long-acting inhalers available. Children need to be supported to use these especially if they have a spacer. Bronchodilators can also be administered via nebuliser mask or mouthpiece: these convert drugs into a fine spray using an oxygen or compressed air nebuliser.

Peak flow meters measure the speed of expelled air (peak expiratory flow test or PEF) as an assessment of lung function – especially used by people with asthma. The test can be used to assess how effective medication is at controlling asthma attacks. Patients should always use the same peak flow device as different peak flow meters might give different readings. The patient should be either sitting upright or standing when they use the device to achieve best lung expansion. A disposable mouthpiece should be used each time the meter is employed. The slide counter should be pulled back to nearest to the mouthpiece, the mouthpiece should be held in a horizontal position, the patient then takes a deep breath, places the meter in their mouth, ensuring the lips make a good seal, then blows hard and fast into the meter. This is repeated three times; the highest reading should then be recorded. Most asthmatics keep a daily diary of their readings. Normal values are dependent on height and age. You can download adult and child values from www.peakflow.com/top_nav/normal_values/index.html

Table 9.7 gives the range of respiration rates.

Table 9.7   Respiration rates

Normal breathing rate at rest	16–20 breaths per minute
Abnormal breathing rate at rest	Under 12 breaths or over 25

OXYGEN SATURATION

Pulse oximetry is a non-invasive method of monitoring the percentage of haemoglobin that is saturated with oxygen. The device clips onto a finger (toe or earlobe) (see Figure 9.3) and uses red and infrared light waves to measure the amount of oxygen in the blood. Red blood cells must carry sufficient oxygen through the arteries to all of the internal organs and tissues to keep you alive. Normally, when red blood cells pass through the lungs, 95–100% of them are saturated with oxygen. If someone has lung disease or anaemia, fewer of the red blood cells may be carrying their usual load of oxygen, and the oxygen saturation level might be lower than 95%. If the reading is below 90%, the patient will need oxygen support. These machines often will give a pulse reading also. It is important to note that the machines may not be accurate if the patient has nail varnish on their fingers or toes. Many people purchased pulse oximetry machines during the time of Covid as falling O_2 levels are an indicator of Covid progression.

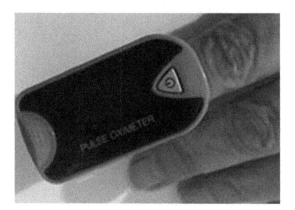

Figure 9.3   Pulse oximeter

BLOOD PRESSURE

This measures the force of the blood pushing against the artery walls. Each time the heart beats, it pumps blood into the arteries. Blood pressure is therefore usually measured in the left arm as the brachial artery is nearest to the heart, although the right arm and the legs can be used if necessary. Blood pressure is measured in millimetres of mercury (mmHg). Blood pressure is affected by caffeine, smoking, exercise, stress, fever, weight, salt intake, alcohol, age, heart disease and medication.

- The force of contraction in the ventricles is called the **systolic** rate
- The resting heart pressure is called the **diastolic** rate

✿ Activity 9.2

Practise taking a blood pressure reading. Raise the person's arm so that the brachial artery is roughly at the same height as the heart. If the arm is held too high, the reading will be artificially lowered, and vice versa. Ensure that the arm and back are supported, and the feet are resting firmly on the floor, not dangling.

The cuff should be applied directly over the skin (tight or thick clothes artificially raise blood pressure). Position the lower cuff border 2.5 cm above the bend in the elbow so the inflatable bladder is over the brachial artery (Figure 9.4). Correct positioning is important to the accuracy of the reading and for the comfort of the patient. Ensure that you use the correct cuff size for the patient.

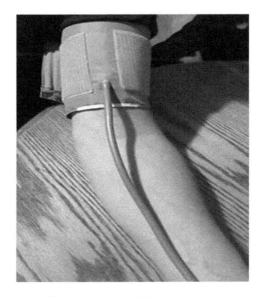

Figure 9.4   Correct position of blood pressure cuff

Usually, blood pressure is measured using digital machines, but it is always useful to know how to take a manual BP. The cuff is placed on the arm as described above, ensuring the bend in the arm is exposed. Inflate the bladder on the cuff to 10% over the last reading, or 160 mmHg. A stethoscope is placed over the antecubital fossa to listen for the blood flow, known as the Korotkoff sounds:

I   Systolic pressure – tapping sound – take reading
II   Sounds become fainter

Ausculttory gap – sounds may disappear

III   Return of clear sounds – diastolic pressure – take a reading
IV   Muffling
V   Sounds completely disappear

Table 9.8 gives the range of blood pressure readings.

Table 9.8   Blood pressure

Normal systolic pressure: which is the heart contracting	90–120 mmHg
Normal diastolic pressure: which is the heart resting	60–80 mmHg
Hypertension	140/90 mmHg or higher
Hypotension	90/60 mmHg or lower

POSTURAL HYPOTENSION

This is also known as postural orthostatic hypotension (POT). If the patient suffers from dizziness or fainting when standing up (postural dizziness), they may have postural hypotension. Postural measurements may be used to determine if the postural dizziness is the result of a fall in blood pressure. Postural hypotension is prevalent in older people, and in conditions such as Parkinson's disease or diabetes, and other ailments which affect the autonomic nervous system (see Chapter 6). People can also develop the condition if they are dehydrated or are taking medications such as tricylic antidepressants or antihypertensives). NICE (2021a) recommend compression garments, increasing hydration, elevating the bed head, and relaxation techniques rather than medication.

First measure the BP and pulse rate when the patient is supine (lying down) and then repeat after the patient has stood for 2 minutes, which allows for equilibration. The patient may need to be supported, with their arm held in the correct position. If there is a decrease in the blood pressure measurement from supine to standing (10–20 mmHg) and simultaneous increase in heart rate (raised by approximately 30 beats per minute), the patient likely has postural hypotension. This should be recorded and escalated for further examination by the medical team.

NEUROLOGICAL ASSESSMENT: LEVELS OF CONSCIOUSNESS

Assessing the level of consciousness of your patient is part of critical clinical care and considers the degree of arousal and awareness. Causes of loss of consciousness include lack of oxygen (hypoxia), stroke, analgesia, overdose (drugs and alcohol), sedatives and subarachnoid haemorrhage. The pupil size and reactivity can indicate arousal or brain injury. When assessing a patient's response to verbal stimulus, it is helpful to know if they have a hearing loss. The states of consciousness are given in Table 9.9.

Table 9.9   Levels of consciousness

1.	Alert and awake
2.	Confusion: Not orientated to time and space
3.	Lethargy: Sleepy but can be roused
4.	Obtundation: Extreme drowsiness, difficult to rouse
5.	Stupor: No response other than to painful stimuli
6.	Comatose: No response

The quick system of AVPU can be used to judge the appropriate response:

A = alert

V = responds to vocal prompts

P = responds to painful stimulus

U = unresponsive

If the patient is unresponsive then an assessment tool such as the Glasgow Coma Scale can be used to gauge the depth of unconsciousness.

PRESSURE AREA RISK ASSESSMENT

Patients need to be assessed for pressure areas. There are several tools available for this, such as the Waterlow Score or the Braden Score, and your employer will have a record of which score tool is used. The purpose of the scoring system is to inform you if your patient is at risk of developing pressure sores (decubitus ulcers) and to develop a plan of care which prevents this from happening. In nearly all instances of pressure area ulcers, poor nursing care is the cause. Patients of ethnic origin with darker skin are just as much at risk of developing pressure ulcers but sometimes the signs are missed.

Remember when assessing darkly pigmented skin that it does not blanch, but may be violaceous (aubergine colour) or purplish blue.

Pressure ulcers occur when the patient cannot move or reposition themselves in the bed (or chair), usually because they are acutely ill, malnourished or have mobility issues such as stroke or paralysis. Some elderly people or patients who are obese may have difficulty in moving around and therefore are at risk. Pressure ulcers are painful, and they can take a long time to heal, and this negatively affects the quality of life of the patient.

The patient's skin should be assessed, especially if they are incontinent, underweight (have bony prominences) and lack mobility. The heels, shoulders and sacrum need regular observation and any redness in the skin needs early preventative treatment by careful washing and drying of susceptible areas and by the application of Cavilon or other recommended preparation. Remember that pressure ulcers can also occur on the back of the head and the ears.

Young children who are receiving interventions such as nasogastric feeding or are in splints or casts also need regular observation to prevent such ulcers occurring.

> ### Go Further 9.2
>
> The NHS have prepared a guidance called SSKIN to prevent pressure ulcers occurring:
>
> **S**urface: make sure your patients have the right support
>
> **S**kin inspection: early inspection means early detection – show patients and their carers what to look for
>
> **K**eep your patients moving
>
> **I**ncontinence/moisture: your patients need to be clean and dry
>
> **N**utrition/hydration: help patients have the right diet and plenty of fluids
>
> You can read a case study here: www.england.nhs.uk/atlas_case_study/preventing-and-managing-skin-tears-in-residential-homes/

The National Wound Care Strategy Framework is supporting a reduction in pressure ulcer prevalence. NHS staff are working with all care settings to raise awareness of pressure sore prevention strategies as over 1300 new ulcers are reported each month (NHS Digital, 2019) at a cost to the NHS of more than £1.4 million every day, not to mention the pain and discomfort to the patient.

In the event of a pressure ulcer forming, remember that you have a duty of candour and clear documentation must be made. Ensure that a specialist tissue viability nurse is consulted, and advice taken as to the type of wound and wound dressing to be used. Care providers should know that pressure sores above grade 3 need to be reported to the CQC (Care Quality Commission).

Also check for rashes: this could be evidence of an allergy to washing products or topical medication. It might also indicate a contagious infection such as childhood diseases (measles, chicken pox, slapped cheek) or might indicate meningitis (rash that does not disappear when rolled over by a clear glass); it might also indicate ring or round worm. Patients can develop sweat rashes where skin surfaces touch each other (under breasts and groin area); this is common in obese patients.

PREPARING THE PATIENT AT THE END OF OBSERVATION

Assist the patient to get dressed again and to return to their chair or bed, if you have moved them. Explain the results: it is not enough to give a generic or soothing answer, if someone has an elevated temperature (hyperthermia/pyrexia), say so and offer a homely remedy such as a cooling drink, and thank them for their cooperation. You should then record your findings and escalate if the patient's readings indicate a deteriorating condition.

Ensure that you clean any equipment used by wiping it down with products recommended by your organisation's convention and replace equipment in a safe place. If need be, put it back on charge in order that it is ready to be used again. Dispose of your PPE to convention and wash your hands thoroughly.

URINALYSIS

Normal urine is pale straw colour (may be darker in the morning), has a non-offensive odour and should be clear with nothing floating in it.

1. Ensure safe working practice and wear personal protective clothing, disposable gloves and apron.
2. Collect urine in a clean, dry, covered container and test it as soon as possible.
3. If testing cannot be done within 2 hours after voiding, refrigerate the specimen immediately for preservation. Do not use a domestic refrigerator used for food.
4. Allow the urine specimen to return to room temperature prior to testing.

To carry out the test, you will need: a box of in-date reagent strips, a timing device and a paper towel (Figure 9.5).

LABELLING SAMPLES

Always label the sample pot in the room you took the sample or at the bedside as this reduces the risk of errors.

Always confirm the patient's name and date of birth before removing the specimen from the room (even if it is someone you know very well).

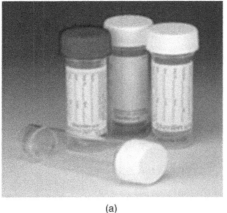

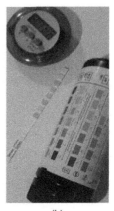

(a)   (b)

Figure 9.5   (a) Urine sample containers. (b) Preparing to test urine

TESTING URINE

1. Remove one reagent strip from the bottle and replace the cap immediately.
2. Completely immerse reagent areas of the strip in FRESH urine and remove immediately to avoid dissolving out reagents.
3. Ensure all of the test pads are wet.
4. After dipping, run the edge of the entire length of the strip against the rim of the urine container to remove excess urine.
5. Hold the strip in a horizontal position to prevent possible mixing of chemicals from adjacent reagent areas and/or contaminating the hands with urine.
6. Blot the strip to remove excess urine by touching the edge to a paper towel. Do not drag the strip across the towel; touch the edge only.

Remember to hold the strip vertically and the bottle horizontally to compare colour readings (Figure 9.6). Ensure no urine comes into contact with the bottle.

Proper read time is critical for an optimal result. The side of the bottle will tell you the time for each reading.

Dispose of the stick per health and safety rules/organisational convention. Table 9.10 gives you the signs and symptoms of a urinary tract infection (UTI).

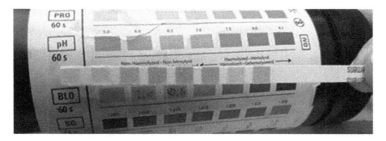

Figure 9.6   Can you spot the mistake?

Table 9.10   Signs and symptoms of a urinary tract infection

Pain on passing urine – burning/stinging sensation
Low abdominal pain
Urine frequency
Urine appearing abnormal – colour, clarity, odour
High temperature
Confusion

STOOL EXAMINATION

The Bristol Stool Chart (Figure 9.7) is pictorial and gives an explanation of what different types of faeces can indicate. Stools are typed 1–7 from hard and compacted to liquid. The stool chart offers diagnostic assistance by suggesting causes and outcomes if the situation is not remedied. For instance, hard and compacted faeces can be caused by poor diet, low fluid intake and a lack of exercise; the passage of such faeces can damage the lining of the bowel and cause anorectal bleeding due to laceration. The exertion of trying to excrete such faeces might cause the development of haemorrhoids (piles), which are swollen blood vessels in the anus.

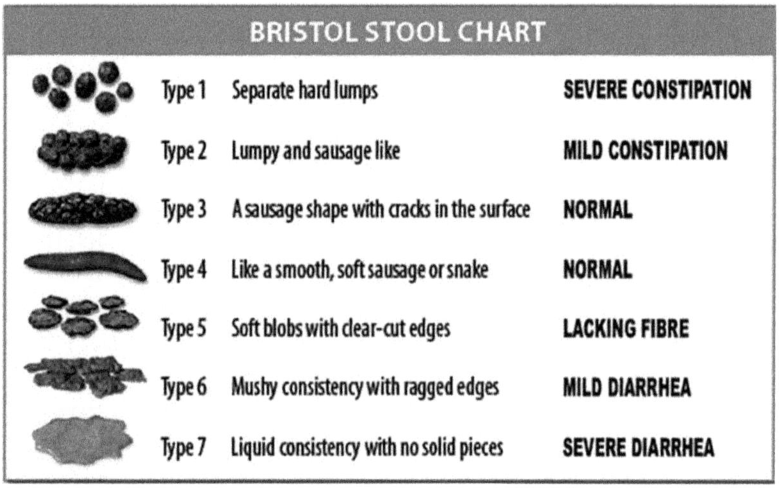

BRISTOL STOOL CHART

	Type 1	Separate hard lumps	**SEVERE CONSTIPATION**
	Type 2	Lumpy and sausage like	**MILD CONSTIPATION**
	Type 3	A sausage shape with cracks in the surface	**NORMAL**
	Type 4	Like a smooth, soft sausage or snake	**NORMAL**
	Type 5	Soft blobs with clear-cut edges	**LACKING FIBRE**
	Type 6	Mushy consistency with ragged edges	**MILD DIARRHEA**
	Type 7	Liquid consistency with no solid pieces	**SEVERE DIARRHEA**

Figure 9.7   The Bristol Stool Chart

Source: Stool Form Scale as a Useful Guide to Intestinal Transit Time, Lewis, S.J & Heaton, K.W, *Scandinavian Journal of Gastroenterology*, July 2009. Available at https://commons.wikimedia.org/wiki/File:BristolStoolChart.png

RECORDING AND REPORTING

Ensure that you chart the results of all clinical observations and escalate any concerns to your senior staff member. Recording results is critical to understanding your patient's health. Gaps in charts lead to frustration by the medical team as they may be making a diagnosis and offering interventions based on misleading or incorrect information.

Residential care settings need to take baseline measurements at least monthly in order to have a good understanding of the general health of their patients, and this should include recording their patients' weight too, to ensure that weight gain or loss is being monitored.

DISCHARGE PLANNING

Transition from hospital to home, a rehabilitation facility, or a nursing home should be planned to achieve an optimal outcome; planning should commence either prior to or when the expected date of discharge (EDD) and clinical criteria for discharge (CCD) is known. The patient, family, caregivers and healthcare providers all play roles in maintaining a patient's health after discharge. Box 9.1 shows what needs to be considered when planning discharge. It is always a good idea to check the patient has had any medical devices such as cannula/Venflon removed (see Figure 9.8).

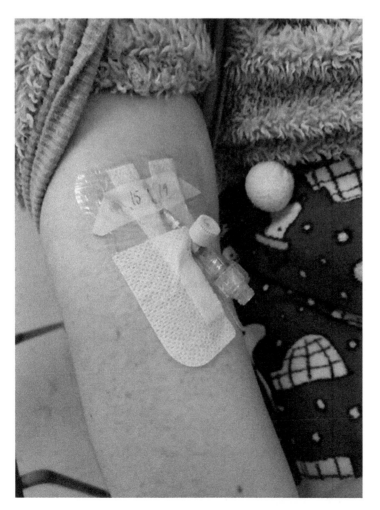

Figure 9.8   Cannula

Source: © Gillian Rowe

Box 9.1

Evaluation of the patient by healthcare professionals

Discussion with the patient and their carers/family/Adult Social Care/social workers

Planning for home or transfer to another care facility

Determining whether caregiver training or other support is needed

Referrals to a home care/domicilary agency and/or appropriate support organisations in the community

Arranging for follow-up appointments or tests

Ensuring any medical devices have been removed

Ensuring any medications have been reconciled, and have been ordered and the patient has received them

Ensuring the patient has contact telephone numbers in case of need

Taken from caregiver.org

---

gov.uk (2022) explains: 'Planning for a patient's discharge from hospital is a key aspect of effective care'. Nurse-led discharge planning and evaluation protocols should be initiated on day 1 of the patient's hospital stay and the plan should include assessment of spousal/relative support systems, home living situation and need for social care support, plus any appointments for post-discharge follow-up.

The plan should include disease-specific patient education. Some patients may be discharged with medical devices such as enteral feeding systems, in which case the family or carers would need to be trained to use the equipment safely. Discharge planning might include signposting to community services such as provided by social services, community care agencies, meals on wheels and community transport for outpatient appointments.

END OF LIFE CARE

End of life usually refers to the last year of life, although many understand this as the last few days. Approximately 500,000 people die each year in the UK; most will die in a hospital, and around three-quarters of these will be 'expected' deaths. End of life care should be holistic: this means that the person should be provided with physical, emotional, psychological and spiritual support. The patient's family will have many questions and will also need support.

As we have only one chance to get this right, it is important to understand how to support those who are dying. You will need to talk to the patient and their families about where they would like their death to take place: some would like to die at home, some would prefer a hospice or other care setting. It is not always possible for their wishes to be met but we should try our best to ensure they have the death they would prefer.

We should maintain the patient's health by ensuring they have adequate nutrition and hydration, that pain is managed effectively and that their natural anxiety and concerns are addressed. Also, their basic physiological needs for bowel and bladder care should be attended to as well as their personal hygiene. Don't underestimate the power of a good wash and clean nightwear for making a patient feel more comfortable. Box 9.2 contains the advice given by the RCN when supporting a patient through the end of their life.

Box 9.2

When providing end of life care, ensure you:

- Treat people compassionately
- Listen to people
- Communicate clearly and sensitively
- Identify and meet the communication needs of each individual
- Acknowledge pain and distress and take action
- Recognise when someone may be entering the last few days and hours of life
- Involve people in decisions about their care and respect their wishes
- Keep the person who is reaching the end of their life and those important to them up-to-date with any changes in condition
- Document a summary of conversations and decisions
- Seek further advice if needed
- Look after yourself and your colleagues and seek support if you need it

---

Go Further 9.3

There are free resources on the RCN website to support your learning; these can be found at: https://rcni.com/hosted-content/rcn/fundamentals-of-end-of-life-care/getting-started

---

After someone has died, the death needs to be certified by a medical practitioner before the body can be moved. A copy of this certificate must be given to the next of kin to take to the local registrar to register the death. The next of kin usually formally identifies the body and gives permission for a post-mortem examination if one is required. In some circumstances, a coroner's post-mortem examination may take place if the death was unexpected or within a short time of surgery or discharge. The body will then be laid out and kept in the hospital mortuary until the next of kin appoints a funeral director who will then take the body to their chapel of rest until the funeral takes place.

ORGAN DONATION

A recent change in English legislation has meant that anyone over the age of 18 will be considered to be in favour of donating their organs and tissues after death unless they 'opt out'. Families will be consulted as to their loved one's wishes, and if the deceased would not have agreed, then donation would not take place.

While anyone can donate organs, generally because of the constraints of time, usually only those dying in hospital are able to donate organs, although tissues can be taken up to 48 hours after death. The team which retrieve organs are not members of the patient's care team. This is to ensure procedures are ethical. Tissue samples are taken and compared with the register of people needing a donated organ to find a match, and priority is given to patients who most urgently need a transplant. The National Health Service Blood and Transplant (NHSBT) operates the UK-wide, 24/7, 365 days a year system. The donor operation is performed as soon as possible as organs deteriorate after a person's death and need to be transplanted quite quickly.

The transplant recipient may be given some brief details about their donor and may send an anonymous letter of thanks to the donor family. The donor family may also receive some brief details about the recipient. This is something that families decide about: if they do not want to know about the recipient, the specialist nurses supporting the family will not pass on any message.

POST-QUALIFICATION

Once you are a qualified NA there is a huge array of clinical skills that can be undertaken (depending on setting), such as IV drug administration, vaccination, insertion of catheters, wound care, doppler/ultrasound for continence care and smear tests. Training and competence assessment takes place in the setting and under the supervision of qualified nurses. You too will be supervising other trainee NAs and student nurses, so it is important you are able to correctly demonstrate your skill set and evidence your underpinning theoretical knowledge.

CHAPTER SUMMARY

- This chapter has discussed the importance of gaining consent prior to engaging in taking observations and shown you how to take the observations.
- We have discussed safe working practice in both acute and care settings.
- We have also considered health and safety and the legislation that you need to be aware of when monitoring vital signs. This chapter has guided you to consider how to prepare yourself and your patient so that you are both safe and comfortable with the activity.
- You must ensure that you are properly trained and that you are judged competent by a professional assessor to engage in these activities before you undertake them with your patients.

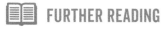 FURTHER READING

WEBSITES

Researching these websites will enhance your understanding and deepen your knowledge of the issues covered in this chapter:

- Care Quality Commission: www.cqc.org.uk/guidance-providers/adult-social-care/administering-medicines-covertly
- Health data: www.hdruk.ac.uk/
- Medical devices: www.gov.uk/topic/medicines-medical-devices-blood/medical-devices-regulation-safety
- NEWS2: www.rcplondon.ac.uk/projects/outputs/national-early-warning-score-news-2
- Resuscitation Council life support guidelines: www.resus.org.uk/public-resource
- Wound management: Hewish, J., Online lecture notes: www.oxfordhealth.nhs.uk/wp-content/uploads/2015/08/Fundamentals-of-Wound-Management-2014.pdf

BOOKS

The following books will help you to deepen your understanding of essential skills:

- Delves-Yates, C. (2015) *Essential Clinical Skills for Nurses: Step by Step*. London: Sage.
- Starkings, S. (2015) *Passing Calculations Tests for Nursing Students* (Transforming Nursing Practice Series). London: Sage.
- Whelan, A. and Hughes, E. (2016) *Clinical Skills for Healthcare Assistants and Assistant Practitioners*. Chichester: Wiley.

JOURNAL ARTICLE

- Bennett, M.A. (1995) Report of the task force on the implications for darkly pigmented intact skin in the predication and prevention of pressure ulcers. *Advances in Wound Care*, 8(6): 34–5.

VIDEOS

- Skills for Health: NHS training: www.youtube.com/watch?v=enWD6SETL04
- Proper Patient Care – Communication Techniques: www.youtube.com/watch?v=e9U-r9D6oVw
- Introducing the NHS Patient Safety Strategy: www.youtube.com/watch?v=nN0ZCOjxSe4
- NMC OSCE NEWS2 / National Early Warning Scoring System Explained / How to Chart in the NMC OSCE: www.youtube.com/watch?v=AFY2yUOjYP4
- How to Pass your OSCEs | Nurse Zara UK: www.youtube.com/watch?v=YXtyZclUe8o

REFERENCES

Foucault, M. (1963) *The Birth of the Clinic: An Archaeology of Medical Perception*. London: Tavistock.
gov.uk (2022) Hospital discharge and community support. Available at: www.gov.uk/government/publications/hospital-discharge-and-community-support-guidance/hospital-discharge-and-community-support-guidance
HSE (Health and Safety Executive) (2016) *Healthcare infection rates*. Available at: www.hse.gov.uk/biosafety/healthcare.htm
HSE (Health and Safety Executive) (2021a) *Infections at Work*. Available at: www.hse.gov.uk/biosafety/infection.htm
HSE (Health and Safety Executive) (2021b) *Work-related Ill Health*. Available at: www.hse.gov.uk/statistics/overall/hssh1920.pdf
HSE (Health and Safety Executive) (2021c) *Musculoskeletal Disorders*. Available at: www.hse.gov.uk/statistics/overall/hssh1920.pdf
NHS Digital (2021) Pressure ulcers: applying All Our Health. Available at: www.gov.uk/government/publications/pressure-ulcers-applying-all-our-health/pressure-ulcers-applying-all-our-health
NICE (2021a) Postural hypotension. Available at: www.nice.org.uk/advice/esuom20/ifp/chapter/What-is-postural-hypotension
NICE (2021b) NICE recommends range of effective treatments for people with chronic primary pain. Available at: www.nice.org.uk/news/article/nice-recommends-range-of-effective-treatments-for-people-with-chronic-primary-pain-and-calls-on-healthcare-professionals-to-recognise-and-treat-a-person-s-pain-as-valid-and-unique-to-them
NMC (Nursing and Midwifery Council) (2018) The Code: Professional standards of practice and behaviour for nurses, midwives and nursing associates. Available at: www.nmc.org.uk/globalassets/sitedocuments/nmc-publications/nmc-code.pdf
RCN (Royal College of Nursing) (2019) Are you glove aware? Available at: www.rcn.org.uk/get-involved/campaign-with-us/glove-awareness
Unison (2018) Cleaners at the forefront of needlestick injuries. Available at: www.unison.org.uk/news/article/2018/10/hns-week-needles/

10

ESSENTIAL SKILLS: MEDICINES MANAGEMENT AND ADMINISTRATION

GILLIAN ROWE

STANDARDS OF PROFICIENCY FOR NURSING ASSOCIATES (2018)

Relevant Platforms include:

Platform 1:1.12 Recognise and report any factors that may adversely impact safe and effective care provision.

Platform 1:1.13 Demonstrate the numeracy, literacy, digital and technological skills required to meet the needs of people in their care to ensure safe and effective practice.

Platform 1:1.14 Demonstrate the ability to keep complete, clear, accurate and timely records.

Platform 3:3.2 Demonstrate and apply knowledge of body systems and homeostasis, human anatomy and physiology, biology, genomics, pharmacology, social and behavioural sciences when delivering care.

Platform 3:3.4 Demonstrate the knowledge, communication and relationship management skills required to provide people, families and carers with accurate information that meets their needs before, during and after a range of interventions.

Platform 3:3.7 Demonstrate and apply an understanding of how and when to escalate to the appropriate professional for expert help and advice.

Platform 3:3.16 Demonstrate the ability to recognise the effects of medicines, allergies, drug sensitivity, side effects, contraindications and adverse reactions.

(Continued)

Platform 3:3.17 Recognise the different ways by which medicines can be prescribed.

Platform 5: 5.7 Understand what constitutes a near miss, a serious adverse event, a critical incident, and a major incident.

Annex B 10.1–10.10.

INTRODUCTION

For both trainee nursing associates and qualified nursing associates and healthcare practitioners, it is essential that you understand and apply the legislative framework that governs medicines management. Your work needs to be accurate in practice and therefore this chapter will support your medicine management studies. It will guide you through the legislation, consider why and how medicines work, how medication is categorised, safe administration and the patient's rights. You are given examples of the use of maths in medication administration, and you are advised to ensure your calculations are correct by practising using both commercial packages available through your training organisation and those found online. It is always better to be safe than sorry. Medicines optimisation covers such things as the cost of drugs and their effectiveness. It is predicated on person-centred care and supporting the patient to participate in their care. Medicines optimisation looks at the value which medicines deliver, making sure they are clinically effective and cost-effective. It is about ensuring people get the right choice of medicines, at the right time, and are engaged in the process by their clinical team (NHS England, 2019). An informed patient is more likely to comply with the prescribed treatment regime and prevents waste. The 2021/2 drugs bill for the NHS is estimated to be £2 billion. According to NHS England and the Medicines Value Programme (NHS England, 2021a) between 5 and 8% of all hospital admissions are due to adverse medicines incidents, many of which are preventable, and up to half of patients do not take medicines as intended. Therefore, appropriate medicine reviews together with supporting the patient to get the benefits they need from their medicines should improve compliance and reduce waste. Your role as a nursing associate or healthcare practitioner is to use your knowledge and skills to support and advise your patients with their medication.

Glossary

- **Contraindication** A medicine should not be used because it may be harmful to the patient
- **Drug interaction** A substance (e.g. another medicine, food) which affects the activity of a drug when both are administered together

- **Pharmacokinetics** The study of the way in which drugs move through the body during absorption, distribution, metabolism and excretion
- **Pharmacodynamics** The effect that drugs have on the body
- **Pharmacology** The study of the biological effect of chemicals administered in living organisms
- **Side effects** An effect that can be harmful or unpleasant (or occasionally beneficial)

WHY DO WE USE MATHS IN HEALTHCARE?

The leading cause of medication errors is difficulty in undertaking drug calculations. When reconstituting medicines, safe practice would indicate a second checker before administration; the second checker should always challenge when unsure. A good rule is to never administer medication you have not witnessed being prepared. Managing risk and near misses is good organisational culture, as is supporting staff when errors occur.

It is probable that you have already undertaken functional skills level 3 or GCSE maths. Many students will have struggled with abstract ideas such as algebra (something you will use if you specialise in orthopaedic trauma), fractions and percentages. However, you will be using maths regularly in your day-to-day work. Here are a few examples to remind you and some drug calculations to work through.

1. Mrs Jones is on a strict fluid balance chart. Today she had IV fluids 1300 ml and oral fluids 450 ml. Her catheter bag contained 1250 ml, she vomited twice today, judged approximately 200 ml, her wound drainage bag contained 50 ml. What was her fluid balance total?

IN	OUT
1300 ml	200 ml
450 ml	1250 ml
	50 ml
Total 1750 ml	Total 1500 ml

2. Mr Smith weighed 76.20 kg when he was admitted to your unit, he now weighs 74.18 kg. How much weight has he lost?

   76.20
   −74.18
   = 2.02 kg

You might have to convert stones and pounds into kilos. Table 10.1 gives you the conversion table for doing this.

Table 10.1   Converting stones to kilograms

1 stone (14 pounds)	6.35 kilograms
1 pound	0.45 of a kilogram
1 kilogram	2.2 pounds (approximately)

DRUG CALCULATIONS

1. Mrs Baker is taking OxyNorm liquid (OxyContin) 5 milligrams (mg) (dose) in 5 millilitres (ml) (volume) of liquid for pain relief. She can take 2.5 mg every 3 hours. What is her maximum total dose in any 24 hours?

   24 hours ÷ 3 hours = 8 doses

   8 doses × 2.5 mg = 20 mg/ml daily total

2. Mrs Jones weighs 14 stone (88.90 kg). Her medication dose is 2.5 micrograms (mcg) per kilo, how many micrograms should she receive?

   88.90 kg

   ÷ 2.5

   = 222.25 mcg

You need to ensure that you know the conversions for micrograms, milligrams and grams. Table 10.2 gives you these.

Table 10.2   Conversions

1,000,000 micrograms (mcg)	1 gram (g)
1000 micrograms (mcg)	1 milligram (mg)
1000 milligrams (mg)	1 gram (g)

3. Mr Turner needs 6 mg of his medication, but the stock cupboard has only 10 mg (dose) in 5 ml (volume). What volume are you going to give him?

$$\frac{\text{Doses required}}{\text{Doses available}} \times \frac{\text{Volume}}{1} = \frac{6}{10} \times \frac{5}{1} = 3 \text{ millilitres}$$

4. Mrs Rooney needs heparin, which is available as 4000 units/5 ml. What volume is needed to give her 20,000 units?

$$20,000 \div 4000 = 5$$

therefore 5 × 5 ml = 25 ml

5. Miss Woodman is prescribed saline 500 ml over 6 hours. What percentage would be administered after 3 hours?

$$\frac{3}{6} \times \frac{100}{1} = \frac{300}{6} \qquad\qquad 6\,\overline{)\,300}$$

= 50 therefore she has received
50% which equals 250 ml

6. Adam needs a transfusion of packed cells; 1 unit contains 250 ml of packed cells. The giving set delivers 15 drops per ml, the packed cells need to be given over 4 hours, calculate the drip rate

$$\frac{\text{Volume}}{\text{Hours}} \times \frac{\text{Drops}}{60} \quad \frac{250}{4} \times \frac{15}{60} \qquad 60\,\overline{)\,3750} = 16 \text{ drops per minute}$$

= 62.5
÷ 4
= 15.62

7. Tom needs 1 gram of antibiotics daily to be taken in 4 equally divided doses, however, the pharmacy has dispensed in 125 mg tablets, how many tablets should he take at each dose?

$1000 \div 125 = 8$ therefore 2×125 mg tables at each dose

Go Further 10.1

If you struggle with fractions and percentages, download an app to your phone and practise doing them. If you are not sure, always get someone to check your calculation – it is always better to be safe than sorry. You can find some really good resources to help you at: https://unihub.mdx.ac.uk/_data/assets/pdf_file/0031/187654/Nursing-Calculations-Help-Sheets.pdf
    Look at Table 10.3 and ensure that these never events do not happen.

Table 10.3   Safety first: never events

Always check you have the right patient, the right medication, and the right dose
Never give someone another patient's drugs, even if they are the same dose
Never cut tablets into 2, even if they are scored and you have a pill cutter

LEGISLATION AND REGULATORY BODIES

Medicines management law is contained in many pieces of legislation such as the Human Medicines Regulations (2012), which give the scope, provisions and classifications of medicinal products and the regulations for prescribing and pharmaceutical practice (among many other things). The Medicines and Healthcare Products Regulatory Agency (MHRA) regulates medicines, medical devices and blood components for transfusion and oversees the issuing of yellow cards and adverse warnings (see Go Further 10.3); it also hosts various advisory committees and the Clinical Practice Datalink (CPRD) database and the National Institute for Biological Standards and Control (NIBSC).

LEGISLATION

The Medicines Act 1968 is the overarching and enabling legislation that governs the supply of medications in the UK. This covers such things as the licensing of drugs and is regulated via the MHRA. The Misuse of Drugs Act 1971 superseded the Dangerous Drugs Act 1920 and divides classification of drugs into schedules and classes. Class A is opiates such as diamorphine, class B is the intermediate drugs such as codeine and class C would include the least harmful drugs such as zopiclone. The five schedules range from schedule 1, which includes drugs seldom used in medicine such as LSD, schedule 2 which contains the opiates and schedule 3 the synthetic opiates, to schedule 4 drugs such as benzodiazepines and schedule 5, minor analgesics. This is further regulated by the (2001) Misuse of Drugs Regulations, which govern controlled drugs; these are classified into schedules by potential for misuse. This was amended in 2018 by the Misuse of Drugs (Designation) to allow the prescription of cannabis products under certain controlled conditions.

Medication is prescribed for a specific individual; this is called a patient-specific direction (PSD) and includes the dose, route and frequency or appliance to be supplied or administered to a named patient. These drugs are the property of the patient and to use it (or them) for someone else is theft. Nursing associates should therefore refer to the Department of Health (2006) publication *Medicines Matters: A Guide to Mechanisms for the Prescribing, Supply and Administration of Medicines*. Section 18 of the NMC Code (2018) specifically refers to medicines administration. Section 18.2 states 'keep to appropriate guidelines when giving advice on using controlled drugs and recording the prescribing, supply, dispensing or administration of controlled drugs'; therefore, you should familiarise yourself with local convention and guidelines for safe practice.

The prescription form is a legal document and is classified as 'secure stationery'. Suitably qualified registered nurses can prescribe and are governed by the Medicinal Products: Prescription by Nurses Act 1992, and they can prescribe from the BNF nurses formulary.

HOW DO MEDICINES WORK?

Medication can be delivered orally (and sublingually), aurally, rectally (PR), in the vagina (PV), optically, nasally, rubbed in, injected, implanted and transdermally. It can also be administered through a cannula and drips. The chosen route affects absorption, distribution, metabolism and elimination (ADME). Routes are chosen depending on the tissue being targeted, severity of illness, urgency of the problem and the patient's general state of health.

Medication is absorbed via the bloodstream to the liver, where drug metabolism occurs (the first-pass effect). The drug metabolites may be more or less potent and may pass through the liver several times before being eliminated. Capsulated oral medication is protected from gastric acid and releases the dose into the intestine for absorption. Dissolved drug metabolites are distributed into the cells and function through biochemical reactions; they then pass back to the liver, are metabolically deactivated and then excreted.

The brain is generally protected from drug activity by the brain blood barrier unless the brain has inflammation, in which case, large molecule antibiotics can pass through (see Chapter 6, Bioscience, and Chapter 8, Prevention and Control of Infection). Some medication is designed to take advantage of weakness in the blood brain barrier (such as L-Dopa); these need to be fat soluble to be effective. Neurotransmitters can be modified by specific psychoactive substances such as opiates and benzodiazepines acting on cell receptors.

Adjuvants are medicines that are designed for a specific ailment but have beneficial side effects which allow them to be prescribed for pain relief. An example of this is tricyclic antidepressants, which help with psychological ailments but also offer pain relief.

PHARMACOKINETICS

Most drugs either inhibit or mimic physiological/biochemical actions or pathological processes by depressing or stimulating agonist receptors. The binding of drugs (ligands) requires numerous biomolecular processes. Absorption rates vary with age, weight, fat and muscle mass and delivery system; also the time the drug is taken such as before/after/with food will have an impact on metabolism and elimination, thus pharmacokinetics seeks to understand the interactions between drugs and the biological environment (such as between the bloodstream and oily cell surfaces) in order to predict the bioavailability (the therapeutic window) of the drug.

This was first understood by Claude Bernard in the 1880s when he discovered how curare causes paralysis by blocking the neurotransmitter acetylcholine. Some drugs can be considered broad spectrum as they can fit into many cell receptors (and thus possibly cause side effects). Occasionally, metabolism causes an inactive compound to become pharmacologically active, or innocuous drugs to create a toxic chemical.

There is a correlation between the quantity of drug administered and the drug response (the dose–effect relationship); all drugs have a threshold range where the intended effect is greater than unintended off-target effect (side effects). Those with narrow therapeutic ranges are difficult to manage and need frequent monitoring (such as thyroxine and digoxin). Pharmacologists use blood (and urine) to calculate drug processing time and adjust dosage accordingly.

DRUG NOMENCLATURE

It is important that you recognise the names of a medication: both branded and its international non-proprietary (generic) name. NICE prefers prescribers to use non-proprietary products as they are cheaper. Non-proprietary products are named for the active ingredient in the medicine and that is decided by an expert committee and is understood internationally (WHO, 2013).

> An example: class of drug HMG-CoA reductase inhibitors (statins). Brand name: Lipitor. Generic name: atorvastatin

Prescribers will usually prescribe by the generic name and the pharmacy will dispense whatever brand they have in stock. It may well be cheaper for a patient to buy certain drugs such as paracetamol and clotrimazole in a supermarket or chemist as a prescription currently costs over £9.

PLACEBO EFFECT

You may have heard of the placebo effect; a placebo is inactive substance (sugar pill or saline injection) used in randomised controlled trials to prove an active ingredient is more effective than no drug or a competitor's drug. The placebo effect is a phenomenon where people have experienced a good outcome from an inactive substance. This phenomenon has been extensively researched and has indicated that belief in the efficacy of a medication can positively impact on health outcomes, even when it shouldn't. Dr Ben Goldacre describes how patients fitted with heart pacemakers had improved cardiac performance, but this was *before* the pacemaker was switched on (Goldacre, Ted talk, 2012). A possible explanation for this is that the act of taking a medication triggers the release of endorphins, which act as the brain's own natural painkillers, which can calm a patient. Another explanation is the expectation of a positive result, especially if the prescriber gives the medication a glowing recommendation.

Case Study 10.1

Carla worked as a care practitioner in a care home catering to a mix of elderly residents with physical and mental health issues. Carla was on night shift and was supporting Mrs Grey with her late evening medications. Mrs Grey was an elderly widow with no surviving family, she had mild dementia and had recently suffered a series of transient ischemic attacks (TIAs). Mrs Grey often had difficulty sleeping but was not prescribed any soporific medication. Her GP was reluctant to prescribe sleeping pills as she suffered from early morning confusion and was at risk of falls.

Mrs Grey asked Carla to give her some sleeping pills as she was so tired but could not get to sleep. Carla knew she could not do this, but she was aware that sometimes placebos could help. She had a packet of small breath fresh mints in her pocket. She put one in a medicine pot and offered it to Mrs Grey with a glass of water. Mrs Grey took the mint and enjoyed a good night's sleep. Mrs Grey expected the 'pill' to help her to sleep and so she slept well. Carla explained this in Mrs Grey's notes, and it became routine to give Mrs Grey a small mint if she asked for sleeping medication.

There are ethical considerations here. Mrs Grey was taking the mint in the belief she was taking sleeping medication. Had she been told; it is probable it would have eliminated the desired placebo effect. However, her GP was happy that the placebo effect was working and agreed to the deception.

In contradiction to the placebo effect is the nocebo effect, where the person receiving the placebo experiences adverse side effects such as nausea and headaches. This could be because they have experienced these side effects before and expect to experience them again.

CATEGORIES OF MEDICATION

Medication is graded into three main categories according to the Medicines Act 1968:

1. General sales list (GSL)
2. Pharmacy only (pharmacist must be present)
3. Prescription only (POM) (pharmacist only to dispense)

Drugs used in the UK are collated into the British National Formulary (BNF), which is a pharmaceutical reference book, published twice a year (March and September), that gives information by detailing all medicines that are prescribed in the UK. Box 10.1 explains the information given in the BNF. It is used by all healthcare professionals as a reference for prescribing and information.

Box 10.1

Indications – what the drug is used for

Dosages – mg, drops, tabs, puffs

Contraindications – when not to give

Cautions – give with care

Side effects – unwanted effects

Interaction – with other drugs or food

SAFE STORAGE

The Safe and Secure Handling of Medicines: A Team Approach (RPSGB, 2017) states that nurses must adhere to regulations for the proper storage of medicines, and all drugs should be stored within locked cupboards/drug trolleys/refrigerators. Controlled drugs should be in a locked cupboard, within a locked cupboard and these have a controlled drug register (CDR) which should be signed by at least one registered nurse, and someone assessed as competent to sign the CDR; the CDR should similarly be kept in secure storage. In care settings, quite often the drug trolley is chained to a wall for added security. The keys for drug trolleys should also be secured safely.

When receiving drugs, it is important that they are properly checked in against the prescription to ensure the correct date, drug, dose and route. This job should be performed by at least one registered nurse, in a safe environment without interruptions to prevent errors. Out-of-date drugs should be returned to the pharmacy for safe disposal and stock drugs should be rotated and checked regularly so administration errors do not occur. The NMC Code (2018) affirms 'Take all steps to keep medicines stored securely' (18.4).

Most drugs supplied to care settings come in pre-prepared dose formats. These are additionally regulated by the Health and Social Care Act 2008 (Regulated Activities) Regulations (2014); specifically, 'Safe Care and Treatment' (Regulation 12) ensures 'the proper and safe management of medicines'. Monitored dosage systems (MDS) are promoted as a safe system as it is clearly apparent when a drug has been removed from the packaging; however, it is not suitable for all drugs such as medicines that are susceptible to moisture, e.g. dispersible aspirin or light-sensitive medicines such as chlorpromazine. Care settings that cannot afford the MDS system should not secondary dispense, i.e. decant drugs into compliance systems (such as dosette boxes) (Prescqipp, 2017). When the patient's own medicines are brought into a healthcare setting, it is important to document the patient's consent to remote storage (in a suitable drugs storage facility).

When administering the patient's own supply of drugs kept in their own room or locker, they should still be checked against the prescription and recorded as given on a medication administration record (MARs) sheet or e-recording system.

Many hospitals have adopted e-prescribing systems, the motivation being to improve the safety of medicines used and reduce the unacceptable levels of adverse drug events. According to Westbrook et al. (2009), a systematic review found a clear reduction in prescribing errors when e-prescribing was introduced.

ADMINISTRATION

Workers administering medication need to be accountable for their actions and should be assessed as competent to support the patient in taking medication. You should know the setting's policies and procedures and understand that maladministration carries consequence for all. Before giving drugs, ensure that you have checked the items in Box 10.2 and you have washed your hands and are wearing appropriate personal protection.

Box 10.2

Always check: patient's identity, any known allergies; check the drug matches the prescription (dose, format, delivery route); check the expiry date; do not give the medicine if an adverse reaction has occurred (you should contact the prescriber for advice and complete a yellow card); ensure the drug is administered at the correct time; record accurately if the medication has been taken (or refused).

Never: give a drug you haven't checked against the prescription sheet or an injection/infusion you have not witnessed being prepared. If in doubt, challenge.

NB: If the patient has any cognitive deficiency, a current photograph and/or wristband is an acceptable alternative for identification.

Drugs can be administered orally, topically, optically, aurally, anally, enterally, via inhalation and by injection. Nursing associates and practitioners should know and understand why drug administration routes are chosen and ensure it suits both the medical needs and the patient. It is important that you are properly trained to administer medications by invasive routes. Some patients are terrified of needles and will need support to accept drugs given this way; also, some patients find drugs such as suppositories or enemas less socially accepted or even abhorrent, and they too must have their fears calmed by detailed explanation of the need for the procedure. Go Further 10.2 explains why some routes are chosen.

> ## Go Further 10.2   Understanding why administration routes are chosen
>
> Someone experiencing an asthma attack may be given aminophylline suppositories, this is because while theophylline relaxes the smooth muscle of the trachea and bronchus, it irritates the gastric mucosa and can cause nausea, so a fast-acting dose with greater bioavailability can be delivered by suppository as a preventative and for symptom relief. Suppositories are underused in the UK as means of drug delivery; in Europe, it is the preferred mechanism as it prevents many side effects, and a lower dose can be given. There has been some debate as to which end of the suppository goes in first, we can only assume there is a reason the manufacturer gives it a pointed end.

PAIN RELIEF

Pain is a biochemical and neurological event; it is unpleasant sensation and an emotional experience. How people deal with pain depends on their emotional response and expectation. Athletes and combat sportspeople have a higher tolerance to pain as minor injury is expected, people who are depressed or suffer anxiety tend to have a lower tolerance to pain. Recent research has shown that redheads have a lower tolerance to pain and that they need greater anaesthesia for dental pain, this is because the gene for red hair (MC1R) also encodes for pain receptors in the brain. Pain can be culturally mediated, and age mediated, and there are tools to measure pain (see Chapter 9). An aware nursing associate should also be mindful of their own beliefs and attitude to pain relief. An understanding of pain can contribute to pain management – if a nursing associate thinks the patient is malingering or 'putting it on', they are less likely to offer pain relief. Pain should always be recorded and reported and escalated if the patient is experiencing discomfort.

Pain relief does not always require medication: many devices are available such as heat patches, TENs machines and implantable neuromodulators. Psychological techniques such as meditation, breathing and relaxation techniques can support people with chronic pain. Quite often, people underestimate the power of paracetamol as it is widely available. Paracetamol is effective for joint pain, headaches and muscle pain, although how the drug works is poorly understood.

There are different types of pain:

- Acute pain such as appendicitis
- Chronic pain such as arthritis
- Neuropathic pain such as neuralgia
- Nociceptive pain such as a sprained ankle
- Radicular pain such as spinal nerve compression, sciatica

As stated earlier, everyone has a different tolerance to pain. Some conditions – such as congenital insensitivity to pain with anhidrosis (CIPA) – can numb pain (hypoalgesia) and this might sound attractive but could result in injury or damage that is unnoticed. Allodynia is extreme sensitivity (especially to touch) and basic activities can cause severe pain.

The WHO devised a pain relief (analgesic) ladder, as part of their palliative care programme (Anekar and Cascella, 2021). Pain relief begins with the lowest amount of drug that is effective. The ladder has three steps:

1. First step. Mild pain: non-opioid analgesics such as non-steroidal anti-inflammatory drugs (NSAIDs) or acetaminophen with or without adjuvants
2. Second step. Moderate pain: weak opioids (hydrocodone, codeine, tramadol) with or without non-opioid analgesics, and with or without adjuvants
3. Third step. Severe and persistent pain: potent opioids (morphine, methadone, fentanyl, oxycodone, etc.) with or without non-opioid analgesics, and with or without adjuvants

Anekar and Cascella critique the programme and you can read their points if you click on the links on the reference page or type their names into your browser.

Pain relief for end-of-life care is usually by battery-powered syringe drivers; this is currently only administered by specially trained end-of-life care registered nurses, although syringe drivers can be used to support nausea during chemotherapy.

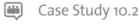

Case Study 10.2

Alesha has suffered from epilepsy since a childhood stroke, due to atrioventricular malformation in her brain. Over time, Alesha's seizures have become more severe and more frequent and less predictable. This has had an impact on her mental and emotional wellbeing as Alesha had several grand mal type (generalised tonic-clonic) seizures during social events and this caused her extreme embarrassment. Alesha became socially withdrawn and began suffering generalised social anxiety. Her consultant neurologist offered her levetiracetam (Keppra) medication. This medication is not suitable for all epilepsy sufferers, but Alesha agreed to try the drug. She had a 6-month review with the epilepsy nurse and Alesha reported that the drug is working well, her seizures are less frequent and less severe. However, she has many side effects: she has developed mild allergies to foods or products she was not previously allergic to, weight gain, some hair loss and increased loss of balance and coordination. After discussing the side effects with the nurse, Alesha decided to remain on the drug as it was so good at controlling her seizures, and this allowed her to resume her social life.

In this case study, Alesha was able to make an informed choice. Some of the side effects were problematic as hair loss is not a known side effect but may be a result of the interactions with her other anti-convulsant medication. Her allergies need to be monitored as levetiracetam can cause severe allergic reaction (anaphylaxis) requiring urgent medical intervention.

NURSING ASSOCIATES AND CONTROLLED DRUGS

The guidance for nursing associates regarding controlled drugs is, to say the least, ambiguous. The onus is placed on the employing organisation and their conventions. The Health Education England advice (HEE, 2018) is 'employers should not focus purely on controlled medicines but consider all safety critical medicine' and further states that 'employers should have local policies detailing the remit, responsibilities and activities of nursing associates'. If you feel you need further training, refuse to administer CDs until you feel fully confident in your role, under standard 5.8 you should understand when to seek appropriate advice to manage a risk and avoid compromising quality of care and health outcomes. The NMC Code (2018) recommends that you 'keep to appropriate guidelines when giving advice on using controlled drugs and recording the prescribing, supply, dispensing or administration of controlled drugs' (18.2). Therefore, do not feel under pressure to engage in practice until you are competent and safe.

ADMINISTRATION ERRORS

The RCN (2018) states that 'medication errors can occur at any stage of the medicines process, this includes prescribing, dispensing, preparation and administering medicines and monitoring their effects'. Errors in administration need to be reported and recorded, however the MHRA has indicated its concerns that this does not happen often enough or in any meaningful way and suggests changes need to be made to the clinical governance of medication error reporting. The MHRA states: 'Incident reports are not always reviewed locally by staff with medication safety expertise to check quality and to initiate action before being submitted to the National Reporting and Learning Systems (NRLS)' (MHRA, 2017). Standard 24 of the NMC Standards for Medicines states: 'As a registrant, if you make an error, you must take any action to prevent any potential harm to the patient and report as soon as possible to the prescriber, your line manager or employer (according to local policy) and document your actions'. The NMC Code also states:

> 14.1 Act immediately to put right the situation if someone has suffered actual harm for any reason or an incident has happened which had the potential for harm
>
> 14.2 Explain fully and promptly what has happened, including the likely effects, and apologise to the person affected and, where appropriate, their advocate, family or carers
>
> 14.3 Document all these events formally and take further action (escalate) if appropriate so they can be dealt with quickly

The professional duty of candour is about openness and honesty when things go wrong. 'Every healthcare professional must be open and honest with patients when something goes wrong with their treatment or care which causes, or has the potential to cause, harm or distress' (Joint statement from the Chief Executives of statutory regulators of healthcare professionals, cited in the NMC Code, 2018).

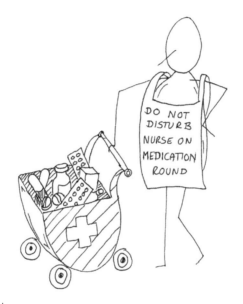

Figure 10.1   Drug round

All errors are classed as 'patient safety incidents' and should be reported through local risk management systems. The National Patient Safety Improvement Programmes include the Medicines Safety Improvement Programme (MedSIP), which offers training to prevent maladministration. Research by NHS Improvement found that 7% of patients suffered harm by maladministration, mainly caused by interruptions while nurses were on the drug round. Table 10.4 details causes of medication errors, incident, and frequency.

Table 10.4   Causes of medication errors

Wrong dose, strength, frequency	28.7%
Omitted medicine	17%
Wrong medicine	11.5%
Wrong patient	5%
Patient allergic	3.2%
Wrong formulation	2.4%
Wrong route	2.1%

Your duty of candour means you must be open and honest when errors occur; you must report and escalate if maladministration happens.

Box 10.3   Remember the six rights of medication

- Right individual
- Right medication
- Right dose
- Right time
- Right route
- Right documentation

When patients are transferred from settings, for example from a care setting to a hospital, or between wards, NICE recommend that you accurately list all of the person's medicines (including prescribed, over-the-counter and complementary medicines) and carry out medicines reconciliation within 24 hours or sooner and that this should be recorded (e-prescribe or paper-based system).

EVIDENCE-BASED PRACTICE

Nurses and nursing associates are primarily responsible for safe medication administration; TNAs give medication under the supervision of registered nurses, and they are assessed for safe practice.

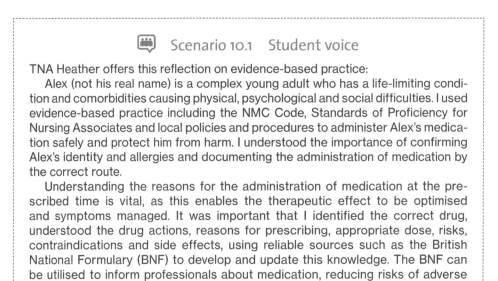

Scenario 10.1   Student voice

TNA Heather offers this reflection on evidence-based practice:

Alex (not his real name) is a complex young adult who has a life-limiting condition and comorbidities causing physical, psychological and social difficulties. I used evidence-based practice including the NMC Code, Standards of Proficiency for Nursing Associates and local policies and procedures to administer Alex's medication safely and protect him from harm. I understood the importance of confirming Alex's identity and allergies and documenting the administration of medication by the correct route.

Understanding the reasons for the administration of medication at the prescribed time is vital, as this enables the therapeutic effect to be optimised and symptoms managed. It was important that I identified the correct drug, understood the drug actions, reasons for prescribing, appropriate dose, risks, contraindications and side effects, using reliable sources such as the British National Formulary (BNF) to develop and update this knowledge. The BNF can be utilised to inform professionals about medication, reducing risks of adverse events and toxicity, thus promoting safe practice. This information should be discussed with patients when requesting consent to administer medications, and the effects of medication monitored.

Alex has capacity, giving informed consent for medication administration, and he understands the purpose, benefits, risks and side effects of his medication. He complained of pain after administration of his regular medications. Non-pharmaceutical interventions including a position change, reassurance and distraction were provided, and no further action was necessary as Alex's pain reduced. Evidence suggests that non-pharmaceutical interventions should be considered as well as pharmaceutical symptom relief. Alex informed me he suffers from this pain most nights and it is usually relieved by changing his position, but he does sometimes require extra pain relief medication.

If Alex's pain had continued, I could have checked which other medications were prescribed on an as required basis. I could have completed a set of observations on Alex to compare to his baseline observations and requested advice and a review from the doctor to ensure Alex's pain did not have another cause. Alex's medications should also be reviewed regularly by a doctor to check they are being taken as prescribed and remain effective, ensuring troublesome side effects are minimised, and are therefore having a positive impact on the patient's life. NAs should assess and work in partnership with patients, using their professional judgement, clinical observation skills and a problem-solving approach, to maximise the benefits of medications for patients, thus optimising outcomes and quality of life.

Heather's reflection on evidence-based practice has included legislation and local regulations and she has a good background knowledge of her patient and his condition; this allows her to consider the best therapeutic options. She also demonstrates her awareness of the needs for medicines optimisation and regular medicines reviews in order to support her patient in consultation with the medicine's prescriber.

RIGHT TO CONSENT

Chapters 4 and 9 detail the patient's rights in giving and withholding consent. Before giving medication, especially before giving medication via an invasive procedure, always seek consent. Patients have fundamental legal and ethical rights to determine what happens to their own bodies, and, to be honest, seeking consent is a matter of common courtesy. Compliance with a treatment regime is based on mutual respect, giving the patient the information they need, in a format they understand, in order for them to give informed consent. If the patient is incapable of giving consent to medicate, remember that any medication should be in their 'best interests', and you should seek permission (written and recorded) from a family member or mental capacity advocate.

RIGHT TO REFUSE

Patients have the right to refuse medication, and you must respect the patient's rights and record this to convention, the NMC Code (2018) states 'respect, support and document a person's right to accept or refuse care and treatment' (2.5). It is important to gain consent to treat from the patient as invasive devices such as drips and cannulas should not be interfered with (see above for rights of consent). NICE offers advice considering that 'If a patient is not taking their medicines, discuss with them whether this is because of beliefs and concerns or problems about the medicines (intentional non-adherence) or because of practical problems (unintentional non-adherence)' (NICE, 2017). Unintentional refusal might be due to inability to remove the drug from its packaging, or forgetfulness. Patients suffering poor mental health should be assessed using the Mental Capacity Act 2005, and in some instances, such as a Community Treatment Order (Mental Health Act 1983, 2007), medication is enforced. Ensure that the outcome of any conversation is documented if the patient refuses their medication and escalate if the medication is safety critical.

COVERT DRUG ADMINISTRATION

Decisions made regarding covert medication are guided by the Mental Capacity Act 2005. The patient has the right to refuse medication. Accordingly, CQC (2022) states, 'The medicines could be hidden in food, drink or through a feeding tube without the knowledge or consent of the person receiving them. As a result, the person is unknowingly taking a medicine. Every person has the right to refuse their medicine, even if that refusal appears ill-judged to staff who are caring for them' (CQC, 2022). Guidance should be given to the patient and a risk assessment should be included within the plan of care. Therefore, when considering disguising medication, the treatment must be necessary to save life, prevent deterioration and ensure improvement in the individual's physical and mental health. If the prescriber gives consent for 'disguising' or covert medication this should be documented, and advice sought from the pharmacist for the best means.

SUPPORTING PEOPLE WITH MEDICATION

Before supporting people with medication, ensure you understand any instructions such as timing of dose, should the medication be taken before, with or after food and drink. Sometimes, the prescriber can give ambiguous directions such as 'take one or two', you will need to seek clarification if the dose is dependent on pain, anxiety, or something else. You will need to know if the patient has other difficulty in taking their own medicine such a blindness, arthritis (which can stop patients from opening containers), memory loss or other mobility issues. Dropped tablets need to be recorded and destroyed as there will be cross-infection issues.

If the patient is vomiting or has diarrhoea, they may not be able to take their medication; this should be recorded and escalated for alternative medication delivery if the medication is critical.

MEDICATION RISKS

The risk of overdose or accumulation occurs when patients cannot remember if they took their medication and take another dose, or they feel the dose they took is not working and take more. Another risk lies with the drug formulation, many tablets come in different dosages but look similar. An example of this is some brands of carbamazepine (Tegretol): the 200 mg and 400 mg tablets are both pink capsules. Overdose can lead to loss of balance, steadiness or coordination.

Patients can develop tolerance for drugs, meaning they become less effective over time. This is true of a range of opioid pain relief and requires careful management to prevent both tolerance and dependence.

Missed doses tend to occur when the treatment is four times per day as ward and care home drug rounds routines tend to be three times a day. This is especially so for antibiotic administration, which is particularly prone to error with doses being missed over the course of treatment.

ADVERSE DRUG EVENTS

Adverse drug reactions (ADRs) are an 'unwanted or harmful reaction experienced following the administration of a drug or combination of drugs under normal conditions of use' (NHS.gov, 2017). Some side effects are known and documented; others may be previously unrecognised. Detection and reporting are important as it is vital drugs are safe to use. Reporting systems are hosted by the MHRA through the 'yellow card' scheme, which can be downloaded from the MHRA website (see Go Further 10.3) Many people taking the Covid-19 vaccine have used the system to report side effects, this has allowed a picture to develop between the various vaccines and likely side effects that people need to know about. Pharmacovigilance systems monitor drugs in everyday use.

Medically significant events are those that are fatal, life threatening, disabling, or lead to congenital abnormalities. An example of this is the repurposing of the drug thalidomide intended for patients suffering leprosy or cancer (myeloma). It has a sedative effect and was thus marketed to pregnant women suffering morning sickness (hyperemesis) (it was sold over-the-counter in Europe). It caused congenital deformities such as malformation of the limbs (phocomelia) and organ deformities if taken in the first trimester. Another example is the OxyContin scandal (Van Zee, 2009) in America where over prescribing of the drug has led many to become addicts. Drug companies have been fined and had their products removed from the market if they have been proven to cause serious side effects.

SIDE EFFECTS AND ALLERGIES

Unwanted side effects can act as a preventative to patient compliance. Some are minor inconveniences: for instance, diphenhydramine (Benadryl) eases allergy symptoms but it also suppresses acetylcholine which can lead to drowsiness and a dry mouth. Side effects also occur when patients mix drugs with alcohol (accidental overdose) or when the patient inadvertently takes too much of a drug (for example warfarin dissolves blood clots but in overdose can cause internal bleeding). Drinking grapefruit juice when taking antihypertensive medication can affect its potency, as can mixing prescription medication with folk (herbal) remedies.

Mild side effects should be explained to the patients to help with medicines compliance: if they know what to expect, they can mentally prepare and manage them. Patients also need to know the difference between a mild side effect and a more severe side effect, such as a mild rash itch as opposed to blisters, peeling, hives and pain which require medical attention. Antibiotics and diuretics are known to cause skin reactions and the patient should be forewarned.

Allergic reaction treatment includes:

1. Antihistamines to relieve mild symptoms such as rash, hives and itching
2. Bronchodilators such as salbutamol to reduce asthma-like symptoms (moderate wheezing or cough)
3. Corticosteroids applied to the skin, given by mouth, or given intravenously
4. Epinephrine by injection to treat anaphylaxis

It is important to discuss any concerns with the patient so they can make an informed choice regarding their medication. It is remarkable how many patients leave the clinic or GP surgery with no clear idea of what drug they are taking or why, and this lack of understanding leads to erratic or non-compliance in medication regimes.

Go Further 10.3

Medicines yellow card details and advice can be found at: www.gov.uk/government/organisations/medicines-and-healthcare-products-regulatory-agency/about
Medicines optimisation guide from NICE: www.nice.org.uk/guidance/ng5

MEDICATION ADMINISTRATION AND CHILDREN

Children's nurses need to work closely with the child's family and carers to support them with the child's care. A sick child is always distressing for a family. They need to be fully informed about treatment and medications with explanations of the intended therapeutic goal – an engaged and informed family are more likely to adhere with regimes and can spot unintended side effects if they are taught what to look for. Verbal information should always be supported with written information to consolidate their knowledge and understanding; also the family can consult written instructions when needed after discharge. This should include specific information such as when to give and when to cease giving medication and where to go for further advice.

When administering medication to children, it is essential that errors of dose are not made as this can have significant consequences. The child's weight should be accurately measured as dose is often weight related (mg/kg). This should be recorded on the prescription chart, which should ensure the medication is appropriate in dose, format and route for the child's age.

Children's nurses should have a good understanding of the signs and symptoms of adverse medicine reactions and be able to respond appropriately.

MEDICATION ADMINISTRATION AND LEARNING DIFFICULTIES

People with learning difficulties (LD) are just as likely as anyone else to have somatic conditions which need prescribed medication; however, the prescriber needs to work with the patient and the patient's carers to discuss treatment goals for best therapeutic outcomes. The NMC Code (2018) explains that you should 'use a range of verbal and non-verbal communication methods, and consider cultural sensitivities, to better understand and respond to people's personal and health needs' (7.3). The prescriber needs to ensure the patient has understood the need for the medication and gives valid consent to take it. The drug should be prescribed in a formula that the patient can readily take – most medications can be offered in dispersible forms for those who cannot swallow tablets or capsules.

Go Further 10.4

To support people with swallowing difficulties, you can improve your knowledge and get advice at: https://swallowingdifficulties.com/

The four principles of medicine optimisation explain how healthcare personnel can enable LD patients to improve their quality of life and outcomes from medicine use. These are:

1. Patient experience: Allow time for consultation and use the patient's preferred communication strategy.
2. Appropriate medication: Ensure medication is in a formulation the patient can take.
3. Safe and effective: Ensure the medication is appropriate and be mindful of polypharmacy.
4. Medicines optimisation as part of routine practice: an example of this would be a Medicines Use Review (MUR) which is an examination of the patient's actual use, understanding, beliefs and experience of taking drugs.

Further information can be found at the Royal Pharmaceutical Society and Mencap websites:

www.rpharms.com/Portals/0/RPS%20document%20library/Open%20 access/Policy/learning-disability-mo-article-160324.pdf

www.mencap.org.uk/sites/default/files/2016-07/Mencap_DP_Pharmacy_ resource_v2.pdf

MEDICATION AND THE ELDERLY

Older patients tend to suffer from impairment of function in the liver and kidneys (see Chapter 6), therefore important pharmacokinetic and pharmacodynamic changes occur in old age. A reduction in renal and hepatic function has pharmacokinetic consequence in terms of drug metabolism and clearance, leading to a longer drug half-life (such as digoxin). Pharmacodynamic change might include increased sensitivity to drugs such as anticoagulants and cardiovascular and psychotropic drugs (Mangoni and Jackson, 2004). Ageing is associated with a reduction in first-pass metabolism, probably due to reduction of liver mass and reduced blood flow in the cardio compromised. Malnourished older patients (and those with protein deficiency disorders such as protein-energy malnutrition [PEM]) have reduced bioavailability for drugs such as diazepam and warfarin; also a reduction in renal function affects the clearance of many drugs such as water-soluble antibiotics and diuretics. Mangoni and Jackson (2004) consider that elderly patients 'are particularly vulnerable to adverse effects from neuroleptics' (p. 7) and can develop postural hypotension and cardiac arrhythmias as a result. The observant healthcare worker will note and report adverse effects to the prescriber.

Elderly people are at a greater risk for adverse drug reactions (ADRs) because of the above-described metabolic changes and this iatrogenic risk is exacerbated by the increasing number of drugs prescribed for the elderly (polypharmacy). Drug to drug reactions and interactions can cause off-target side effects that cause decreased alertness, loss of appetite, confusion, constipation, or diarrhoea, weakness, tremors, and dizziness. These side effects could be misinterpreted as a new disorder leading to a prescribing cascade, with further medications added to treat the new condition. Therefore, frequent medication reviews should be undertaken to avoid unwanted effects.

MEDICAL DEVICES

Medical devices are regulated by the MHRA and Department of Health and are usefully defined by the World Health Organization (2017) as 'any instrument, apparatus, implement, machine, appliance, implant, reagent for in vitro use, software, material or other similar or related article, intended by the manufacturer to be used, alone or in combination, for human beings', and can be used for diagnosis, prevention, monitoring, treatment or alleviation of disease. This includes infusion pumps and enteric feeding systems.

Medical technology is a rapidly developing arena: it is now common for cardiac function to be supported by implants which regulate and stimulate the heartbeat, or to relieve atherosclerosis by stent; there are contraceptive implants, prosthetic blood vessels, hearing implants, renal dialysis and prosthetic limbs (to name but a few). AI robotic surgery has successfully taken place and there are artificial laboratory grown organs to replace worn out or diseased ones. Technology is used in the laboratory for diagnostic purposes, and MRI/PET/CAT scanners are now in every major hospital (and shopping malls in America) making X-ray machines nearly redundant. On wards, computers and tablets (such as iPads) are used for daily health recording and monitoring systems, patient records and drug management. Even before the patient arrives at A&E, paramedics will have used computerised systems to inform medical staff of the prospective patient's condition. You might have used computer software for training (such as Safemedicate), and medical staff have used virtual reality devices for training surgeons. The current 'Transformation and Sustainability' programme will promote remote/virtual GP appointments, with the patient wearing devices which record and transmit vital signs. However, protecting electronic data from 'hacking' or unethical use is a major issue.

PROTECTING E-DATA IN THE WORKPLACE

The Data Protection Act 1988, General Data Protection Regulation 2016 and the Data Protection Act 2018 together protect digital personal data against misuse of personal information. The Department of Health hosts the Guidance for Reporting, Managing and Investigating Information Governance and Cyber Security Serious Incidents, with a digital helpdesk to report security breaches requiring investigation using an e-notification form. If you use an electronic device which stores patient data, it must be password protected and safely kept where it is not easily accessible for theft. Your employer will have e-safety protocols about information sharing and confidentiality, and you should familiarise yourself with them to protect your patients' data.

CHAPTER SUMMARY

This chapter has introduced you to some of the calculations you need to be safe and effective as a nursing associate and care practitioner. Always remember, if you are in any doubt, seek help and support. Do not undertake any medicines administration method or delivery that you feel unsure about. The Code supports you here 'raise your concerns immediately if you are being asked to practise beyond your role, experience and training' (16.2). And states that for safety you can 'ask for help from a suitably qualified and experienced professional to carry out any action or procedure that is beyond the limits of your competence' (13.3).

This chapter has discussed the legislation that governs medicines administration and the regulatory framework for safe medicines management from storage to transportation and dispensation. We then considered pain and pain management and the use of alternative methods of pain control. We then considered adverse, off-target effects and how these can be reported.

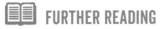

We discussed patients' right both to accept and refuse medication and the legal approach to disguised medication, which links with Chapters 4 and 9.

We also looked at medicines and specific groups: children, people with LD and elders. We considered the pharmacologic implications of ageing and medication; this has a relationship with Chapter 6, Biosciences, and the impact of ageing on the body systems.

We had a brief look at medical devices; this is a rapidly changing landscape as many new devices are being created for specific ailments, medical and surgical training, IT monitoring systems and general IT use on wards and in the community. Covid presented challenges for the whole nursing team and new practices have emerged such as pain relief delivery systems, remote monitoring and teleconferencing.

FURTHER READING

WEBSITES

- Advisory Guidance Administration of Medicines by Nursing Associates: www.hee.nhs.uk/sites/default/files/documents/Advisory%20guid ance%20-%20administration%20of%20medicines%20by%20nurs ing%20associates.pdf

- Managing medicines in care homes: www.nice.org.uk/guidance/sc1 and www.england.nhs.uk/wp-content/uploads/2018/03/medicines-opti misation-in-care-homes-programme-overview.pdf
- Medicine optimisation guide: www.nice.org.uk/guidance/ng5
- NHS England: www.england.nhs.uk/medicines/medicines-optimisation/
- Controlled drugs: safe use and management: www.nice.org.uk/guidance/ng46
- Secure and safe handling of medicines: a team approach: www.rpharms.com/recognition/setting-professional-standards/safe-and-secure-han dling-of-medicines

VIDEOS

- Why is Antimicrobial Stewardship Important? www.youtube.com/watch?v=gEM8JbwZquM
- Lewisham Integrated Medicines Optimisation Service (care homes/hos pitals): www.youtube.com/watch?v=rJWVqC42FhE
- Medication Error Training Video: www.youtube.com/watch?v=qMuN-MV6Z9Q

BOOKS

- Harris, M. (2021) *Understanding Person-centred Care for Nursing Associates.* London: Sage/Learning Matters.
- Roulston, C. and Davies, M. (2021) *Medicines Management.* London: Sage/Learning Matters.

JOURNAL ARTICLES

- Medicines management. Available at: https://journals.rcni.com/nurs ing-standard/medicines-management-ns.29.33.36.e9194
- Medicines management for the transition of care from hospital to home: a study. Available at: www.mdpi.com/journal/pharmacy/spe cial_issues/medicines_management

REFERENCES

Anekar, A.A. and Cascella, M. (2021) WHO analgesic ladder. *StatPearls [Internet].* Treasure Island, FL: StatPearls Publishing. Available at: www.ncbi.nlm.nih.gov/books/NBK554435/

Build Back Better: Our Plan for Health and Social Care (2021). Available at: www.gov.uk/government/publications/build-back-better-our-plan-for-health-and-social-care

Care Quality Commission (2022) Covert medication. Available at: www.cqc.org.uk/guidance-providers/adult-social-care/covert-administration-medicines

Department of Health (2006) *Medicines Matters: A Guide to Mechanisms for the Prescribing, Supply and Administration of Medicines.* Available at: www.sps.nhs.

uk/articles/medicines-mattersa-guide-to-mechanisms-for-the-prescribing-sup ply-and-administration-of-medicines-in-england/

Goldacre, B. (2012) What doctors don't know about the drugs they prescribe, TEDx talk. Available at: www.youtube.com/watch?v=RKmxL8Vyy0M

HEE (Health Education England) (2018) *Advisory Guidance: Administration of Medicines by Nursing Associates.* Available at: www.hee.nhs.uk/sites/default/files/ documents/FAQs%20-%20administration%20of%20medicines%20by%20nurs ing%20associates.pdf

Mangoni, A. and Jackson, S. (2004) Age-related changes in pharmacokinetics and pharmacodynamics: Basic principles and practical applications. *British Journal of Clinical Pharmacology, 57*(1), 6–14.

MHRA (Medicines and Healthcare Regulatory Authority) (2017) Medicines and healthcare products regulatory agency annual report and accounts 2016 to 2017. Available at: www.gov.uk/government/publications/medicines-and-healthcare-products-regulatory-agency-annual-report-and-accounts-2016-to-2017

NHS England (2019) Medicines optimisation. Available at: www.england.nhs.uk/ medicines-2/medicines-optimisation/

NHS England (2021a) Medicines: Improving outcomes and value (Medicines Value Programme). Available at: www.england.nhs.uk/medicines-2/

NHS England (2021b) Medicines optimisation found at www.england.nhs.uk/ medicines-2/medicines-optimisation/

NHS.gov (2017) Adverse drug reaction reporting. Available at: www.nhstaysideadtc. scot.nhs.uk/netFormulary/PDF/Adverse%20drug%20reaction%20reporting.pdf

NICE (National Institute for Health and Care Excellence) (2017) Medicines management. Available at: www.nice.org.uk/guidance/health-and-social-care-delivery/ medicines-management

NMC (Nursing and Midwifery Council) (2018) The Code: Professional standards of practice and behaviour for nurses, midwives and nursing associates. Available at: www.nmc.org.uk/globalassets/sitedocuments/nmc-publications/nmc-code.pdf

Prescqipp (2017) *Care Homes – Reviewing the Use of Monitored Dosage Systems (MDS).* Available at: www.prescqipp.info/media/1235/b174-care-homes-use-of-moni tored-dosage-systems-20.pdf

RCN (Royal College of Nursing) (2018) Medicines management: Professional resources. Available at: www.rcn.org.uk/clinical-topics/medicines-management/ professional-resources

RPSGB (Royal Pharmaceutical Society of Great Britain) (2017) Secure and safe handling of medicines: A team approach. Available at: www.rpharms.com/what-we-re-working-on/safe-and-secure-handling-of-medicines.asp

Van Zee, A. (2009) The promotion and marketing of oxycontin: Commercial triumph, public health tragedy. *American Journal of Public Health, 99*(2): 221–27.

Westbrook, J., Reckman, M., Li, L., et al. (2009) Effects of two commercial electronic prescribing systems on prescribing error rates in hospital in-patients: A before and after study. *PLoS ONE, 9*(1): e1001164.

WHO (World Health Organization) (2013) Guidance on INN (Ladder of analgesia) Available from: https://professionals.wrha.mb.ca/old/professionals/files/PDTip_ AnalgesicLadder.pdf

WHO (World Health Organization) (2017) Medical devices. Available at: www. who.int/health-topics/medical-devices#tab=tab_1

11

PUBLIC HEALTH

MICHELLE HENDERSON
AND GILLIAN ROWE

STANDARDS OF PROFICIENCY FOR NURSING ASSOCIATES (2018)

Relevant Platforms include:

Platform 2:2.1 Understand and apply the aims and principles of health promotion, protection and improvement and the prevention of ill health when engaging with people.

Platform 2:2.2 Promote preventative health behaviours and provide information to support people to make informed choices about their mental, physical, behavioural health and wellbeing.

Platform 2:2.3 Describe the principles of epidemiology, demography and genomics and how these might influence health and wellbeing outcomes.

Platform 2:2.4 Understand the factors that may lead to health inequalities in health outcomes.

Platform 2:2.6 Understand and explain the contribution of social influences, health literacy, individual circumstances, behaviours and lifestyle choices to mental, physical and behavioural health outcomes.

Platform 2:2.7 Explain why health screening is important and identify those who are eligible for screening.

Platform 2:2.8 Promote health and prevent ill health by understanding the evidence base for immunisation, vaccination and herd immunity.

Platform 2:2.9 Protect health through understanding and applying the principles of infection prevention and control, including communicable disease surveillance and antimicrobial stewardship and resistance.

Annex A 2.2, 2.2, 2.3.

Most of us cherish the notion of free choice, but our choices are constrained by the conditions in which we are born, grow, live, work and age.

Sir Michael Marmot (2010)

Glossary

- **Incidence** Number of new cases in a given population in a given time period (usually per year or per quarter)
- **Prevalence** All cases in a given population in a given time period (usually per year) or the number of cases in a given population at a point in time (point prevalence)
- **Hazard** Something that has the potential to cause harm
- **Risk** The likelihood of causing harm

INTRODUCTION

WHY IS PUBLIC HEALTH IMPORTANT?

Public health is a partnership effort through statutory and voluntary organisations, and those in the community and wider society to promote and protect health. The remit is wide ranging but the importance of tackling public health issues is very clear. A public health approach to health in the current climate is essential where financial pressures require not just a reactive, but a preventative, approach to reduce future burden on health services and reduce mortality and morbidity. The Wanless Report (2002) identified that disease prevention should be a priority and if not tackled would place huge pressure on the future health service. Over 20 years later in 2010, the Marmot Review, *Fair Society, Healthy Lives*, identified that health inequalities were still key factors, with people living longer in poorer health and those in the most deprived areas of the England most affected (Marmot, 2010). Public health is essential in tackling social inequality and ensuring all have a chance to live a healthy life across the life course, regardless of where you are born. Indicators suggest that those living in the most deprived areas at birth have 19.3 fewer healthy life years if female than their least deprived counterparts; for males it was almost 19 years fewer (Office for National Statistics, 2021a). It is estimated that the burden of health inequalities costs the NHS £4.8 billion per year (Asaria et al., 2016). Marmot (2010) argued that reducing health inequalities is not just important for health service provision, but for social justice and fairness. Therefore, public health is about addressing and promoting health across the life span by ensuring that children have the best start in life, and adults have the opportunity to live in healthy, sustainable communities, and that people can also age well.

This chapter will focus on the two main areas of public health practice: improving and protecting health. Health improvement is the addressing of inequalities, working with health, housing, education and communities, for example, to improve lifestyle and health outcomes. Health protection tackles issues such as infectious disease and environmental hazards: examples include immunisation and health screening, and management and surveillance of infectious disease. Often public health is proactive, such as campaigns to prevent deaths from cancer or promoting the National Immunisation Schedule. Sometimes public health is reactive and is required to respond to acute events such as flooding or an outbreak of an infectious disease, such as the recent global pandemic associated with Covid-19.

HEALTH INEQUALITIES

Health inequalities are defined as differences in health across the population. Health inequalities can be because of the conditions in which people are born, grow, live, work and age. These conditions can impact on an individual's health, and can shape mental health, physical health and wellbeing (NHS England, 2021b). We also sometimes talk about the wider and social determinants of health that can impact on a person's health and wellbeing, including housing, education, employment and air quality for example, a lot of which are out of an individual's control. Marmot recognised the impact of the conditions in which people are born, grow, work, live and age, and the wider set of forces and systems shaping the conditions of daily life. These forces and systems include economic policies and systems, development agendas, social norms, social policies and political systems (WHO, 2019).

Whilst life expectancy in general has risen in the UK due to medical advances and treatments, the population is living longer and is therefore faced with chronic diseases, like obesity, diabetes and heart disease, which impact on quality of life. These often also affect the poorest people, living in the most deprived areas. This means greater demand for health and social care services. Therefore prevention is key. *Build Back Better: Our Plan for Health and Social Care* (2021) identified this is crucial for a fairer society.

The Covid-19 pandemic has also shone a light on the importance of infectious and communicable disease as a public health threat. The Covid-19 global pandemic has refocused how we survey, control and manage emerging infections. Public health does not just focus on health promotion and promoting healthy lifestyles, nor just on social equity to achieve better health outcomes. Protection from communicable disease and other environmental threats is also important. Whilst deaths and disability from communicable diseases have reduced over the last century (through better understanding of diseases and immunisation programmes for example), communicable disease control is still an important part of public health. The surveillance of infections is vital to monitor and observe trends, reduce transmission of infectious disease, and to plan for future threats. This has never been more evident than in the global Covid-19 pandemic (which will be discussed further in this chapter).

Public health is everybody's business and is not just local but nationally and sometimes internationally driven. Organisations such as the World Health Organization (WHO), NATO and the United Nations (UN), for example, can sometimes shape policy which affects us here in England. Nationally, the public health field comprises multi-professional teams, which include: the UK Health Security Agency and the Office for Health and Improvement and Disparities (previously part of Public Health England), the NHS services, other health providers, local authorities (LAs), health workers, police, teachers, pharmacy workers, housing officers and the voluntary and charity sector and communities themselves.

DELIVERING PUBLIC HEALTH IN ENGLAND: THE NEW LANDSCAPE AND NEW WAYS OF WORKING

A review of how the wide remit of public health is delivered was addressed in the Health and Social Care Act 2012, which moved significant responsibility for tackling a population's health to LAs. It was identified that LAs were best placed to understand public health in locales and to determine what affected their local populations. This saw the creation of Public Health England (PHE), a national organisation with regional teams to support and advise government, local government and the NHS as a specialist body. The government paid a ring-fenced grant to local authorities for public health expenditure to change the focus from treating sickness to actively promoting health and wellbeing. Localities are deemed best placed to understand their local community health needs and work across sectors to provide a response. Each LA promotes health and social wellbeing in different ways. Each locality should address the needs of minorities such as refugees, asylum seekers and the street homeless. These groups are vulnerable and outreach services can support their health and wellbeing. Each council has mandatory duties such as sexual health services, NHS health checks and child measurement programmes. There is much more of a focus on population health and population health management. NHS England define population health as 'an approach that aims to improve physical and mental health outcomes, promote wellbeing and reduce health inequalities across an entire population' (NHS England, 2021a). This cannot be achieved in isolation and requires multiple statutory and non-statutory organisations working together.

Go Further 11.1

Go to your local council's website and search for public health. This should lead you to the things your local authority are addressing around public health and what services they offer. What kinds of things are their priorities and focus? How might some of these measures impact on the patients and clients you look after in your area as a nursing associate or assistant practitioner?

The landscape of public health is changing however, following the impact of the global pandemic of Covid-19. The functions of PHE were reviewed as part of the ongoing response and as of 1 October 2021 PHE has been disbanded and its functions split with the formation of two new national organisations with regional teams: the Office of Health Improvement and Disparities (OHID) and the UK Health Security Agency (UKHSA). The formation of Integrated Care Systems (ICS) as statutory bodies across regions from July 2022 onwards will also play a key role in public and population health at a local level.

OHID is part of the Department of Health and Social Care (DHSC) and will lead and drive the prevention agenda. The UKHSA remit will focus on preparing, preventing and responding to threats to public health such as infectious disease and environmental hazards. UKHSA will be focused on a science and research-based approach, working on a global scale to bring together the functions of the PHE health protection remit, the Joint Biosecurity Centre, and Test and Trace.

PARTNERSHIP WORKING IN PUBLIC HEALTH

Partnership working is key within public and population health across both statutory private and voluntary sectors but also with public involvement. The King's Fund (2016) defines cross-boundary working as reaching across structures to build relationships, interconnections and interdependencies. Therefore, an appreciation of the value of the wider public health workforce means the core of this workforce cannot work in silos. It is clear from emerging evidence that aside from traditional health and social care services, it is factors such as lifestyle and where we live and work that have impacts on our health, and that wider thinking is now occurring on how public health can be addressed in many of these arenas (Health Foundation, 2017; Marmot 2010).

The Office for Civil Society (2010) identified the importance of work between public and private sectors, and voluntary organisations and wider cross-boundary working to achieve public health outcomes by harnessing experience and skills. The Marmot Review in 2010 suggested the challenge of delivering public health was going to lie far beyond the NHS (Marmot, 2010), with NHS England (2014) later identifying that those services should be around those they serve, and not restricted by professional boundaries and systems. The Public Health Skills and Knowledge Framework (PHSKF) recognises that public health is system wide and requires interdisciplinary working with those in the wider workforce and across organisations (PHE, 2019).

Whilst the literature is clear on why cross-boundary working is important, it is recognised that it is not necessarily easy to achieve. It is acknowledged that there can be conflict with collectivism and that a complex range of issues can impact on the success of cross-organisational and professional boundary working (The King's Fund, 2017). This includes a myriad of values, organisational cultures and ways of working which can hamper individuals or groups working in an interdisciplinary manner.

Research clearly identifies leadership skills as important in managing some of these challenges (PHE, 2016a, 2016b, 2019). The PHSKF recognises the importance of leadership at all levels in the public health workforce in delivering the public health agenda, and it is clear from the components of the framework that leadership skills are required regardless of grade or position (PHE, 2019). The King's Fund (2016) argues that there is often emphasis on individual leadership development, but a collective organisation approach may be more fitting through shared leadership and collectivism, to address wider system challenges which apply to public health. Moreover, it identifies that cross-boundary working has outcomes for the people it is serving at its heart. It also recognises that leadership is much broader than those running or heading up services, and rightly considers those delivering the work on the frontline to be effective change makers in ways of going forward.

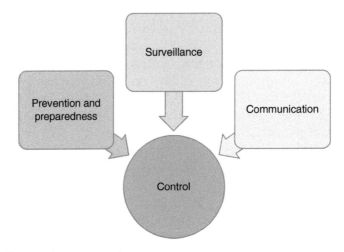

Figure 11.1   Infectious disease control

THE BURDEN OF PREVENTABLE DISEASE

OBESITY

Mortality and poor health from non-communicable disease are increasing. The UK has one of the largest obesity problems in Europe, with just over half of the population estimated as being overweight or obese, and one in three year 6 school children measuring overweight (PHE, 2020a). There were 10,780 hospital admissions directly attributable to obesity in England in 2019/20 (NHS Digital, 2021). Obesity is highest in those from the most deprived areas. With children in these areas more than twice as likely to be obese as their peers living in the richest areas (DHSC, 2020).

Obesity is also associated with reduced life expectancy as it is linked to many chronic diseases, including heart disease, type 2 diabetes, some forms of cancer, and liver and respiratory disease. Obesity can also impact on quality of life and mental health (DHSC, 2020).

A report by the Obesity Health Alliance (2021) has made several recommendations on how tackling the issues leading to obesity can be further addressed, including:

- Reviewing how unhealthy food products are advertised
- Effectiveness and take-up of weight management support and interventions for families
- Intensifying structured and unstructured physical activity in primary schools
- Invest more in obesity-related research

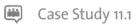 Case Study 11.1

Rachel is a nursing associate working in primary care. She is seeing one of her patients, Mr Jones, who has had recent surgery on his leg following an injury at work. He has been referred to his GP surgery for a wound dressing review and Rachel has been assigned to follow him up as per his care plan. Mr Jones is aged 50; he states he rarely accesses healthcare as he is normally well and has no health problems. During conversation he mentions he knows he is very overweight and should really do something about it. As he rarely attends health services there is no record of his weight in his notes.

What might Rachel do next?

Jot down your thoughts then read the model answer at the end of the chapter.

TYPE 2 DIABETES

Data suggest 1 in 10 people over 40 in the UK have type 2 diabetes (Diabetes UK, 2021). The number affected by type 2 diabetes is expected to grow further. In 2019, the expenditure associated with this preventable illness was estimated to cost the NHS £10 billion each year, which has doubled from 2010 (Diabetes

UK, 2019; Marmot, 2010). Those with diabetes are twice as likely to be admitted to hospital than those without type 2 diabetes and over 80% of the costs of managing someone with type 2 diabetes is managing complications (Diabetes UK, 2019). A study during the global Covid-19 pandemic also found that those with type 2 diabetes were at increased risk of death, demonstrating the significant impact the condition can have on people's mortality (Barron et al., 2020). The World Health Organization recognises that a healthy diet, regular physical activity, maintaining a normal body weight and avoiding smoking are key to prevent or delay the onset of type 2 diabetes (WHO, 2021b).

EXCESS ALCOHOL

Excess alcohol is linked to increased risk of certain cancers, high blood pressure and heart disease, cirrhosis of the liver and mental illness.

There were over 7000 alcohol-related deaths recorded in 2020 in England and Wales. This had grown by over 19% since 2019 (Office for National Statistics, 2021b). Males living in deprived areas were 4.2 times more likely to be part of these numbers, again linking the impact that can be seen with many preventable diseases of health and social inequalities. Alcohol deaths rates in England and Wales have been consistent, suggesting much work still needs to be done to prevent premature death and disability.

🗨 Case Study 11.2

Nursing associate Jane has been tasked to produce some information for the ward notice board about Dry January – a campaign that encourages people to give up alcohol during the month of January. Imagine you are Jane, where would you begin with this task?

Engage in some research and compare with the model answer at the end of the chapter.

SEXUAL HEALTH AND SEXUAL HEALTH SERVICES

The number of STIs (sexually transmitted infections) diagnosed in England decreased by 32% between 2019 and 2020. However, it should be noted that this could be linked with a 25% decrease in sexual health screening over the same period caused by the disruption in service provision during the Covid-19 pandemic, therefore it is difficult to understand the picture for 2020 (PHE, 2020b). Despite the overall decrease in recent years for STI diagnoses, STIs continued to disproportionately impact young people aged 15–24 years, and especially the black, Asian and minority ethnic (BAME) community (PHE, 2020c). However, government plans to establish 'Relationships Education' in primary schools, and 'Relationships, Sex and Health Education' in all secondary schools aim to help to educate young people about their sexual health.

Vaccination is now given to young adolescents before they become sexually active in order to prevent human papillomavirus (HPV), which causes genital warts and can be a precursor to cervical cancer as well as cancer in the vagina, vulva, anus, mouth and throat. C Card or Get It On (GIO) schemes are available in many counties, offering free condoms to (mainly) young people. Young people register for the card, and the settings that offer them also offer sexual health advice.

Sexual health services are also offered to those engaging with vulnerable groups such as sex workers. These services are often offered as outreach, as sex workers are likely to be hard to reach for safe sex services as prostitution is illegal. They are also less likely to engage in prevention services such as AIDS/HIV services, cervical smears and breast mammograms. Sex workers are also at risk of domestic violence and self-protection advice is offered.

Sexual health services are not just reactive, dealing with infections and following up cases, they also undertake a proactive approach in promoting health at local events, for example attending Pride festivals each year.

MENTAL HEALTH AND SUICIDE PREVENTION

Mental illness is a significant concern and cause of disability. In terms of employment, poor mental health impacts reduce productivity, which resulted in 17.5 million days lost at work in 2019 (Office for National Statistics, 2019). Recognition has grown over recent years that mental health services need greater parity of esteem to tackle the impact mental illness has on people's health and wellbeing (Department of Health, 2013; Mental Health Taskforce Strategy, 2016; Royal College of Psychiatrists, 2013). Rates of mental disorders in those aged 5–16 years are increasing, from 1 in 9 in 2017 to 1 in 6 in 2020 (NHS Digital, 2020). Between 2019 and 2020 2,878,636 people were known to be in contact with secondary mental health services such as community mental health teams (CMHTs) and crisis resolution teams; 763,888 of these were under 18 years of age.

Social inequalities impact on someone's risk of mental illness exacerbation, such as homelessness, unemployment, poverty and those in prison and those with drug and/or alcohol problems.

In England in 2020 4912 people took their own life: 75% were male and 25% were female, a trend that has continued for a number of years

Males aged 45–49 continue to have the highest suicide rates and the Northeast of England has the highest rates per 100,000 population (Samaritans, 2021). Suicide in those under 25 has been increasing for over a decade. A national cross-government strategy has been developed. The strategy outlines two principal objectives: to reduce the suicide rate in the general population and provide better support for those bereaved or affected by suicide. There are six areas for action:

1. Reduce the risk of suicide in key high-risk groups
2. Tailor approaches to improve mental health in specific groups
3. Reduce access to the means of suicide
4. Provide better information and support to those bereaved or affected by suicide
5. Support the media in delivering sensitive approaches to suicide and suicidal behaviour
6. Support research, data collection and monitoring

HM Government (2019)

In England, responsibility for the suicide prevention action plan and strategy usually lies with local government through health and wellbeing.

Go Further 11.2

Read this report from March 2021 on the progress of the government's suicide prevention strategy: https://assets.publishing.service.gov.uk/government/uploads/system/uploads/attachment_data/file/973935/fifth-suicide-prevention-strategy-progress-report.pdf

- Summarise the key themes from the report.
- What has gone well and where are improvements still required?

Go Further 11.3

Sign up to the e-learning for health suicide prevention module: www.e-lfh.org.uk/programmes/suicide-prevention/

HEALTH IMPROVEMENT AND PREVENTION APPROACHES

Health improvement is an area of public health that aims to improve the health and wellbeing at individual, community and population level by promoting healthy lifestyles. It addresses some of the wider underlying causes of poor health that can lead to some of the preventable illnesses discussed previously in this chapter. Health improvement is often tackled at scale through national campaigns or by changes in the law. Under the Health and Social Care Act 2012 local authorities have responsibility at a local level to tackle health inequalities by working together with the NHS, social care, housing, environmental health, leisure and transport sectors.

Examples of public health national campaigns that continue to date include:

- Change4Life – Aimed at healthy eating and living to reduce obesity and launched in 2009 as part of a national strategy set out by government's Healthy Weight, Healthy Lives (Parliament.uk 2008) document
- Frank – A national anti-drug advisory service jointly established by the Department of Health and Home Office of the British government in 2003
- Keep Antibiotics Working – This national campaign was first launched in 2017 across England and aimed to decrease antimicrobial resistance

The Department of Health launched the Change4Life campaign in January 2009, which focuses on prevention and aims to change the behaviours leading to weight gain. A survey undertaken by PHE found that 97% of mothers with children aged 5–11 associated the Change4Life brand with healthy eating (PHE, 2019).

As well as national campaigns, national policy can be set in law to improve public health.

An example of this is tobacco use.

The Tobacco Advertising and Promotion Act was introduced in 2002. This started with a ban on print media and billboard advertising in 2002. In 2007, smoking was banned in all indoor public places and from 2009 point-of-sale displays in shops had to remove tobacco products from public view. In 2016, plain packs with graphic images were introduced. This along with other initiatives has seen a steady decline in smokers in the last decade and the reduction is one of the key public health success stories of the last century.

POPULATION SCREENING

Screening is the process of targeting healthy people who may have an increased chance of a disease or condition based on their age, sex or health conditions. This enables early treatment or an awareness of susceptibility.

Screening can have many benefits:

- Screening can detect something early
- Finding out if they have a health condition, or an increased risk of a health problem can help people make better informed decisions about their health

However, there are risks and limitations to screening; screening tests are not always 100% accurate. A 'false positive' may occur and may lead to some people having unnecessary further tests or treatment as a result of screening. A screening test could also miss something – this is called a 'false negative' and could lead to people having a lower threshold for risk of a condition if they perceived a screening test did not detect anything. Screening can cause anxiety whilst people await test results, and some screening may lead to difficult decision making, such as antenatal tests that show a foetus has an abnormality for example. See Chapter 7, Advanced Health Science, Case Study 7.2 for a case in point.

The UK National Screening Committee is responsible for reviewing and advising on all aspects of screening, including the case for introducing new population screening programmes and for continuing, modifying or withdrawing existing population programmes. The current screening programme within the United Kingdom can be found in Table 11.1.

Table 11.1   UK screening programmes

Stage	Screening programme
Antenatal	• Screening for infectious diseases (hepatitis B, HIV and syphilis) • Screening for Down syndrome, Patau's syndrome and Edwards' syndrome • Screening for sickle cell disease and thalassaemia • Screening for physical abnormalities (mid-pregnancy scan)
Newborn babies	• A physical examination, which includes the eyes, heart, hips and testes • A hearing test • A blood spot test to check if the baby has any of the following – sickle cell, cystic fibrosis, congenital hypothyroidism, inherited metabolic disease, severe combined immunodeficiency (SCID)
Adults	• Diabetic eye screen (all those with diabetes aged 12 and over) • Cervical screening is offered to women aged 25–64 to check the health of cells in the cervix. It is offered every 3 years for those aged 26–49, and every 5 years from the ages of 50 to 64. • Breast screening is offered to women aged 50–70 to detect early signs of breast cancer; women over 70 can self-refer • AAA screening is offered to men in their 65th year to detect abdominal aortic aneurysms; women over 65 can self-refer • Bowel cancer screening (there are two types of screening for bowel cancer)

Source: Information taken from www.gov.uk/topic/population-screening-programmes

A FOCUS ON A NATIONAL SCREENING CAMPAIGN: CERVICAL CANCER SCREENING

The NHS cervical screening campaign is targeted at women aged 25–64 in England. Cervical screening aims to try to prevent cancer by detecting and treating abnormalities of the cervix. Cervical screening involves collecting samples of cells from the cervix.

Human papillomavirus (HPV) is a common virus transmitted through sexual contact; in most cases, a woman's immune system will clear the infection without the need for treatment. HPV has hundreds of different subtypes, most of which do not cause serious disease. If left untreated, these abnormal cells may go on to develop into cervical cancer. It is estimated that cervical screening in England for example prevents 70% of cervical cancer deaths (PHE, 2017).

However there have been debates over at which age cervical screening should take place and a parliamentary debate took place in 2019 following a petition for the age to be lowered from 25 years to 20 years. The motion was not passed and the lowest age eligible for a cervical screening remains at 25 years old following the advice of the National Screening Committee.

⚙️ Activity 11.1   Critical debate

Gather into two groups:

- A group who is petitioning for the age limit to be lowered. From your group's perspective put arguments forward as to why you think the age limit should be lowered for cervical screening.
- A group representing the UK Screening Committee. From your group's perspective put arguments forward as to why you think the age limit should remain unchanged for cervical screening.

Use the links below and carry out independent research to support your argument:

www.gov.uk/topic/population-screening-programmes/cervical

www.cancerresearchuk.org/about-cancer/cervical-cancer/getting-diagnosed/screening

https://obgyn.onlinelibrary.wiley.com/doi/pdf/10.1111/1471-0528.13720

https://researchbriefings.files.parliament.uk/documents/CDP-2021-0113/CDP-2021-0113.pdf

www.manchestereveningnews.co.uk/news/greater-manchester-news/woman-given-devastating-cervical-cancer-20855523

MAKING EVERY CONTACT COUNT (MECC)

Some factors such as smoking, lack of physical exercise, excessive alcohol intake and poor diet are known to increase the risk of illnesses such as stroke, coronary artery disease and cancers. Therefore, making changes to one's lifestyle can greatly reduce the risks of developing such illnesses and conditions. MECC is an approach to tackling this through everyday interactions and contacts with people through our line of work. MECC is not just aimed at those who traditionally may have contact with clients or service users such as hospital staff and those working in GP surgeries for example. The MECC approach is encouraged in all those who may have contact with the public across health and social care and beyond; this can include statutory authorities such as social services, charities serving the voluntary sector and private sector retail outlets such as chemists and pharmacies.

Go Further 11.4

Investigate the free online training resources of All Our Health, which offer bitesize learning around a range of public health topics: www.e-lfh.org.uk/programmes/all-our-health/

Health Education England (2019) recognises that staff across health and social care, public services, local authorities and voluntary sectors have a lot of contact every day with individuals and are ideally placed to promote health and healthy lifestyles. This links in with the All Our Health campaign, which focuses on healthcare professionals and those working with patients and the public and encourages them to think about how they can help to prevent illness, protect health and promote wellbeing through their interactions with people and through brief interventions that promote health messages.

Go Further 11.5

Using the links provided to increase your knowledge and understanding of MECC, take each case scenario and discuss how MECC could be implemented by the healthcare worker.

    www.makingeverycontactcount.co.uk/
    www.makingeverycontactcount.co.uk/search-results?term=case+studies
    www.hee.nhs.uk/our-work/better-training-better-care

A. Amanda is a nursing associate working on a medical ward. Most patients are admitted with acute medical illness such as chest pain or respiratory conditions.

B. Rachel is an assistant practitioner working with the community district nursing team. Her role is varied and involves going into people's home to support with wound dressings, blood pressure monitoring and chronic illnesses.

C. Hassan is a trainee nursing associate working in a nursing care home for clients with both physical and mental health needs.

SOCIAL PRESCRIBING

It is recognised that there are many factors that can impact on an individual's health that cannot necessarily be resolved or improved by traditional medical approaches.

Examples may include:

- Feelings of isolation
- Little or no family or few friends
- Feeling lonely
- Lacking a focus in life
- Few or no hobbies
- Living alone and little social contact

Current methods to improve health outcomes in individual mental health and wellbeing are implementing non-clinical or medicalised ways of achieving better health outcomes. It is recognised that people's health is impacted on by a range of social and environmental factors. The principle of social prescribing is to support an individual to access voluntary services and other support services which may help to improve their social connections and interactions. The NHS Long Term Plan (2019) has a commitment to personalised care and increasing access to social prescribing for the whole population. The General Practice Forward View (2016) emphasised the role of voluntary sector organisations to reduce pressure on GP services. In June 2016, NHS England appointed a national clinical champion for social prescribing to advocate for schemes and share lessons from successful social prescribing projects (The King's Fund, 2017) which will help with mental and physical health conditions. Examples may include referral to a local gym, education or training courses, community groups or signposting to voluntary work.

Social prescribing is seen to potentially have many benefits including:

- Meeting new people and making new networks
- Learning a new skill
- Increasing self-esteem and worth
- Improved fitness
- Increasing wellness
- Reducing need for more traditional clinical services

Go Further 11.6

Read more about social prescribing at: www.gov.uk/government/publications/social-prescribing-applying-all-our-health/social-prescribing-applying-all-our-health

DIGITAL APPROACHES TO HEALTH IMPROVEMENT

Technological changes such as how data and information technology are used to support the delivery of the public health agenda have been significant over the last decade and are increasingly evolving, as in other areas of health. How we communicate health improvement messages is vital to ensure we reach the people intended. The rise in social media has been notable since the introduction of Facebook in 2004 and Twitter in 2006, followed by Instagram in 2010 and TikTok in 2016. One of the greatest advantages of social media is reach, with the opportunity of potential targeted health promotion programmes. Where traditionally an individual may have to search for information on a health concern, social media can use opportunistic pop ups on people's accounts or shares from friends or acquaintances. This may also bring something to an individual's attention they may not have previously thought about.

Moorhead et al. (2013) found that social media can:

- Provide information on a range of issues at scale
- Facilitate dialogue between patients and health professionals
- Collect data on patient experiences and opinions
- Help in direct health intervention, for health promotion and health education
- Help to reduce illness stigma

However, using social media in the field of public health is something of a double-edged sword as the quality of information can vary greatly and there is much disinformation, which can be shared 'virally' and is more difficult to control.

The benefits of digital approaches include access to online training which can be done at the user's convenience outside of traditional learning or workplace settings. This also means that the training provided is standardised and can be assessed using standardised measures. Digital platforms also allow for simultaneous group sharing so communities of practice can share knowledge and debate through, for instance, podcasts and group chat. An added benefit is reduced costs for training.

Text messages are being used to support health, including reminders to take medication, health service appointment reminders, monitoring and self-management of chronic disorders such as diabetes. This method of contact and delivery has been found to be cost-effective and has scalability to large populations. Another example of utilising technology could be with patients who require direct observed therapy. The treatment of tuberculosis often requires a multi-drug regime that if not taken correctly, and for an appropriate timeframe, may mean the infection is not treated and possibly multi-drug resistance could occur. Therefore, in groups who may be deemed as unlikely to comply with their treatment, direct observed therapy is initiated. This often involves visiting the patient at their home or attendance at a clinic to observe medication has been taken. This is costly and can have a huge impact on resources. Newer ways of carrying out observed therapy are being trialled such as video observed treatment using smartphones.

The NHS Long Term Plan includes increasing the range of digital health tools and services. These allow people to interact with the NHS through apps that will offer the ability to see medical records, make appointments and view test results. So far, over 70 apps are available in the NHS apps library and more will come onstream over time. Indeed, the Health Secretary's document *Prevention is Better Than Cure* identifies that we must think about how we can harness technology to improve health. It acknowledges it can be difficult to monitor and review how these newer approaches to health and wellbeing work, and accessing their effectiveness will be something that will need to be monitored and evaluated as they move forward (DHSC, 2018).

Go Further 11.7

Current apps and digital tools used in public health include:

- Sugar smart app
- Couch to 5k
- Heart Age tool

Research the above apps/tools and think about:

- What are the benefits to this app/tool?
- What could be the negatives to this app/tool?
- Who may these apps/tools be aimed at?
- What channels on the internet/social media may be best to promote such apps/tools?

ASSET-BASED APPROACH TO PUBLIC HEALTH

In this chapter so far, we have talked about how health systems work with local authorities and the voluntary sector to meet the wider remit of public health challenges. It is also important to consider the role that communities themselves play in improving public health.

The King's Fund (2021) argues that community roles in improving health are receiving increasing and long-overdue attention, and that systems need to appreciate the role communities can play in tackling health improvement.

Asset-based approaches to public health can be defined as a 'bottom-up' strategy where a community's life experience, skills and knowledge are used to tackle issues and problems. It looks at harnessing those assets and empowering communities for sustainable change and working with them in partnership to achieve this. The role of co-production in health, where health services work with service users to develop, review and improve services, is not a new concept. This is also important in public health, and the voice of those most affected by issues should be heard. The Health Foundation (2017) identifies that this approach challenges the historical view of the health professional or those in authority being the expert and considers the service user as an equal expert in lived experience. This way of working balances power platforms and allows those driving services to learn and understand things from the service user's perspective.

PREVENTION AND PROTECTION AGAINST COMMUNICABLE DISEASE AND ENVIRONMENTAL AGGRESSORS

Health protection involves the management of communicable disease and managing outbreaks and incidents which could threaten the health of the public. On 1 April 2013, the Health Protection Agency was abolished, and its responsibilities and duties were transferred to PHE (Public Health England). Health protection teams were created to provide specialist public health advice and operational support to the NHS, local authorities and other agencies. There are eight centres outside London, along with an integrated regional centre in London. Local teams lead response to all health-related incidents alongside their local authority and NHS colleagues, providing support to prevent and reduce the impact of infectious diseases, chemical and radiation hazards, and major emergencies. On 1 October 2021 during the global Covid-19 pandemic, PHE was disbanded, and the health protection element was moved to the UK Health Security Agency (UKHSA).

Health protection teams work to protect the public by:

- Local disease surveillance
- Maintaining alert systems
- Investigating and managing health protection incidents and outbreaks
- Implementing and monitoring national action plans for infectious diseases at local level

COMMUNICABLE DISEASE

A communicable disease is one that is spread from one person to another through a variety of ways:

- **Directly** through body fluids such as sexual contact (e.g. syphilis, HIV)
- **Person-to-person** by inhalation of infected airborne droplets or particles (e.g. Covid-19, influenza, TB)

- **Indirectly** via surface or other contamination (e.g. hepatitis C from contaminated needles, HIV from blood products)
- By **ingestion** of contaminated food or water (e.g. salmonella, hepatitis A)
- Through an intermediate **animal host or vector** (e.g. malaria)

Important factors include:

- Severity: Is the illness self-limiting? Could it lead to severe complications? Is it treatable?
- Transmission: Directly person-to-person (faecal/oral); indirectly (needlestick injury); ingestion (food/water); vector or animal (bite)
- Susceptibility: Exposed people/person, are they person immune? Are they at greater risk?

People at risk of being *more* susceptible to infection *and/or* more likely to become severely ill include:

- The very young
- The very old
- Pregnant women
- People with comorbidities
- People who are immunosuppressed
- IV drug users

INCUBATION PERIOD VS INFECTIOUS PERIOD

The incubation period is the timeframe from being exposed to the infection to developing symptoms yourself. Some infections have a very short incubation period such as salmonella, which can be 12–72 hours. Other infections have much longer incubation periods such as hepatitis A, which has a range of 15–50 days.

The infectious period is the timeframe someone can be contagious and pass infection on to others. Again, the infectious period differs from infection to infection. For example, mumps is infectious a couple of days before swelling to 5 days after swelling, whereas measles is 4 days before the rash and 4 days after.

Infectious period timeframes are essential when dealing with cases where contact tracing is important and people at risk may need follow-up or isolation.

WHAT ARE NOTIFIABLE DISEASES?

Certain diseases and infections are notifiable (see Table 11.2), meaning the diagnosing clinician or those working in laboratories have a responsibility to report to their local consultant in Communicable Diseases Control (CDC), usually because an additional public health action is required.

Table 11.2   Schedule 1 of the Notification Regulations 2010 (NOIDs)

Measles	Diphtheria	Malaria	Scarlet fever
Acute infectious hepatitis	Enteric fever (typhoid or paratyphoid fever)	Severe Acute Respiratory Syndrome (SARS)	Meningococcal septicaemia
Mumps	Food poisoning	Smallpox	Tetanus
Acute poliomyelitis	Haemolytic uraemic syndrome (HUS)	Infectious bloody diarrhoea	Invasive group A streptococcal disease
Anthrax	Acute meningitis	Plague	Typhus
Botulism	Tuberculosis	Rabies	Leprosy
Brucellosis	Legionnaires' disease	Rubella	Whooping cough
Cholera	Viral haemorrhagic fever	Acute encephalitis	Yellow fever

Source: www.gov.uk/guidance/notifiable-diseases-and-causative-organisms-how-to-report

1. Prevention – stopping infection happening in the first place by:
    - Immunisation
    - Food hygiene
    - Clean water supply
    - Sexual health advice

2. Prevention – stopping more cases occurring by:
    - Treatment
    - Contact tracing and advice about reducing risks

IMMUNISATION

The two public health interventions which have had the greatest impact on the spread of communicable disease are the provision of clean water and immunisation. Herd immunity occurs when enough people in a community are vaccinated: it is harder for a disease to pass between people who have been vaccinated. This is particularly important for the protection of people who cannot be vaccinated because they are too ill, or they are having treatment that damages their immune system or they are too young.

ISSUES FOR POLICY MAKERS AND IMMUNISATION

The Joint Committee on Vaccination and Immunisation (JCVI) is an independent departmental body made up of experts which advises UK health departments on immunisation following due consideration of the evidence on:

- The burden of disease
- Vaccine safety and efficacy
- Cost of the programme vs benefit
- Population accessibility
- Cultural attitudes and practices
- Facilities available for delivery

The government considers the JCVI's advice to inform, develop and make policy. The UK immunisation policy, 'Immunisation against Infectious Diseases', is also known as the Green Book. The details and statistics are ascertained by surveillance and through published literature and special studies.

Go Further 11.8

Choose one of the following infections:

- Measles
- Polio
- Meningitis C

Using the Green Book as a reference (see link below) find out for your chosen infection:

What symptoms can it cause?

How common is it?

How is it spread?

What is the infectious period?

What is the incubation period?

What vaccination is available (if any) and how many times is it given and when?

www.gov.uk/government/collections/immunisation-against-infectious-disease-the-green-book

---

COVID-19 GLOBAL PANDEMIC

On 11 March 2020, the World Health Organization declared a global pandemic caused by a novel emerging coronavirus named SARS-CoV-2 causing coronavirus disease 19 (or Covid-19 as it is commonly known). This followed an emerging situation of increased respiratory illness and deaths in China in December 2020.

The first case in the UK was reported on 31 January 2021, and there have been over 150,000 UK deaths (UKHSA, 2022). On a global scale there have been well over 5 million deaths (WHO, 2021a), but figures are likely to be lot higher than this due to reporting mechanisms in some parts of the world.

Coronavirus disease (Covid-19) is an infectious disease caused by the SARS-CoV-2 virus.

There are different kinds of coronavirus that usually cause mild illness like the common cold. However, there are three which are known to have caused more severe illness in recent years (Table 11.3).

Table 11.3   Coronavirus case numbers

	First cases	Case numbers
SARS-CoV (severe acute respiratory syndrome)	First outbreak in 2002. Emerged in China. Smaller outbreak in 2004	8098 cases in 29 countries
MERS-CoV (Middle East Respiratory Syndrome)	First identified in 2012 in the Middle East. Linked to camels and transfer to humans	2580 cases across 27 countries
SARS -CoV 2	December 2019 emerged in China	220 million cases – global

People usually experience symptoms within 2–14 days of exposure to the virus (incubation period). A person infected with coronavirus can be contagious (infectious period) to others for up to 2 days before symptoms appear, and they can remain contagious to others for 10–20 days, depending upon their individual immune system and how severe their illness is.

PUBLIC HEALTH MEASURES TO CONTROL THE PANDEMIC

The government has used a variety of physical and social controls to try and reduce the spread of Covid-19 and its severity of illness including:

- Mass vaccination
- Mask wearing and other PPE
- Social distancing and advice to stay at home
- Changes to public buildings and workplaces to make them 'Covid secure'
- Contact tracing and isolation advice

This next section will look at some of these key interventions

VACCINES

Over 76% of the UK population have received two doses of Covid-19 vaccination (Gov.uk, 2021), and over 60% of the global population has had at least one vaccination.

The Covid-19 vaccines currently approved for use in the UK are:

- Moderna vaccine (mRNA)
- Oxford-AstraZeneca vaccine (viral vector)
- Pfizer-BioNTech vaccine (mRNA)
- Janssen vaccine (available in 2021/22) (viral vector)

There are two main types of vaccines. Viral vector vaccines use an unrelated harmless virus (the viral vector) to deliver SARS-CoV-2 material into the person. The body then uses the material to produce a specific viral protein, which is recognised by the immune system and triggers an immune memory response. mRNA vaccines contain a piece of genetic material of the SARS-CoV-2 virus, which causes Covid-19. When administered, the body uses the genetic material to make the protein, which is recognised by the immune system and triggers a specific immune memory response.

The vaccination campaign in England saw a huge scaling up and delivery en masse at a scale not seen in previous immunisation programmes. Whilst the introduction of the vaccines in such a small timeframe was seen as a scientific and systemic success, it has brought some issues and controversies.

A survey by Mavron (2021) found that some people were hesitant to receive the vaccine due to perceived unknown immediate and long-term side effects. Some raised concerns about the short timeframe the vaccine had taken to be developed in comparison to vaccinations in the past. This was further impacted by a small number of people receiving the AstraZeneca vaccination developing fatal bloods clots. However, studies have since found the risk of life threatening clots is higher for those who develop Covid-19 infection (Taquet et al., 2021). Others stated they did not need the vaccine due to age, or that they did not have an underlying health condition that would put them at risk. There were also members of the public who perceived the vaccination as being forced on them by the state and removing freedom of choice. There are also groups who believe the disease does not exist and therefore no interventions are needed.

The Covid-19 vaccination remains a key means of controlling the significant symptoms and spread of the disease. Ongoing research continues to monitor its effectiveness and need for future (booster) vaccinations. It is also important that the global challenges of ensuring fair distribution of vaccination remain on the agenda, as control cannot work in isolation: to tackle a global pandemic and the vaccination side of control will require a continued global approach going forward.

TESTING

Testing during the Covid-19 pandemic has been targeted at both those with symptoms and those without (asymptomatic). Testing at scale:

- Allows monitoring of the infection rates
- Detection of clusters or outbreaks associated with a particular area or setting
- Identifies positive cases who can then isolate appropriately avoiding further transmission

Rapid growth of both NHS and private laboratories was undertaken to meet the demand of Covid testing. Pillar one laboratories are NHS local laboratories and pillar two are the national laboratories commissioned by the government to support testing.

There are currently two main types of testing taking place in the UK (Table 11.4).

Table 11.4   Types of testing for Covid-19

Test	How is it done	Pros	Cons
Polymerase chain reaction (PCR) tests	PCR tests can be ordered and done at home or at a specialist drive through. A swab is taken and then sent away to a lab to diagnose	Most accurate test available to test for Covid-19	Must be sent away to a lab and can take 24–48 hours for results Can show a false negative if sample not of good quality
Lateral flow tests (LFTs) are antigen tests. They look to detect the proteins rather than RNA	LTFs can be ordered and done by individuals at home. A swab is taken and then using a specific piece of equipment is tested immediately. Results can be read within 30–60 minutes	LFTs are antigen tests that can diagnose Covid-19 quickly. Can be done at home	Are not as accurate as PCR tests. Should not be used on those with symptoms

The UKHSA has intervened when laboratories have failed quality standards and suspended testing due to reliability issues.

CONTACT TRACING AND ISOLATION ADVICE

Other key means the government has attempted to control the spread of Covid-19 have been through contact tracing, isolating cases and contacts, and encouraging social distancing among the general public.

Test and Trace is a government initiative that aimed to track and prevent the spread of Covid-19 through contact tracing, surveillance and advice. It initially involved calls and texts to members of the public and included the introduction of an app which was received with mixed reception; the app experienced technical issues which impacted on public trust in its use.

Contact tracing is not a new tool used in controlling infectious disease; it has been used for a long time by public health teams. The principles are simple: to identify cases and give advice on isolation periods and to identify the contacts during the infectious period to give them advice about risk, and sometimes treatment to prevent onward spread of disease. Contact tracing and isolation advice has evolved during the pandemic, governed by case numbers and the introduction of the vaccination programme.

The latest guidance has removed the need for contacts of cases to isolate if they have received two Covid-19 vaccines (except in special circumstances such as health workers).

There have been debates over how the Test and Trace service will look going forward, with some crossover of work between health protection teams and the local authorities. The National Audit Office (2021) reviewed the Test and Trace system and identified that there needs to be a clear evaluation of its purpose and the outcomes it is achieving to determine its value for money.

IMPACTS OF COVID-19 ON HEALTH AND SOCIAL CARE

Following the the Health and Social Care Act 2012, public health in England was moved into local authorities. Public health teams in LAs delivered a wide range of services before the pandemic. However, public health budgets have been cut significantly since 2015/16. Data from the Health Foundation (2021b) show that 6 million fewer people completed elective care pathways between January 2020 and July 2021 compared to pre-pandemic. This meant a lot of routine and elective care was postponed. The way that patients accessed care changed during this time, with some services moving to virtual or digital approaches and other, non-urgent and routine procedures being cancelled.

Directors of public health (DsPH) have a key role in protecting their communities, and they have played a significant role in England's response to the Covid-19 pandemic. Their knowledge and expertise (and that of their teams) in population health have been vital in addressing the immediate impacts of Covid-19 on health, as well as understanding and mitigating the economic and social impacts of the pandemic that will affect the health of their populations well into the future.

In April 2020, a third of all deaths associated with Covid-19 in England were in care homes. Social care workers also had some of the highest death rates during the first phase of the pandemic and sickness absence rates *more than doubled* between February and October 2020 (Health Foundation, 2021a). The demographics of social care staff is considered to be a factor. A quarter are aged 55 and older and 21% are from black and minority ethnic backgrounds (Health Foundation, 2021a).

The social care system was both underfunded and understaffed entering the pandemic, thus ensuring a poor response to the additional pressures placed upon it (Health Foundation, 2020). There have been sharp criticisms that the government did not do enough in the early stages of the pandemic to protect care home residents and staff – particularly poor access to PPE and the failure to test prior to discharging residents back to care homes from hospitals. The majority of care homes are provided by private companies. This brings difficulties in terms of control and management of a system that is already fragile and not under public service control.

The Department of Health and Social Care made an amendment to the Health and Social Care Act 2008, which means from 11 November 2021, all care workers who work in Care Quality Commission (CQC) registered homes must be vaccinated. The rationale for this is that of the greater public health benefit of protecting those who are most vulnerable (the care home residents) from severe illness and death from Covid-19.

Registered home managers and providers will be responsible for monitoring this and, in turn, will be monitored by the CQC. This has been a controversial subject, balancing individual rights with that of the wider benefit of others. There are concerns this could cause a staffing crisis (Unison, 2021), especially as the care sector has seen an exodus of staff (Skills for Care, 2021).

The government funded seven Nightingale hospitals in preparation for NHS hospitals becoming overwhelmed with unwell patients, but without experienced staff available to operate them, they were an expensive white elephant.

HEALTH IMPACTS OF COVID-19 ON THE INDIVIDUAL

Shielding recommendations for those with underlying health conditions meant many experienced isolation. In an ONS poll, 35% reported an increase in poor mental health (Office for National Statistics, 2020).

A study by Health Protection Scotland found that 87% felt that shielding had impacted their quality of life, with 85% reporting their physical activity had reduced (Public Health Scotland, 2020).

The demographics of those who were significantly impacted by Covid-19 are similar to what we have talked about earlier in the chapter around preventable disease – those from the most deprived areas, including:

- Those living in cramped, overcrowded housing often with no outdoor space or room to isolate.
- Children being home schooled by parents who struggled due to their own educational attainment.
- Those without broadband or access to IT equipment.
- Lack of access to transport in the early days of the pandemic meant accessing testing without a car was difficult (this was soon adapted with walk-in testing centres and kits being sent to people's homes). This was especially noticeable in rural areas.
- Often those working in low-income jobs had no option to work from home, for example: care workers, retail workers, bus drivers, refuse collectors.

PHE (2020c) reported a strong association between economic disadvantage and Covid-19 diagnoses, incidence and severe disease.

A study by PHE (2020c) also found that the highest rates of Covid-19 per 100,000 population were in people belonging to black, Asian and ethnic groups. Many of the reasons found to be contributing factors to this linked to inequalities that had existed prior to the pandemic such as discrimination and lack of trust in health services resulting in delayed assessment and communication difficulties.

WHAT DOES THE FUTURE HOLD FOLLOWING THE GLOBAL PANDEMIC OF COVID-19 FOR PUBLIC HEALTH?

VARIANTS OF INTEREST AND CONCERN

The nature of viruses is they can mutate over time. This is called a variant. This means that the original virus changes slightly, and sometimes the mutation makes it more transmissible or causes more serious illness.

PHE (now UKHSA) has been responsible for monitoring variants during the pandemic. They are categorised as follows:

- VUI – variant under investigation. This is where scientists are monitoring the effects of a new emerging variant.
- VOC – variant of concern. This is where a VUI has been identified as being of concern due to its increased risks.

In May 2021, WHO announced a new naming system for the Covid-19 variants of concern (VOC):

- Alpha variant – originally named the Kent variant. It was discovered in the South East of England in December 2020.
- Beta variant – originally termed the South African variant.

- Gamma variant – this variant was first identified in Brazil, and is less prevalent in the UK.
- Delta variant – first classified as a VOC in May 2021. Originally termed the Indian variant.
- Omicrom variant – classified in November 2021.

The Delta variant was the most dominant variant in the UK, found in almost 90% of samples, as of September 2021, but by December 2021 the Omicron variant became the dominant virus, a demonstration of the changing nature of variants.

Further monitoring of emerging variants is important to detect how the virus evolves and to review if current vaccines are as effective for emerging variants of concern.

TACKLING INEQUALITIES HIGHLIGHTED BY THE PANDEMIC

The Marmot Covid-19 review 'Build Back Fairer' looked at the impact Covid-19 had on inequalities; this was part of the government initiative 'Build Back Better'. It identified that the inequalities that already existed before the pandemic contributed to the increased death toll in those from areas of deprivation and hard to reach and marginalised groups. Marmot highlighted that there needs to be a strong investment from government as health and the economy are intrinsically linked, but also from a justness perspective (Marmot, 2020). This follows from another Marmot report in 2020, which found the gap between health inequalities has been widening and life expectancy plateauing since Marmot did his original review a decade earlier (Marmot, 2010).

LONG COVID

The impact on the health system has not only meant a backlog in non-urgent and elective procedures, it has also seen the emergence of individuals who are suffering long-term effects of Covid-19. These effects are impacting on quality of life and ability to work and participate in normal activities in society. As we are continuing to learn and understand more about the virus, there is emerging evidence that some people are experiencing debilitating symptoms long after expected recovery times.

WHO announced a definition of long Covid in October 2021. 'Post COVID-19 condition occurs in individuals with a history of probable or confirmed SARS-CoV-2 infection, usually 3 months from the onset of COVID-19 with symptoms that last for at least 2 months and cannot be explained by an alternative diagnosis. Common symptoms include fatigue, shortness of breath, cognitive dysfunction but also others which generally have an impact on everyday functioning. Symptoms may be new onset, following initial recovery from an acute COVID-19 episode, or persist from the initial illness. Symptoms may also fluctuate or relapse over time' (WHO, 2021a).

Emerging evidence has suggested that between 88 and 97% of those with Covid-19 in England will recover within 12 weeks and have no significant long-lasting complications. The Office for National Statistics (ONS) suggested, however, that as of September 2021 there could be as many as 643,000 people living in England with long Covid-19, and with symptoms ranging in severity in terms of impact on quality of life and activities of daily living (Office for National Statistics, 2021c). National research is ongoing into the symptoms and effects, and special long Covid clinics with specialist teams are being set up within the NHS to support those facing the ongoing effects of Covid-19 well beyond the pandemic.

NON-INFECTIOUS HAZARDS TO HEALTH

Non-infectious hazards can be just as detrimental to human health as infectious disease.

ANTIMICROBIAL RESISTANCE (AMR)

Antibiotics are generally used to treat bacterial infections, but there is a growing issue with bacteria becoming resistant to many of the antibiotics that would normally be used to treat them. This means infections may be difficult to treat or take longer to treat. Sepsis is already a significant cause of death in the UK (see Chapter 8 for more details about sepsis). If more common bacteria become further resistant to antibiotics, the number of deaths will increase. Many people undergoing routine surgery or those receiving chemotherapy for cancer, for example, may be even more vulnerable.

Resistant bacteria can also spread to other people both in and out of healthcare settings. Antibiotic resistance is a global problem. Globally antibiotic resistance has been developing due to:

- Over prescribing of antibiotics
- Patients not taking or completing their treatments correctly
- Poor infection control principles in healthcare settings
- Overuse of antibiotics in the farming and fishing industries
- Lack of development of any new antibiotics in the last few decades

WHO has identified things that can be done by individuals to prevent AMR:

- Only use antibiotics prescribed by a health professional
- Always take the antibiotics as instructed and do not give them to anyone else
- Practise good infection control, which can help to prevent some infections in the first place, such as washing hands, practising safe sex and attending

for vaccinations as per national schedule, and practise good food hygiene and preparation

The WHO (2015) Global Action Plan on Antimicrobial Resistance has five strategic objectives:

- To improve awareness and understanding of antimicrobial resistance
- To strengthen surveillance and research
- To reduce the incidence of infection
- To optimise the use of antimicrobial medicines
- To ensure sustainable investment in countering antimicrobial resistance

The UK government has also developed its own strategy to tackle antimicrobial resistance and has set out its aims to achieve reduction by 2040.

Go Further 11.9

To enhance your knowledge, try this World Health Organization quiz:

How Much Do You Know About Antimicrobial Resistance?

www.emro.who.int/world-antibiotic-awareness-week/2019/test-your-knowledge.html

Read the UK government's strategy here: www.gov.uk/government/publications/uk-5-year-action-plan-for-antimicrobial-resistance-2019-to-2024

AIR POLLUTION

There are growing concerns about the impact of air pollution, not just on our planet, but also on human health. There is evidence of its link to respiratory and cardiovascular disease, low birth rates and more recently conditions such as dementia (PHE, 2018). Many things contribute to air pollution, including transport using fuel such as diesel and petrol, industrial and farming processes and the fuels we use to heat our homes.

PHE (2018) estimates that air pollution is likely to be linked to between 28,000 and 35,000 deaths each year in England. Those who are particularly at risk include: young children, those with underlying health conditions, older persons and those living in heavily polluted areas, such as on traffic dense urban roads or near busy junctions.

Local authorities have a responsibility to review the impact of air pollution on their populations and find strategies to reduce it. For example, London's response to traffic pollution has been to charge cars to enter the city, and to extend its transport infrastructure (crossrail projects and nightlink buses). Other cities have invested in trams, electric buses and cycle lanes.

The UK government response includes its strategy to end the sale of diesel and petrol vehicles by 2040 and it is looking at ways to:

- Support the agricultural industry and other industries to reduce emissions
- Reduce the use of wood, coal and solid fuel sources to heat homes

Air pollution is also a wider part of climate control change and our need to look after our planet to ensure it is sustainable for the future.

CHAPTER SUMMARY

This chapter has introduced you to the role of public health regionally, nationally and internationally.

You have learned how health surveillance informs policy and how policy is implemented locally by local authorities to meet community needs.

We examined how public health has responsibility for critical emergency planning, identifying emerging threats and recognising national health issues and promoting measures to tackle inequalities to support people to live longer, healthier lives.

📖   Case study model answers

Case Study 11.1

- What information and knowledge would Rachel need to signpost Mr Jones to the right support?

Knowledge of local weight reduction sessions include those provided by the health sector via Nurse Associate clinics, social prescribing clinics, local non-profit activities and private for-profit providers (such as commercial weight loss clubs). She could explain to Mr Jones the dangers of obesity such as diabetes, Cardiovascular disorder and dementia and explore the health benefits of weight loss such as increased life expectancy with fewer disabilities and offer him an appointment at a well man clinic for a well man check.

Case Study 11.2

You have been tasked with producing materials on Dry January for the ward noticeboard. Begin with general reading around the subject and look at drink aware websites where you might find resources and then decide what key things you want to put on the noticeboard about the impact of alcohol on health such as heart and liver damage, a higher cancer risk, a weakened immune system, memory issues and mood disorders. Alcoholchange.org website offers a list of reasons to do Dry January; they offer an app, a booklet and blogs. You could utilise some of their materials and make a QR code link to the website and the social media pages. You could include the hashtag #stopsobershaming as awareness raising of the problems people who give up alcohol face from friends and family.

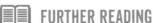 **FURTHER READING**

WEBSITES

- Department of Health and Social Care: www.gov.uk/government/organisations/department-of-health-and-social-care
- UK Health Security Agency: www.gov.uk/government/organisations/uk-health-security-agency
- Office for Health Improvement and Disparities: www.gov.uk/government/organisations/office-for-health-improvement-and-disparities
- Royal Society for Public Health: www.rsph.org.uk/
- Royal College of Nursing: Public Health: www.rcn.org.uk/clinical-topics/public-health
- World Health Organization: www.who.int/health-topics/health-promotion#tab=tab_1

VIDEOS

- Public Health Surveillance – A Brief Overview: www.youtube.com/watch?v=3IpE8dE4cVc
- Epidemiological Studies – Made Easy!: www.youtube.com/watch?v=Jd3gFT0-C4s
- The Urgent Action Needed to Tackle Health Inequalities: www.youtube.com/watch?v=dfBLaZbROJo

REFERENCES

Asaria, M., Doran, T. and Cookson, R.J. (2016) The costs of inequality: whole-population modelling study of lifetime inpatient hospital costs in the English National Health Service by level of neighborhood deprivation. *Journal of Epidemiology and Community Health.* Available at: www.england.nhs.uk/publication/the-costs-of-inequality/

Barron, E., Bakhai, C., Kar, P., Weaver, A., Bradley, D. and Ismail, H. (2020) Associations of type 1 and type 2 diabetes with COVID-19-related mortality in England: a whole-population study. *The Lancet: Diabetes and Endocrinology.* Available at: www.thelancet.com/journals/landia/article/PIIS2213-8587(20)30272-2/fulltext

Data.gov UK (2022) *Covid Vaccinations UK.* Available at: https://coronavirus.data.gov.uk/details/vaccinations

Department of Health (2013) Achieving parity of esteem between mental and physical health. Available at: www.gov.uk/government/speeches/achieving-parity-of-esteem-between-mental-and-physical-health

Department of Health and Social Care (2018) *Prevention is Better than Cure: Our Vision to Help You Live Well for Longer.* Available at: www.gov.uk/government/publications/prevention-is-better-than-cure-our-vision-to-help-you-live-well-for-longer

DHSC (Department of Health and Social Care) (2020) Tackling obesity: empowering adults and children to live healthier lives. Available at: www.gov.uk/government/publications/tackling-obesity-government-strategy/tackling-obesity-empowering-adults-and-children-to-live-healthier-lives

DHSC (Department of Health and Social Care) (2021) Covid-19 vaccination of people working or deployed in care homes: operational guidance. Available at: www.gov.uk/government/publications/vaccination-of-people-working-or-de ployed-in-care-homes-operational-guidance

Diabetes UK (2019) Statistics on people living with diabetes. Available at: www. diabetes.org.uk/about_us/news/new-stats-people-living-with-diabetes

Gov.uk (2020,2022) UKHSA data series on deaths in people with COVID-19: tech- nical summary. Available at: www.gov.uk/government/publications/phe-data- series-on-deaths-in-people-with-covid-19-technical-summary

Health Education England (2019) Making every contact count. Available at: www. hee.nhs.uk/our-work/making-every-contact-count

Health Foundation (2017) *Healthy Lives for People in the UK*. Available at: www. health.org.uk/publications/healthy-lives-for-people-in-the-uk

Health Foundation (2020) New analysis lays bare government's failure to pro- tect social care from COVID-19. Available at: www.health.org.uk/publications/ reports/adult-social-care-and-covid-19-after-the-first-wave

Health Foundation (2021a) How is COVID-19 impacting people working in adult social care? Available at: www.health.org.uk/news-and-comment/blogs/ how-is-covid-19-impacting-people-working-in-adult-social-care

Health Foundation (2021b) Elective care: how has COVID-19 affected the waiting list? Available at: www.health.org.uk/news-and-comment/charts-and-infographics/ elective-care-how-has-covid-19-affected-the-waiting-list

HM Government (2019) Suicide prevention: cross-government plan. Available at: www. gov.uk/government/publications/suicide-prevention-cross-government-plan

Marmot, M. (2010) *Fair Society, Healthy Lives (The Marmot Review)*. London: UCL Institute of Health Equity. Available at: www.instituteofhealthequity.org/ resources-reports/fair-society-healthy-lives-the-marmot-review

Marmot, M. (2020) Health equity in England: the Marmot review 10 Years On. Available at: www.health.org.uk/publications/reports/the-marmot-review- 10-years-on

Mavron, N. (2021) COVID-19 vaccine refusal, UK: February to March 2021: explor- ing the attitudes of people who are uncertain about receiving, or unable or unwill- ing to receive a coronavirus (COVID-19) vaccine in the UK. Office for National Statistics. Available at: www.ons.gov.uk/peoplepopulationandcommunity/ healthandsocialcare/healthandwellbeing/bulletins/covid19vaccinerefusaluk/ februarytomarch2021

Mental Health Taskforce Strategy (2016) *The Five Year Forward View for Mental Health*. London: NHS England.

Moorhead, S.A., Hazlett, D.E., Harrison, L., Carroll, J.K., Irwin, A., et al. (2013) A new dimension of health care: systematic review of the uses, benefits, and lim- itations of social media for health communication. *Journal of Medical Internet Research*, 15(4): e85.

National Audit Office (2021) Test and trace in England – a progress update. Available at: www.nao.org.uk/report/test-and-trace-in-england-progress-update/

NHS Digital (2020) Mental health of children and young people in England, 2020: Wave 1 follow up to the 2017 survey. Found at https://digital.nhs.uk/ data-and-information/publications/statistical/mental-health-of-children-and- young-people-in-england/2020-wave-1-follow-up

NHS Digital (2021) Statistics on obesity, physical activity and diet, England 2021. Available at: https://digital.nhs.uk/data-and-information/publications/statistical/ statistics-on-obesity-physical-activity-and-diet/england-2021#summary

NHS England (2014) *The Five Year Forward View*. London: NHS England.

NHS England (2016a) *General Practice Forward View*. Available at: www.england. nhs.uk/gp/gpfv/

NHS England (2016b) New NHS leadership framework – developing people improving care. Available at: www.england.nhs.uk/2016/12/new-nhs-leadership-framework/

NHS England (2021a) Population health and the population health management program. Available at: www.england.nhs.uk/integratedcare/what-is-integrated-care/phm/

NHS England (2021b) Health inequalities. Available at: www.england.nhs.uk/about/equality/equality-hub/

NHS Long Term Plan (2019) Available at: www.england.nhs.uk/long-term-plan/

Obesity Health Alliance (2021) Turning *the Tide: A 10-year Healthy Weight Strategy*. Available at: https://aso.org.uk/sites/default/files/news/2021-09/Turning-the-Tide-Strategy-Report.pdf

Office for Civil Society (2010) *Supporting a Stronger Civil Society: A Strategy for Voluntary and Community Groups, Charities and Social Enterprise*. London: Cabinet Office.

Office for National Statistics (2019) Mental health. Available at: www.ons.gov.uk/peoplepopulationandcommunity/healthandsocialcare/mentalhealth

Office for National Statistics (2020) Coronavirus and shielding of clinically extremely vulnerable people in England: 28 May to 3 June 2020. Available at www.ons.gov.uk/peoplepopulationandcommunity/healthandsocialcare/conditionsanddiseases/bulletins/coronavirusandshieldingofclinicallyextremelyvulnerablepeopleinengland/28mayto3june2020

Office for National Statistics (2021a) Health state life expectancies by national deprivation deciles, England: 2017 to 2019. Available at: www.ons.gov.uk/people-populationandcommunity/healthandsocialcare/healthinequalities/bulletins/healthstatelifeexpectanciesbyindexofmultipledeprivationimd/2017to2019

Office for National Statistics (2021b) Quarterly alcohol-specific deaths in England and Wales: 2001 to 2019 registrations and Quarter 1 (Jan to Mar) to Quarter 4 (Oct to Dec) 2020 provisional registrations. Available at: www.ons.gov.uk/peoplepopulationandcommunity/birthsdeathsandmarriages/deaths/bulletins/quarterlyalcoholspecificdeathsinenglandandwales/2001to2019registrationsandquarter1jantomartoquarter4octtodec2020provisionalregistrations

Office for National Statistics (2021c) How common is long COVID? *That depends on how you measure it*. Available at: https://blog.ons.gov.uk/2021/09/16/how-common-is-long-covid-that-depends-on-how-you-measure-it/

Office for National Statistics Mental Health data. Available at: www.ons.gov.uk/peoplepopulationandcommunity/healthandsocialcare/mentalhealth

Parliament.uk (2008) *Healthy Weight, Healthy Lives: Six Months On*. Available at: http://data.parliament.uk/DepositedPapers/Files/DEP2008-2168/DEP2008-2168.pdf

Public Health England (2016a) *Diabetes prevalence models estimates for local authorities*. Available at: www.gov.uk/government/publications/diabetes-prevalence-estimates-for-local-populations

Public Health England (2016b) *Fit for the Future: A Review of the Public Health Workforce*. London: PHE.

Public Health England (2017) *Health Matters: Making Cervical Screening More Accessible*. Available at: https://ukhsa.blog.gov.uk/2017/08/30/health-matters-making-cervical-screening-more-accessible/

Public Health England (2018) *Health Matters: Air Pollution*. Available at: www.gov.uk/government/publications/health-matters-air-pollution/health-matters-air-pollution

Public Health England (2019) *Public Health Skills and Knowledge Framework*. London: PHE.

Public Health England (2020a) Obesity profile. Available at: https://fingertips.phe. org.uk/profile/national-child-measurement-programme

Public Health England (2020b) Sexually transmitted infections and screening for chlamydia in England, 2020. Available at: https://assets.publishing.service.gov. uk/government/uploads/system/uploads/attachment_data/file/1015176/STI_NCSP_report_2020.pdf

Public Health England (2020c) Beyond the data: understanding the impact of COVID-19 on BAME groups. Available at www.gov.uk/government/publications/covid-19-understanding-the-impact-on-bame-communities

Public Health Scotland (2020) Shielding survey finds high levels of compliance, but the experience has been hard for vulnerable groups. Available at: www.pub lichealthscotland.scot/news/2020/september/shielding-survey-finds-high-lev els-of-compliance-but-the-experience-has-been-hard-for-vulnerable-groups/

Royal College of Psychiatrists (2013) *Whole Person Care from Rhetoric to Reality: Achieving Parity Between Mental and Physical Health*. Available at: www.basw. co.uk/system/files/resources/basw_103627-6_0.pdf

Samaritans (2021) Suicide prevention. Available at: www.samaritans.org/branches/ballymena/samaritans-ballymena-news/suicide-prevention-help-available-from-samaritans/

Skills for Care (2021) *The State of the Adult Social Care Sector and Workforce in England*. Available at: www.skillsforcare.org.uk/adult-social-care-workforce-data/Workforce-intelligence/publications/national-information/The-state-of-the-adult-social-care-sector-and-workforce-in-England.aspx

Taquet, M., Husain, M., Geddes, J., Luciano, S. and Harrison, P.J. (2021) Cerebral venous thrombosis and portal vein thrombosis: a retrospective cohort study of 537,913COVID-19 cases. Available at: https://osf.io/a9jdq/

The King's Fund (2016) *Supporting Integration Through New Roles and Working across Boundaries*. London: The King's Fund.

The King's Fund (2017) What is social prescribing? Available at: www.kingsfund. org.uk/publications/social-prescribing

The Kings Fund (2021) Communities and health. Available at: www.kingsfund.org. uk/publications/communities-and-health

Unison (2021) Scrap mandatory vaccine deadline or risk decimating the care sec tor, says UNISON. Available at: www.unison.org.uk/news/press-release/2021/09/scrap-mandatory-vaccine-deadline-or-risk-decimating-the-care-sector-says-unison/

UKHSA (2022). Available at: www.gov.uk/government/organisations/uk-health-security-agency

Wanless, D. (2002) *Securing our Future Health: Taking a Long-term View*. Final Report. London: HM Treasury.

World Health Organization (2015) Global action plan on antimicrobial resistance. Available at: www.who.int/publications/i/item/9789241509763

World Health Organization (2019) Social determinants of health. Available at: www.who.int/social_determinants/en/

World Health Organization (2021a) Coronavirus (Covid 19) dashboard. Available at: https://covid19.who.int/

World Health Organization (2021b) Diabetes. Available at: www.who.int/news-room/fact-sheets/detail/diabetes

12

HEALTH PROMOTION

SCOTT ELLIS

STANDARDS OF PROFICIENCY FOR NURSING ASSOCIATES (2018)

Relevant Platforms include:

2.1 Understand and apply the aims and principles of health promotion, protection and improvement and the prevention of ill health when engaging with people.

2.2 Promote preventive health behaviours and provide information to support people to make informed choices to improve their mental, physical, behavioural health and wellbeing.

2.6 Understand and explain the contribution of social influences, health literacy, individual circumstances, behaviours and lifestyle choices to mental, physical and behavioural health outcomes.

4.1 Demonstrate an awareness of the roles, responsibilities, and scope of practice of different members of the nursing and interdisciplinary team, and their own role within it.

4.9 Discuss the influence of policy and political drivers that impact health and care provision.

6.1 Understand the roles of the different providers of health and care. Demonstrate the ability to work collaboratively and in partnership with professionals from different agencies in interdisciplinary teams.

The greatest medicine of all is to teach people not to need it.

cited by Troy Newcome (2021)

INTRODUCTION

To define 'health promotion', students and researchers typically refer to the World Health Organization's (WHO) constitutional definition that health is about a holistic approach to living and not just the prevention of disease. This definition dates back to WHO's inception in 1948 and reflected a bold definition of health for everyone. It is still relevant today of course, but we need a much more responsive and adaptable understanding of health promotion to meet the changing demands on our lives and on our health. People are more mobile than ever before, which brings new challenges in how we address problems such as alcoholism, substance misuse and poor sexual health. This is further exacerbated by the political and economic climates of the Western world, which typically foster elitism and material gain, and vilify the poor and financially vulnerable. This translates into poorer health overall, particularly in relation to obesity, which affects people who live in deprived areas and have lower incomes more frequently than those with a steady income (Royal College of Physicians, 2020).

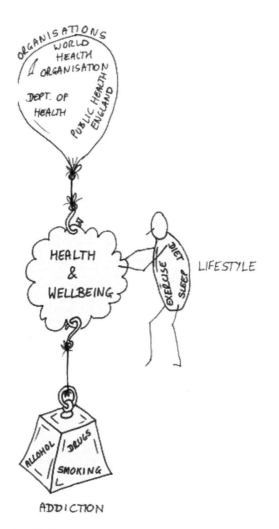

Figure 12.1   Health and wellbeing

Figure 12.1 shows how different factors contribute to an individual's health and wellbeing, including the actions of government departments and lifestyle. Addiction is used in the diagram as an example to show how one element of a person's life can impact on overall health and wellbeing. Of course, not all health promotion work is centred on addiction, and this can be replaced, or supplemented, with issues such as harmful habits, lack of knowledge or specific diseases, to name a few.

In this chapter, we will consider the health outcomes for diverse groups of people who are targeted with health promotion campaigns and discuss the efficacy of our most common methods of health promotion. We will also consider health promotion theory and models of practice utilising my experience as a health promotion professional, practitioner and academic.

Box 12.1   Health promotion – HIV

HIV (human immunodeficiency virus) and AIDS (acquired immune deficiency syndrome) are health challenges that have affected populations regardless of socioeconomic status and decades of prevention efforts since the early 1980s. In 2019, 105,200 people in the UK were living with HIV, of which 6% did not know they were infected (National AIDS Trust, 2021). The lack of a cure or vaccine for HIV and the typically sociosexual basis of transmission has meant progress in reducing new infections has been variable. As such this chapter uses examples of international HIV prevention campaigns to help identify both problematic and successful responses and interventions.

METHODS OF HEALTH PROMOTION

Behaviour modification and harm reduction are the most common aims of health promotion. By improving policy, mobilising community action and using social marketing techniques to communicate with a defined target audience (Gallagher et al., 2021; Melnyk et al., 2020), health promoters can work towards achieving these goals. These three areas coexist to drive health conditions and outcomes for people. On the surface it seems like a lot to ask that a health promotion campaign could address all three. However, with the right methods, we can facilitate changes that impact several areas at the same time. Take the three areas of improvement above. We can use social marketing techniques to better inform people and mobilise a community or population group to take action to improve their health. This can, in turn, improve policy from a local authority because of pressure from their local population.

> ## Box 12.2
>
> Health promotion campaigns and interventions are the most common forms of our work because they help us to engage directly with people at risk of poor health outcomes. This can be because of a range of factors and is not always down to personal lifestyle choices, a common misperception. It is important to consider how people's surroundings, relationships and life circumstances impact on their health. For example, reducing obesity is a common goal of health authorities, which promote the idea that it is a simple matter of choice when it comes to healthy eating. This is often far from the truth and as health promoters we need to consider a range of contributing factors such as whether people have access to affordable healthy food and whether they have the knowledge and skills to prepare such food.

Mass media are a simple social marketing technique that can be used to expose large numbers of people to a targeted message, often by using images to explain. This often takes the form of posters, magazine and newspaper advertising and television and radio adverts. Small media use similar techniques such as print booklets or pocket-sized information cards. Digital media have become increasingly common as a method to reach and engage with a target audience, particularly in sexual health work with young people, who value privacy and efficient access to digital, on-demand advice (Melcher and Torous, 2020).

In all these methods, there are elements that can be tailored to reach individuals within a population group given some extra planning and scoping of an area. The campaign shown in Figure 12.2 was part of a health promotion campaign to empower women to take control of their sexual health as an HIV prevention and education strategy in the US. The focal point of the campaign is a confident black woman and large posters such as this were displayed in neighbourhoods across New York City where HIV incidence rates were high and where census information showed there to be a high proportion of black female residents.

While advertising can be placed in the press based on a magazine or newspaper's known readership, this is far from an exact art. For instance, most of the UK's press aimed at gay men is saturated by HIV prevention work, which makes it difficult for health promoters to know how many people read or understand their work. Similarly, health promotion advertising in bars and clubs is common, including NHS-driven safer drinking campaigns. Such approaches seek to meet WHO's healthy settings approach to health promotion (2021) but do not address the disparity between advertising the risks of excessive drinking in establishments that exist to promote this.

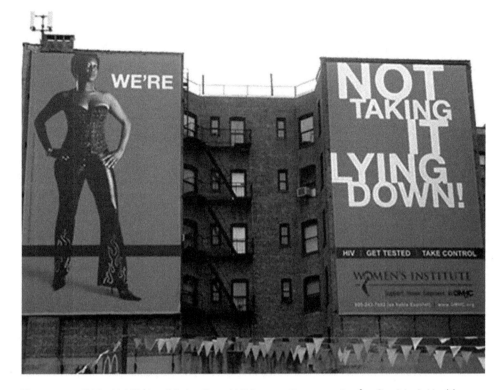

Figure 12.2   *We're Not Taking It Lying Down!* HIV prevention campaign for Gay Men's Health Crisis, Women's Institute at GMHC

Source: Photo courtesy of GMHC

Box 12.3

Good practice in health promotion means looking beyond governmental and health authority publications and data and finding research programmes and outcomes that help us to evaluate the extent to which a campaign or intervention has worked. Such work also helps us to consider very specific elements of a health promotion project that might not be accessible from government or agency reports. For example, above we look at safer drinking campaigns and their placement in bars and clubs. There is little government-level analysis of this practice but by considering broader peer-reviewed research, we can find a wider range of understanding of the importance of the 'where' of health promotion. In this example, research by Phillips et al. (2020) identified that harm reduction media in a bar or club environment can drive positive results because it is delivered in an environment familiar to people and in which they are relaxed and more likely to engage with stimuli.

Using digital techniques to reach and engage with a target audience is becoming increasingly popular, particularly as social media and email provide platforms rich in user behavioural information. Gilbey et al. (2020)

identified digital health promotion methods to have significant potential when working with young people to improve their knowledge of sexual health and risk-taking behaviour. Such methods lend themselves well to planning with established models and theories, such as the behaviour-change theory. However, as is discussed elsewhere in this chapter, the lack of current multi-agency, cross-sector working in the UK's health sector hinders our ability to fully utilise the possibilities of digital health promotion at present. Despite this, some health promotion organisations and NHS centres use digital methods for engagement, including to communicate sexual health screening results and to enable young people to access sexual health advice and condoms.

MODELS AND THEORIES

We use models and theories (often combined and referred to as theoretical models) in health promotion to help us understand how interventions, campaigns and programmes can achieve changes in behaviour and better health outcomes. They work in a few different ways, most commonly:

- **before** a campaign, to help us create materials that are likely to have a degree of success because the model helps us to use evidence of best practice
- **during** or **after** a campaign, to evaluate impact and progress

Most of the theoretical models used in health promotion are adapted versions of their original, some of which can be decades old. Health practitioners and researchers experiment with different applications of models by modifying component parts. This helps us understand how models can adapt to changes in health needs and human behaviour over time, which means we can make use of models created some time ago.

This chapter refers to several theoretical models often used in health promotion. Here I provide a brief overview to help you contextualise them:

- The **medical model of health** views health as the absence of disease, rather than as good holistic health. The model focuses on clinical intervention to treat health problems with medicines. The model is useful for clinical professionals because it enables them to treat large numbers of patients living with disease or health problems. This model can be difficult to apply to health promotion because it views disability as an abnormality to be overcome rather than a difference to be engaged with.
- The **health belief model** focuses on social behaviours relating to health and psychological beliefs about health and lifestyle. This model is often used to improve uptake of health interventions, such as vaccines. The model is unique in that it notes a stimulus, or cue, must be present before a person will consider adopting a health-promoting behaviour.

- The **stages of change model**, also sometimes called the transtheoretical model, describes how people integrate new behaviours and goals into their lives by measuring their readiness to change. The model helps us understand the process of behaviour change, such as when an individual begins to reduce harmful alcohol intake or increase their frequency of exercise.
- The **PRECEDE-PROCEED model** is a cost-benefit evaluation framework still in use since its formal inception in the 1970s. It helps health promotion professionals to assess health needs at a given point in time that help to direct planning towards achieving specific goals, such as a reduction in smoking. The model is written in capitals because it is an acronym; PRECEDE stands for Predisposing, Reinforcing and Enabling Constructs in Educational Diagnosis and Evaluation. PROCEED stands for Policy, Regulatory and Organisational Constructs in Educational and Environmental Development.
- The **nine stages planning model**, sometimes called the nine steps model, helps health promoters to plan a campaign or intervention by considering the preparatory stages that should be completed to facilitate the greatest chance of impact. The model focuses on the role of the health promoter and integrates elements of the target group by asking them to consider factors such as people's readiness to adopt behaviour changes.

The likely success or failure of a health promotion campaign is complex and depends on multiple factors relating to the campaign itself, the environment in which it is operating and the people it aims to help. You should look for evidence of how models are used in your area of health interest and read about how they are used.

Box 12.4

Health promotion models are used to underpin campaigns, communication and intervention work and help healthcare workers and researchers to ensure their work is evidence-based. Laing's (1998) medical model of health represents a clinical model for health improvement but is increasingly criticised by health promoters who acknowledge the holistic benefits of approaching health behaviour from both a physical and psychological standpoint (Sarto-Jackson, 2021). Hochbaum et al.'s health belief model (HBM) (Fish Ragin et al., 2020) and Prochaska et al.'s 1992 stages of change model (SCM) (Ahmad and Singh, 2021) focus on individual decision-making capacity and the ability of individuals to consider the cost/benefit balance of changes in behaviour. For example, we know that smoking rates increase with levels of poverty and hardship (Sattouf, 2020). This is counterintuitive since smoking is expensive and those in hardship have little disposable income. The HBM and SCM, both of which include the importance of social factors, help health promoters to understand that giving up smoking is likely to increase stress amongst population groups that already experience this in abundance such as in lower socioeconomic groups (Cambron et al., 2020).

A number of health promotion theories and models exist and can be used for different purposes, such as planning or evaluation, depending on the desired outcome. There is no one size fits all approach when it comes to choosing a health promotion model and it is easy to find criticism about the failures of each. It is worth remembering that models do not guarantee success, they simply make planning and delivery more robust and help to create understanding so that health promotion work becomes more targeted. Criticism about how health promoters fail to fully utilise the potential of models (Reback et al., 2019) or to implement the model components (Fernandez et al., 2019) is important because it helps us to identify how we can improve our work.

Models range from the simplistic, such as the health belief model (HBM) with its six constructs, to the complex, such as the PRECEDE-PROCEED model (PPM), which has 10 constructs within an eight-phase process. There is no set rule or framework about how complicated or simple a model should be; the most important thing is to choose the model most appropriate to what you are trying to achieve.

I have found few constants in how the hundreds of students I have supervised have chosen their preferred health model or theory, other than they work from the basis of whether they intrinsically believe in a particular medical or social approach to health improvement. A variety of researchers deconstruct this further and believe the choice of model or theory is less important than the need to integrate multiple constructs in health promotion (Hagger and Hamilton, 2021; O'Mara, 2021) in the biopsychosocial model. This model considers multiple influences on the experience, behaviour and health beliefs of individuals, including environment, education and legislative policy. In considering the totality of a person's existence, the biopsychosocial model aims to improve health outcomes by addressing multiple needs in a concurrent approach.

One model I have found to be adaptable to multiple health promotion contexts and which students have found accessible, is the stages of community readiness model (Figure 12.3). Most useful in the early stages of campaign planning, the model has similarities to Corcoran's (2007) nine stages planning model and includes scope for the ongoing development of a campaign into professional fields or long-term responsive placement.

The stages of community readiness model is used as part of a 'community tool box' at the University of Kansas Work Group for Community Health and Development and can be used to position a health promotion campaign within specific communities based on their existing knowledge of a health problem or threat.

One of the model's best attributes is that it can be used for virtually any health promotion campaign or intervention and incorporates both the target group and the health promoter. It begins with the assumption that the target individual or population have no knowledge of the health problem at hand and moves systematically through a process of increasing knowledge. Midway through the stages, the model shifts focus away from the individual and their health knowledge to the health promoter and how they prepare and initiate a campaign or intervention. The final stage, 'professionalisation', refers to how the health promotion work has been implemented and embedded into a health system or programme.

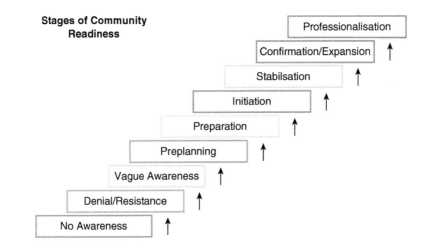

Figure 12.3   Stages of community readiness model, University of Kansas

Aside from the established academic models and theories readily available for health promoters, professional and non-profit organisations often construct their own framework based on their specialist work. Similarly, individual research projects of all sizes often result in new theories or models ready for further testing.

KEY CHALLENGES

Which health problems to prioritise for intervention, and which population groups to target, are often dictated by national epidemiological data. In the UK, the Office for National Statistics (ONS) monitors morbidity and mortality data that show us where problems with disease incidence lie and who is affected most prominently by avoidable poor health outcomes.

Most commonly, this relates to health inequalities such as poor access to healthcare for people with lower levels of education, or those who live in poverty and with unemployment. However, a key challenge for all of those who work in health promotion is how to balance this sensibly with the needs of people who do not live in poverty or in areas of deprivation. This can often be a challenging concept for students to comprehend as the news media and social marketing frequently present minority groups as the most in need.

Indeed, we know that wealth or income are linked on a gradient with health. For instance, as income levels rise, significant health risks decline (Alderwick and Gottlieb, 2019). Similarly, the more income a person has, the more likely they are to describe their own health as good (Health Foundation, 2021). However, some health problems and risks transcend levels of wealth or poverty and by focusing health promotion only on groups most visibly in need, we risk missing an opportunity to engage with people who are in need of urgent intervention. A key example is suicide risk amongst men, regardless of their social background or financial standing.

Suicide is the 7th leading cause of death for men in Canada (Oliffe et al., 2021) and the US (Centers for Disease Control and Prevention, 2019 and the 12th leading cause of death in the UK (ONS, 2020). Societal pressures placed on men that dictate norms of constructed masculinity, including an aversion to showing emotion or demonstrating empathy, contribute significantly to these data (King et al., 2020). There have been recent drives to address the unmet needs of men in general, and young white men specifically in both the US and the UK.

Figure 12.4 is a video still from the Write Home Project and depicts Ben Grenrock, a young man who talks about his experience of serious depression and self-medication with alcohol. This project was set up as a non-profit organisation to help homeless youth in the Berkeley (California) area by utilising art and clinic spaces to provide holistic activities that support well-being. The project's polished, emotionally charged resources have provided effective discussion points for health promotion students in exploring how to move beyond simplistic mass media posters when addressing the most vulnerable in society.

With similarities to the ethos of honesty and transparent communication promoted by the Write Home Project (Figure 12.4), a speaker at TedX Toronto in 2013 spoke candidly about his experience of a suicide attempt. He very clearly describes the events leading up to his attempt to end his own life and forges a clear pathway for health promoters in how to protect those under their care from the same risks. Both examples demonstrate how we can better engage with people at all social, economic and political levels of society whilst avoiding the narrow-mindedness that often occurs naturally when relying excessively on data from a single source or from biased organisations.

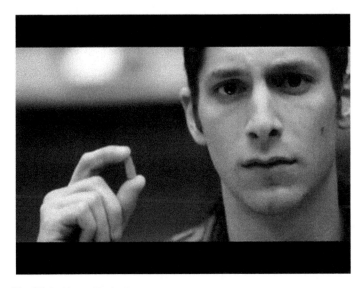

Figure 12.4   The Write Home Project

The risk of young male suicide is shared similarly amongst developed countries and there is therefore significant benefit in triangulating interventions and prevention efforts on an international scale.

APPLICATION OF MODELS

Figure 12.5 shows the HIV epidemiological triangle, a visually evolved representation of Royce et al.'s (1997) research of contributing factors to HIV transmission. The UK's Terrence Higgins Trust, a non-profit organisation, and the US Centre for Disease Control and Prevention have adopted this model. The model assists researchers and health professionals in predicting HIV incidence rates by analysing local population demographics and behaviour patterns. Similarly to the stages of the community readiness model, the epidemiological triangle is particularly useful to scholars as it lends itself well to adaptations to address different areas of health. Addiction, sexually transmitted infections and domestic violence are all conditions that previous students have found useful to frame using this representation.

Rebok et al. (2019) reported on the Experience Corps programme in Baltimore, Maryland that aimed to improve health promotion amongst an ageing population by using a social approach to reduce risk factors that are known to cause disability and other preventable morbidities. The paper suggests the use of the Experience Corps as a social model of health promotion application can be useful in supporting a population with multiple health risks that are often unaddressed. This is a good example of how active, community-based research can generate novel approaches to health promotion to supplement contemporary approaches.

Go Further 12.1

You can read more about the Experience Corps initiative at: www.aarp.org/expe
rience-corps/experience-corps-volunteer/experience-corps-cities-baltimore.html

HIV prevalence and incidence in a population

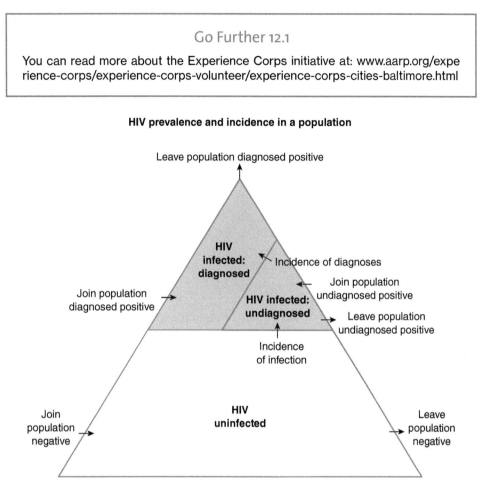

Figure 12.5   The HIV epidemiological triangle

Source: Copyright: © Ford Hickson http://makingitcount.org.uk/england, 2016

📱 Case Study 12.1   Responding to emerging threats

The Conservative Thatcher government of the 1980s released the now infamous
Don't Die of Ignorance campaign in late 1986. Widely criticised since then for its
demonisation of sex, particularly amongst non-heterosexuals, the campaign was
nevertheless instrumental in introducing the concept of AIDS to the British population. Although this served to introduce the emerging threat of AIDS to the country
in a way that made it clear this was not just an American – or gay – problem, it used
'scare tactics' to dramatise a public health problem rather than using structured,
tailored health promotion strategies to raise awareness. Sexual health counsellors
working with young gay and bisexual people are familiar with the damage caused
to sexual development and welfare as a result of the fear and marginalisation cata-
lysed by the campaign. Despite a recorded drop in diagnosed cases of gonorrhoea

(Continued)

during the course of the campaign (Seña et al., 2000), there is little evidence it resulted in the long-term, sustained adoption of safe sex practices. Thirteen years after the campaign launch, the Social Issues Research Centre published evidence to show that campaigns that used shock tactics caused psychological harm to viewers and reduced the likelihood they would act on health advice because such campaigns desensitised them to the problem.

Recent research maintains that health promotion that uses social marketing as a delivery channel typically fails to address longstanding ethical concerns with such tactics, including whether the intended outcome can be justified through means designed to induce fear (Stolow et al., 2020). Activists and social workers have also been vocal about the lack of evidence of measurable impact or efficacy from intentionally scaring people. Johnston (2019) identifies the 'packaging' – or the imagery and language – of health campaigns as particularly problematic for young people, as it simply represents a recycling of concepts that have tenuous links to successful harm reduction. Behaviour change as a result of health promotion campaigns is notoriously difficult to measure, varying based on the source and type of intervention (Gillison et al., 2019) and is rarely attributed to shock tactics.

Although the positioning of shock tactics within health promotion and social marketing strategies remains unresolved, the health sector's failure to address sexually-transmitted HIV and the emergence of related high-risk behaviours translates to repeated experimentation with controversial, eye-catching imagery.

In response to increasing incidence of sexually-transmitted HIV amongst men who have sex with men (MSM) in Canada in 2004, AIDS Vancouver, alongside a number of national health agencies and authorities released the Think Again campaign (Figure 12.6). The campaign designers used sexually graphic, eye-catching imagery to draw attention to the fact HIV is often transmitted because sexual partners are unaware of the other's status. The campaign was based on established knowledge of how men negotiated sexual risk, as well as the outcomes of focus groups facilitated by an expert in the field, but interestingly, did not use a recognised health promotion model in its design. Although some religious and other community groups criticised the sexually graphic imagery, the visual representation of the psychosocial principles of sexual activity developed the more common social marketing approach of delivering a message that communicates an ultimate 'endpoint', such as the menacing threat of AIDS in the 1986 British government campaign.

Box 12.5

An outcome assessment exercise of the Think Again campaign (Figure 12.6) showed promise with the innovative use of explicit graphics without a direct or intentional shock value. The evaluation took into account the views of 417 men to whom the campaign was targeted. In this sample, 73% of men said they found the campaign 'appealing' and 76% said they reconsidered their sexual practices as a result. In addition, 48% said they had changed 'something' about their sexual practices as a result, with men reporting high-risk sexual behaviour more likely to reconsider their behaviour. This suggests renewed health promotion efforts to address well established, longitudinal health problems may well be effective if their use of explicit imagery and messages is socioculturally appropriate, regardless of the potential cause for offence in other social groups. Evaluations such as this can be found by looking for evidence of how health promotions succeed or fail, as we previously discussed. This is particularly important for campaigns that may drive strong opinions about their content, such as Think Again.

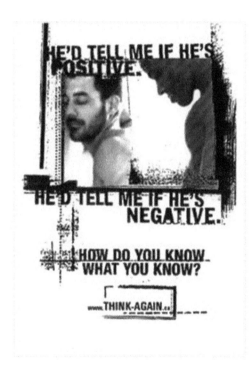

Figure 12.6   Sample poster from the Think Again campaign

Source: © Dr Brian Chidock AIDS Vancouver

   Health promotion researchers, academics, students and practitioners have no shortage of material from which to assess the efficacy of such campaigns. There is little, however, to suggest we can approach all controversial or 'shocking' material from the same point of view. While the judgement that some imagery is inherently distasteful or offensive may well be valid, evaluations of individual campaigns force us to consider potential and impact on a case-by-case basis, as is shown by Think Again. By their very nature, campaigns that force us to consider our sexual behaviour often use explicit imagery and language to get a point across, thus inviting criticism on the grounds of taste and social acceptability. Smoking cessation, mental health and drink driving campaigns have all tried to shock or scare people to engage them and instigate meaningful behaviour change.

During Covid-19 lockdowns in the UK, London's seminal sexual health and HIV clinic, 56 Dean Street, continued the most pressing elements of their health promotion interventions and services. Deployed without judgement for those who were sexually active during lockdowns, the service balanced the risk between Covid-19 infection and an undiagnosed HIV infection by arranging the prescription of HIV-blocking medicine, Pre-Exposure Prophylaxis (PrEP). The service used its existing social media and digital platforms to promote its services, and to ensure they were accessed as urgent care rather than routine care. As lockdown restrictions eased, the service rapidly expanded its media presence and, predicting a rise in risky sex amongst its target population group, prepared health promotion materials, such as that in Figure 12.7.

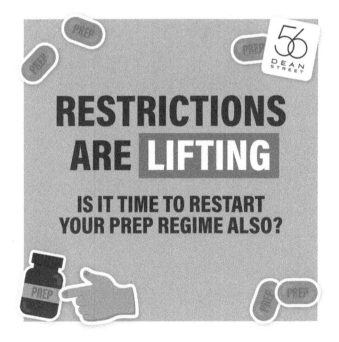

Figure 12.7   Restrictions are lifting

Source: © 56 Dean Street, https://twitter.com/56deanstreet/status/1282644461978255362

56 Dean Street is closely linked with the gay night economy in London and partnered with a nightclub, Heaven, to offer Covid-19 vaccines

alongside new prescriptions for PrEP (see Figure 12.8). This reflected the decades-long relationship between healthcare services and the night-time economy in London. Despite the deconstruction of the gay 'scene' (Nelson, 2019), the service recognised the potential to engage people in a dual approach to health protection.

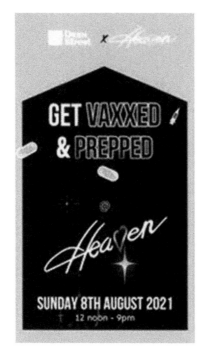

Figure 12.8   Get vaxxed and PrEPped

Source: © 56 Dean Street, https://www.facebook.com/watch/?v=303806744859157

In 2005, the Thomas and Stacey Siebel Foundation and the Partnership for Drug-Free Kids launched The Meth Project in Montana, USA in response to US Department of Justice data that methamphetamine ('meth') use amongst young people was increasing. The project describes its campaign imagery as 'hard-hitting' and typically shows either a teenager at the point of deciding whether to try meth for the first time or in a situation related to their addiction. Scenarios include a boy violently robbing his parents' house with two friends, a teenage girl having sex with a man in a motel, supervised by her boyfriend, and a teenage boy offering a much older man oral sex. All three scenarios centre on the main character trying to steal or earn money to be able to buy meth along with a strapline that tells us that doing so is normal when you are addicted to meth. Figure 12.9 is an example of one of the many engaging, if controversial, images of the project.

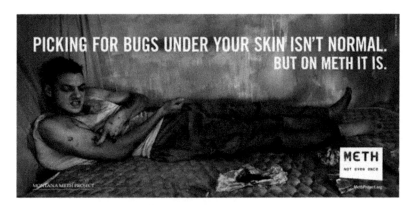

Figure 12.9   Campaign poster from The Meth Project

Source: © Teri Christensen at drugfree.org

The Meth Project partnered with state health authorities and celebrated its 15th anniversary in 2021 (Meth Project Foundation, Inc., 2021). The programme has an impressive track record, including a 77% reduction in teenagers trying methamphetamine in Montana since the campaign's inception and international accolades for anthropological contribution. In 2019, the Montana Youth Risk Behavior Survey joined other statutory organisations to record significant changes in meth use and health outcomes since the project launched. This includes a significant change in meth use amongst communities with funded drug-free community alliances and programmes (Office of National Drug Control Policy, 2021).

I used the digital resources of the campaign in undergraduate and postgraduate discussion groups amongst health promotion and public health students with varying outcomes. Most students agreed the imagery was eye-catching and caught their attention, and most students thought it was an appropriate response to a recreational drug that is highly addictive. Between 2005 and 2011 the project also won 41 media awards and the Stanford Graduate School of Business Center praised the campaign for its philanthropic approach to addressing an urgent social problem. Unlike concerns that shocking consumers of health messages creates a barrier between the individual and the core message, Fitzgerald (2019) found 'disgust' factors in The Meth Project's campaign that related to the representation of pain, such as rotting teeth and infected skin sores, resulted in teenagers establishing a distance between themselves and the use of meth depicted in the images.

Go Further 12.2

You can research this project at www.montanameth.org

HEALTH PROMOTION AND COVID-19

Wilkinson et al. (2020) identified a need for better coordinated messaging from corporate human resource departments, such as liaison with needle exchange programmes to enable employees to take home a greater stock of injecting equipment during lockdowns and work-from-home mandates. Such structured guidance was lacking both in the US and the UK and while respective governments scrambled with compliance-based legislation, researchers found increasing drug use risks and a need for significantly more robust personalised interventions led by physicians (Abramson, 2021; Owens, 2021). Interestingly, countries usually under the global health promotion radar for problematic national meth use reported significantly increased, harmful use levels during lockdowns. Australia (Bade et al., 2021; Parke, 2021), New Zealand (Witton, 2021) and Zimbabwe (Milken Institute, 2021) reported steep rises, leading Australia to sound the alarm for a resurgence of use that 'ravaged' rural areas during government restrictions (Parke, 2021). Data from the UK indicated 43% of regular drug users increased their intake during Covid-19 lockdowns with no barriers to purchasing other than higher prices (Aldridge et al., 2021). Interestingly, over 60% of drug users in the study said their dealers adhered to infection prevention measures when delivering, such as the use of personal protective equipment (PPE) and social distancing.

There were no national, prominent health promotions campaigns dealing with drug use during Covid-19 in the UK or US, although the UK Local Government Association published a typically broad paper on reducing health inequalities alongside the focus on Covid-19 vaccination and other prevention measures. The Canadian Centre on Substance Use and Addiction published a nationwide media campaign (Figure 12.10) to help guide people on less harmful substance practices during the pandemic. Using an infographic, the approach presents useful, important information but may not engage its audience. Post-campaign evaluation would be particularly useful here, to compare impactful/informative approaches.

Fittingly, the WHO attempted to take a lead in Covid-19 health promotion internationally. Their messages were politicised by governments, the media and the public, leading the director general to plead with agencies to deal with the virus outside of political fora (United Nations, 2020). WHO called for a united approach to pandemic response in March 2021, echoing the evidently ignored lessons of the AIDS epidemics previously discussed. The WHO's Regional Office for the Eastern Mediterranean published a mass media health promotion campaign in English and Arabic, targeting migrants at potentially heightened susceptibility to problematic, or fatal, drug use during lockdowns. Oddly, the main message was that illicit drugs do not protect against Covid-19. There is scant evidence drug users commonly hold this belief.

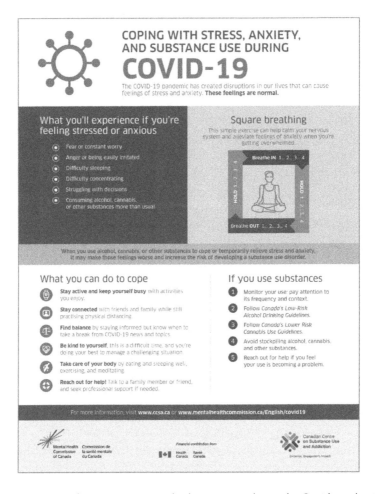

Figure 12.10   Coping with stress, anxiety and substance use during the Covid pandemic

Source: www.ccsa.ca/coping-stress-anxiety-and-substance-use-during-covid-19-infographic
© CCSA/Manon Blouin

Much attention is paid to the design, imagery and content of mass media health promotion campaigns, and there is ample scope for debates on the appropriateness of pictures designed to provoke a response or catalyse a behaviour change. Such debates are important but can distract us from the important analysis of health data that enables us to more accurately assess the need for a campaign and its effects. Anderson (2010) demonstrates this with an analysis of national meth use data using the Youth Risk Behaviour Surveys and concludes that The Meth Project had no discernible impact on meth use. Indeed, the research finds meth use was declining at the start of the project and simply maintained this trajectory. The multiple awards given to the campaign as well as its state-level recognition and substantial funding warn us to consider both the reception a campaign gets, as well as its demonstrable effects.

📇 Case Study 12.2   Autoethnographic experiences in health promotion

The private, statutory and non-profit sectors are unlikely partners in health pro-motion. The disparities between generating a profit, establishing and achieving commissioning targets, and making a difference in a community represent so many competing priorities and goals, that it is surprising multi-sector campaigns ever get off the ground. In 2008 I joined the multi-agency Pan-London HIV Prevention Programme (PLHPP). The UK's Department for Health commissioned the pro-gramme to address rising HIV incidence amongst MSM and Black Africans. As the lead for gay men's mass media, I found myself negotiating media design and messages between the very disparate partners involved.

The first concern was that the project mandate assumed that Black Africans and MSM were mutually exclusive. This made it difficult to justify to budget-holders why mass media should be fully representative of London's very diverse popula-tions. For example, if we showed two black men kissing in a poster, should the billing and evaluation be attributed to the Black African part of the project or the MSM part of the project? A definitive answer was not forthcoming. A private sec-tor firm, with no experience in sexual health, evaluated the project. They heavily criticised the data we could provide based on market saturation of the mass media market. Although we knew how many press adverts we had placed, and what the monthly distribution of the magazines were, we did not know how many people had picked up a magazine, saw our adverts, paid attention to them or understood them.

⚙️ Activity 12.1

Why do you think it was difficult for a non-profit and a private sector organisation to work together on this project? Write some notes before reading the discussion

---

How then, are we to navigate the complex political, economic and social structures that influence health promotion work so closely? Multi-agency working is not something historically equated with statutory agencies and authorities in the UK. Some agencies have begun to recognise the need for more efficient collaborative work in health since the end of the PLHPP in 2011. In 2014, the National Institute of Health and Care Excellence (NICE) released a guidance document for multi-agency working with peo-ple who experience domestic violence and abuse (Cleaver et al., 2019). Also in 2014, the Home Office released guidance on multi-agency working and information sharing for agencies involved in safeguarding. Both doc-uments highlight the need for transparent communication and a shared model of work and practice, although we are reminded to be sceptical of the claims of multi-agency efficacy guidance when this is issued by a government (Waardenburg, 2020). We did not have a shared model of work during the PLHPP, but instead spent a great deal of time locked in discussions about how to interpret behavioural data on the sexual patterns of MSM and Black Africans. This highlighted differences of opinion and professional judgement in how to reach our target groups. We knew that community leaders and church leaders were key to reach Black Africans, and the gay press, bars and clubs were important in reaching MSM. We also based our work on established research and models. Engel's (1977) biopsychosocial model was key to our design and implementation strategy and Dickerson et al.'s (2020) assertion that the most effective campaigns are community-based where they target large groups for intervention. This study also highlighted HIV prevention as the most likely to succeed in behaviour change, compared with health promotion based on cardiovascular disease, cancer, smoking cessation and substance use.

Combining our evidence base with a strategy to engage people involved with African community centres, the managers of gay bars and the editors of magazines were central to a plan to ensure the PLHPP was advertised as broadly as possible. Anecdotally, this was received more positively in African community centres and churches than it was in gay bars and clubs. This seemed to be because it was a novel topic in an environment not usually associated in the African community with discussion of sex, relationships and HIV. However, gay bars are typically saturated with sexualised media and competing messages from numerous health promotion agencies and authorities. As such our messages were somewhat diluted by the environment and it was not clear if they had an impact. As one of the non-profit agencies involved in the PLHPP, we used the gravitas of our brand name to demonstrate to readers within our target group that we were working with the NHS and not with for-profit healthcare services. Participants in focus groups we held to gauge response to the campaign design raised these as important factors and said they would be more willing to trust the message if our branding was used in conjunction with the NHS logo. Working in the PLHPP highlighted the need for more collaboration amongst the various agencies in HIV prevention as well as the need for a more robust model in which private and non-profit sector agencies can work together meaningfully to stimulate behaviour change.

More recently I have been involved in health service regulation. In an effort to establish benchmarks for safe practice and effective patient outcomes, the Care Quality Commission is mandated nationally to inspect all healthcare services using a regulatory and compliance model. This encourages providers of health services to ensure their practice is person-centred and provided in the safest manner possible. It penalises poor performance and rewards the best providers by enabling them to promote their services on the basis of their proven track record. This model provides an interesting context within which to consider how health promotion can be embedded in primary and secondary healthcare services, rather than relying predominantly on community-based interventions led by non-profit agencies. With increasing national recognition that individuals are attending hospitals and their family doctors in reaction to preventable conditions that result from behaviours such as excessive alcohol consumption and obesity, greater focus has been placed on frontline health professionals to engage patients with health promotion messages (WHO, 2021).

The Royal College of Nursing (RCN) recognised the opportunity for their members to become more involved in public health and, in 2012, published a policy document aimed at reducing the reliance on the NHS as a 'sickness service' (2012: 3), a strategy critical to improving care quality (Glasper, 2021). In setting out evidence-based recommendations for national practice, the RCN utilised case studies from nurses in all four UK nations to demonstrate the impact clinical staff can have on health outcomes in areas more commonly associated with health promotion, such as breast and cervical screening and sexual health. In doing so, the organisation has identified how vulnerable or high-risk groups can be reached through a variety of clinical and community settings that extend the basic premise of mass media health promotion. My experiences in regulation have shown many innovative examples of how frontline health staff have tried to combine immediate treatment with longer-term health promotion. This includes decorating a hospital inpatient ward in a dementia friendly style to show relatives how they could adapt their home to make it a safer space, and an emergency department that employed a team of social workers within the department 24 hours a day to meet the needs of a teenage population with escalating substance misuse.

Go Further 12.3

Think about your working environment; how can a health promotion message be integrated into your working day?

A series of child deaths as a result of the failure of different authorities and agencies to work together led to serious case reviews of practice, all of which identified how more collaborative, transparent working could have prevented the deaths of abused children. In a similar way, health promoters must accept that mass media campaigns continually recycled by non-profit agencies could benefit from a multi-disciplinary approach that involves the professionals in the sector responsible for treating the health problems the campaign work seeks to prevent in the first place.

CHAPTER SUMMARY

As we live in ever more diversified communities, so we begin to understand how global movement, behaviour change and sociopolitical conditions affect how we view our health and that of our community. Simple, proven models of health promotion based on perception of risk and rewards for behaviour change do not easily meet the increasingly complex needs of people with multiple health risks or those who accept risky choices as a typical part of their lifestyle. Although existing research frameworks for health interventions rarely indicate that scare or shock tactics are successful in facilitating improved outcomes, health promoters and social marketers are often drawn to recycle such approaches in an anxious attempt to address urgent health problems.

Adaptations of such tactics that include explicit text and images, often around sexual activity, drug use or behaviour likely to cause significant harm to others, are often arguably more successful than approaches that simply induce fear. This may be because visually explicit campaigns attract attention without inherently repelling people with threats. Instead, the reader recognises their own behaviour or lifestyle in the imagery presented, particularly if it delivers a non-judgemental and uncontrived message. In such circumstances, individuals can reflect and consider their risks at their own pace and in the context of the activities and choices that are important to them. In this sense, health promoters should prioritise work that catalyses a thinking reaction from those whose behaviour or risks concern them most.

FURTHER READING

VIDEOS

- Socioeconomic Inequalities in the Use of NHS Care in England: www. youtube.com/watch?v=-i0tiMKzr04
- Better Health – Let's Do This | NHS HP campaign video: www.youtube. com/watch?v=YozNOqbd26Q
- January Smoke Free HP campaign: www.youtube.com/watch?v=wTn8 gjbErjU
- Stoptober Infographic: www.youtube.com/watch?v=FBM-Es7wy3A
- SHINE – What to Expect When You Attend Our Sexual Health Clinic: www.youtube.com/watch?v=dVRgVDvTQyc

REFERENCES

Abramson, A. (2021) Substance use during the pandemic. *American Psychological Association, 52*(2).

Ahmad, A. and Singh, J. (2021) Influence of processes of change on stages of change for smoking cessation. *Journal of Applied Social Science.* doi: 10.1177/ 19367244211036994

Alderwick, H. and Gottlieb, L.M. (2019) Meanings and misunderstandings: a social determinants of health lexicon for health care systems. *The Milbank Quarterly, 97*(2): 407–19.

Aldridge, J., Garius, L., Spicer, J., Harris, M., Moore, K. and Eastwood, N. (2021) *Drugs in the Time of COVID: The UK Drug Market Response to Lockdown Restrictions.* London: Release.

Anderson, D.M. (2010) Does information matter? The effect of the Meth Project on meth use among youths. *Journal of Health Economics, 29*(5): 732–42.

Bade, R., Tscharke, B., O'Brien, J., Magsarjav, S., Humphries, M., Ghetia, M., Thomas, K., Mueller, J., White, J., and Gerber, C. (2021) Impact of COVID-19 controls on the use of illicit drugs and alcohol in Australia. *Environmental Science & Technology Letters 8*(9): 799–804. doi: 10.1021/acs.estlett.1c00532

Canadian Centre on Substance Use and Addiction (2021) Coping with stress, anxiety, and substance use during Covid-19 [infographic]. Available at: www.ccsa.ca/coping-stress-anxiety-and-substance-use-during-covid-19-infographic

Cambron, C., Hopkins, P., Burningham, C., Lam, C., Cinciripini, P. and Wetter, D.W. (2020) Socioeconomic status, mindfulness, and momentary associations between stress and smoking lapse during a quit attempt. *Drug and Alcohol Dependence*, 209.

Centers for Disease Control and Prevention (2019) Leading causes of death in males, United States. Available at: www.cdc.gov/healthequity/lcod/index.htm

Cleaver, K., Maras, P., Oram, C. and McCallum, K. (2019) Review of UK based multi-agency approaches to early intervention in domestic abuse: lessons to be learnt from existing evaluation studies. *Aggression and Violent Behavior, 46*: 140–55.

Corcoran N. (ed.) (2007) *Communicating Health: Strategies for Health Promotion.* London: Sage.

Dickerson, D., Baldwin, J.A., Belcourt, A., Belone, L., Gittelsohn, J., Kaholokula, K., Lowe, J., Pattent, C.A. and Wallerstein, N. (2020) Encompassing cultural contexts within scientific research methodologies in the development of health promotion interventions. *Prevention Science, 21*: 33–42.

Engel, G. (1977) The need for a new medical model: a challenge for biomedicine. Available at: https://pubmed.ncbi.nlm.nih.gov/847460/

Fernandez, M.E., ten Hoor, G.A., van Lieshout, S., Rodriguez, S.A., Beidas, R.S., Parcel, G., Ruiter, R.A.C., Markham, C.M. and Kok, G. (2019) Implementation mapping: using intervention mapping to develop implementation strategies. *Frontiers in Public Health, 7*: 158.

Fish Ragin, D., Hussein, Y., Fichera, A. and Awai, J. (2020) Applying theories in health psychology. In D. Fish Ragin and J. Keenan (eds) (2020) *Handbook of Research Methods in Health Psychology.* London: Routledge.

Fitzgerald, J.L. (eds) (2019) Etched in the skin: pain, methamphetamine violence and affect. In *Life in Pain*. Singapore: Springer.

Gallagher, C.A., Keehner, J.R., Hervé-Claude, L.P. and Stephen, C. (2021) Health promotion and harm reduction attributes in One Health literature: a scoping review. *One Health*, 13.

Gilbey, D., Morgan, H., Lin, A. and Perry, Y. (2020) Effectiveness, acceptability, and feasibility of digital health interventions for LGBTIQ+ young people: systematic review. *Journal of Medical Internet Research, 22*(12): e20158.

Gillison, F.B., Rouse, P., Standage, M., Sebire, S.J. and Ryan, R.M. (2019) A meta-analysis of techniques to promote motivation for health behaviour change from a self-determination theory perspective. *Health Psychology Review, 13*(1): 110–30.

Glasper, A. (2021) Raising and escalating concerns about patient care: RCN guidance. *British Journal of Nursing, 30*(2).

Hagger, M.S. and Hamilton, K. (2021) Effects of socio-structural variables in the theory of planned behavior: a mediation model in multiple samples and behaviors. *Psychology & Health, 36*(3): 307–33.

Health Foundation (2021) Relationship between income and health. Available at: www.health.org.uk/evidence-hub/money-and-resources/income/relationship-between-income-and-health

Home Office (2014) *Multi Agency Working and Information Sharing Project.* Available at: www.gov.uk/government/uploads/system/uploads/attachment_data/file/338875/MASH.pdf

Johnston, G. (2019) The kids are all white: examining race and representation in news media coverage of opioid overdose deaths in Canada. *Sociological Inquiry, 90*(1): 123–46.

King, T.L., Shields, M., Sojo, V., Daraganova, G., Currier, D., O'Neil, A., King, K. and Milner, A. (2020) Expressions of masculinity and associations with suicidal ideation among young males. *BMC Psychiatry, 20*: 228.

Laing, R.D. (1998) *The Politics of the Family and Other Essays.* London: Routledge.

Local Government Association (2021) Public health annual report 2021: rising to the challenges of COVID-19. Available at: www.local.gov.uk/publications/public-health-annual-report-2021-rising-challenges-covid-19#summary-of-key-themes-and-priorities

Melcher, J. and Torous, J. (2020) Concern for privacy and quality of current offerings. *Psychiatric Services, 71*(11): 1114–19.

Melnyk, B.M., Kelly, S.A., Stephens J., Dhakal, K., McGovern, C., Tucker, S., Hoying, J., McRae, K., Ault, S., Spurlock, E. and Bird, S.B. (2020) Interventions to improve mental health, well-being, physical health, and lifestyle behaviors in physicians and nurses: a systematic review. *American Journal of Health Promotion, 34*(8): 929–41.

Meth Foundation Project (2021). Available at: www.methproject.org/

Milken Institute (2021) We forget our troubles: Crystal meth use rises during lockdown in Zimbabwe. Available at: https://covid19africawatch.org/we-forget-our-troubles-crystal-meth-use-rises-during-lockdown-in-zimbabwe/

National AIDS Trust (2021) HIV in the UK statistics. Available at: www.nat.org.uk/about-hiv/hiv-statistics

Nelson, J.A. (2019) *'It Should Be Your Utopia': LGBTQ Perspectives of L.A. Gay Bar Culture and the Straight Takeover.* Thesis, University of California. Available at: https://scholarworks.calstate.edu/downloads/8049g807x

NICE (National Institute for Health and Care Excellence) (2014) Domestic violence and abuse: multi-agency working: guidance (PH50). Available at: www.nice.org.uk/guidance/ph50

Office for National Statistics (2020) Suicides in England and Wales: 2019 registrations. Available at www.ons.gov.uk/peoplepopulationandcommunity/birthsdeathsandmarriages/deaths/bulletins/suicidesintheunitedkingdom/2019registrations

Office of National Drug Control Policy (2021) Drug-free communities support program. Available at: www.whitehouse.gov/ondcp/dfc/

Oliffe, J.L., Kelly, M.T., Montaner, G.G., Links, P.S., Kealy, D. and Ogrodniczuk, J.S. (2021) Segmenting or summing the parts? A scoping review of male suicide research in Canada. *The Canadian Journal of Psychiatry, 66*(5): 433–45.

O'Mara, S. (2021) Biopsychosocial functions of human walking and adherence to behaviourally demanding belief systems: a narrative review. *Frontiers in Psychology*, *12*: 654122.

Owens, M. (2021) Substance use during the pandemic: how clinicians can help. *Addictions, Drug & Alcohol Institute, University of Washington*. Available at: https://adai.uw.edu/substance-abuse-during-the-pandemic-how-clinicians-can-help/

Parke, E. (2021) Crystal meth is resurgent and 'ravaging' regional Australia. *Where it's coming from is a mystery*. Available at: www.abc.net.au/news/2021-05-16/regional-meth-market-booming-despite-covid-impact-addicts/100098682

Phillips, G. II, McCuskey, D.J., Felt, D., Raman, A.B., Hayford, C.S., Pickett, J., Shenkman, J., Lindeman, P.T. and Mustanski, B. (2020) Geospatial perspectives on health: the PrEP4Love campaign and the role of local context in health promotion messaging. *Social Science & Medicine*, 265.

Reback, C.J., Fletcher, J.B., Swendeman, D.A. and Metzner, M. (2019) Theory-based text-messaging to reduce methamphetamine use and HIV sexual risk behaviours among men who have sex with men: automated unidirectional delivery outperforms bidirectional peer interactive delivery. *AIDS and Behavior*, *23*: 37–47.

Rebok, G.W., Parisi, J.M., Barron, J.S., Carlson, M.C., Diibor, I., Frick, K.D., Fried, L.P., Gruenewald, T.L., Huang, J., McGill, S., Ramsey, C.M., Romani, W.A., Seeman, T.E., Tan, E., Tanner, E.K., Xing, L. and Xue, Q. (2019) Impact of Experience Corps® participation on children's academic achievement and school behavior. *Prevention Science*, *20*: 478–87.

Royal College of Nursing (2012) Going upstream: nursing's contribution to public health. Available at: https://books.google.co.uk/books/about/Going_Upstream.html?id=X3jAnQAACAAJ&redir_esc=y

Royal College of Physicians (2020) Health inequalities and obesity. Available at: www.rcplondon.ac.uk/news/health-inequalities-and-obesity

Royce, R.A., Sena. A., Cates, W., Jr and Cohen, M.S. (1997) Sexual transmission of HIV. *The New England Journal of Medicine, 336*: 1072–78.

Sarto-Jackson, I. (2021) Narratives in health care: a case for psychoeducation drawing on the biopsychosocial model. *Balkan Journal of Philosophy*, *1*: 67–76.

Sattouf, Z. (2020) Socioeconomic status impact on smoking rates in Ohio in 2019. Wright State University. Available at: https://corescholar.libraries.wright.edu/scholarship_medicine_all/15/

Seña, A.C., Bachmann, L., Johnston, C., Wi, T., Workowski, K., Hook, E.W., Hocking, J.S., Drusano, G. and Unemo, M. (2020) Optimising treatments for sexually transmitted infections: surveillance, pharmacokinetics and pharmacodynamics, therapeutic strategies, and molecular resistance prediction. *Lancet Infect Dis., 20*(8): e181–e191. doi: 10.1016/S1473-3099(20)30171-7.

Stolow, J.A., Moses, L.M., Lederer, A.M. and Carter, R. (2020) How fear appeal approaches in COVID-19 health communication may be harming the global community. *Health Education and Behavior, 47*(4): 531–35.

The Body (n.d.) HIV prevention poster from 'Think Again' campaign from AIDS Vancouver [image online]. Available at: www.thebody.com/index/whatis/gay-men_prevent.html

The Meth Project (2011) Project overview. Available at: http://foundation.meth-project.org/documents/Meth%20Project%20Fact%20Sheet%2012-15–11.pdf

United Nations (2020) No need to politicize COVID-19: UN health agency chief. Available at: https://news.un.org/en/story/2020/04/1061392

Waardenburg, M., Groenleer, M., de Jong, J. and Keijser, B. (2020) Paradoxes of collaborative governance: investigating the real-life dynamics of multi-agency collaborations using a quasi-experimental action-research approach. *Public Management Review, 22*(3): 386–407.

Wilkinson, R., Hines, L., Holland, A., Mandal, S. and Phipps, E. (2020) Rapid evidence review of harm reduction interventions and messaging for people who inject drugs during pandemic events: implications for the ongoing COVID-19 response. *Harm Reduction Journal, 17*: 95.

Witton, B. (2021) Covid-19: meth users add pressure to busy emergency departments during lockdown. Available at: www.stuff.co.nz/national/health/coronavirus/126537881/covid19-meth-users-add-pressure-to-busy-emergency-departments-during-lockdown

World Health Organization (2021) What role do health workers at the frontline of service provision play towards universal health coverage? Available at: www.who.int/workforcealliance/media/qa/10/en/

Write Home Project (2014) Broken Bottles [video online]. Available at: www.youtube.com/watch?v=O2senVu65JQ

PART THREE

WORKING WITH DIFFERENT GROUPS OF PEOPLE

13

INTRODUCTION TO MENTAL HEALTH AND WELLBEING

GILLIAN ROWE

STANDARDS OF PROFICIENCY FOR NURSING ASSOCIATES (2018)

Relevant Platforms include:

Platform 1:1.5 Understand the demands of professional practice and demonstrate how to recognise the signs of vulnerability in themselves or their colleagues and the actions required to minimise risks to health.

Platform 1:1.8 Understand and explain the meaning of resilience and emotional intelligence, and their influence on an individual's ability to provide care.

Platform 1:1.9 Communicate effectively with a range of skills and strategies with colleagues and people at all stages of life and with a range of mental, physical and cognitive and behavioural health challenges.

Platform 2:2.1 Understand and apply the principles of health promotion, protection and improvement and the prevention of ill health when engaging with people.

Platform 2:2.4 Understand the factors that may lead to inequalities in health outcomes.

Platform 3:3.3 Recognise and apply knowledge of commonly encountered mental, physical, behavioural and cognitive health conditions when delivering care.

Platform 3:3.19 Demonstrate an understanding of comorbidities and the demands of meeting people's holistic needs when prioritising care.

Annex A 1.0-1.7, 1.9, 1.10.

St Mary's of Bethlehem Hospital was described in 1450 by the Lord Mayor of London as a place where may 'be found many men that be fallen out of their wit. And full honestly they be kept in that place; and some be restored onto their wit and health again. And some be abiding therein for ever.' (Allderidge, 1979)

This chapter is an introduction to mental health and wellbeing. You will consider what factors make us think that someone is unwell and how we categorise ailments, and then we will examine how those categorisations can lead to people being labelled. We live in a multicultural society and, as has been considered in other chapters, people from other ethnicities are overrepresented within the mental healthcare system and this will be considered. Historically, mental health sufferers have been stigmatised as lacking moral fibre and the quote by the Lord Mayor of London (1450) shows how historically there was no real treatment other than containment. While we still have secure wards, medical interventions and therapies are preferred options – although we still have a long way to go in combating the stigma that is attached to poor mental health. Included within this chapter are scenarios given by trainee nursing associates; as they have been taken from experiences within their practice, patient confidentiality has been respected.

Glossary

- Depot injections Long-acting medications
- Interventions Any treatment
- Sectioning Detention under one of the sections of the Mental Health Act 1983, (updated 2008, 2017 and currently under review)
- Stigma A negative attitude towards mental health sufferers

INTRODUCTION AND DEFINITIONS

The current model of mental health considers that mental disorders are disorders of brain circuits caused by developmental processes shaped through a complex interplay of genetics and experience. The word 'mental' is viewed as a negative, but we are mental as well as physical entities, and our mental makeup defines who we are. The World Health Organization defines this by stating 'Mental health is the emotional resilience which enables us to enjoy life and to survive pain, disappointment and sadness. It is a positive sense of wellbeing and an underlying belief in our and others' dignity and worth' (WHO, 2014). Developing poor mental health is characterised by changes in our thinking, mood and behaviours; this chapter will introduce you to explanations or models of mental health, why mental health is stigmatised, treatment options for sufferers and how we can support ourselves when suffering from stress.

⚙ Activity 13.1

Think for a moment of all the words to describe mental health. Draw two boxes: in one write positive and the other negative words. Positive words might include sane, mentally healthy, and your negative box might include such words as mad, bonkers, loopy, etc. Is there a difference between the number of positive and negative words?

What is being mentally healthy? The Mental Health Foundation (2017) says if you can manage all these things, you are mentally healthy:

- Make the most of your potential
- Cope with life
- Play a full part in your family, workplace, community and among friends
- Learn
- Feel, express and manage a range of positive and negative emotions
- Form and maintain good relationships with others
- Cope with and manage change and uncertainty

⚙ Activity 13.2

Write your own definition of being mentally healthy in the space below.

One of the drawbacks of being mentally unwell is that it has few physical symptoms. Mental health can be explained in terms of behaviours and expressed emotions. What is or is not acceptable behaviour is culturally mediated and Thomas Szasz (1961) argued that mental illness is a metaphor for the 'problems in living', that mental ill health was a myth and that the description 'mental ill health' is a euphemism for behaviours that are socially disapproved of.

⚙️   Activity 13.3

Look up the disease 'drapetomania'. Now also consider 'oppositional defiant dis-order'. Do you think they are mental health disorders? Or are they behaviours that society disapproves of?

CATEGORISING MENTAL HEALTH

The lack of a universally agreed cut-off point between normal behaviour and behaviour associated with mental illness means that a diagnosis is usu-ally made after a recognition of personal distress, either by the person or by the person's family/friends. The *Diagnostic and Statistical Manual* is a diagnostic handbook created by the American Psychiatric Association. It is the awkward child of the needs of the medical insurance industry for reimbursement and the need of the medical profession to categorise and label signs and symptoms. DSM 1 was published in 1952, it was 145 pages long and contained 106 disorders; the latest iteration is DSM 5 (2013), it is 947 pages long and contains an indeterminate number of disorders (157–300 depending on who you read). The health professions in the UK also use the International Classification of Diseases (ICD), which is hosted by the World Health Organization. The current iteration is ICD 11 (2018). The ICD is not restricted to mental health but identifies all diseases and disorders. DSM 5 also removed the Global Assessment of Function (GAF scale) for assessing people in terms of their ailments and have adopted the WHODAS 2.0 scale (2018). This is based on, and reflects, the assessment of impairment and disability and is separate from diagnostic considerations, its utility being that it can reflect any medical illness, psychiatric illness or comorbid condition.

For many people, the existing systems of categorising illnesses do not relate closely enough to their experiences. Those with enduring complex mental health issues struggle to identify their feelings and emotions with their diagnosis. Recall the explanation of the sick role given in Chapter 5, Applied Health Sciences. Parsons (1951) felt the function of the sick role is necessary to maintain social order, but the reality is more complex. Gabe et al. (2006) discussed the work of Zola (1973) and considered the not-so-obvi-ous question of why a person seeks medical attention. Zola suggested it was as a result of the person's inability to cope with the symptoms, such as when the symptoms begin to impact on a person's ability to get on with their life, work and relationships. Table 13.1 gives some examples of behaviours that have been named or labelled. Wakefield and Horwitz (2006: 149) state, 'What makes a medical disorder mental rather than (exclusively) somatic or physical?' Psychiatry to some extent depends for its existence as a medical

Table 13.1   Behaviours associated with mental health issues

Disconnection from reality and detachment from social rules
Self-neglect
Attention-seeking behaviours including self-harm
Loss of inhibition such as inappropriate sexual behaviours
Suicidal ideation
Obsessive-compulsive activities
Voice hearing
Panic attacks
Anxiety
Depression

specialty on the distinction between mental and somatic disorders, yet the history of this distinction presents a bewildering array of puzzling judgements, radical shifts, and seemingly arbitrary distinctions.

THE MAIN MODELS OF MENTAL HEALTH

THE MEDICAL MODEL

In Western medical thinking, the medical model is the prevailing explanation. It considers the body to be an organism that consists of natural functions designed by nature, and illness is the breakdown of some of these functions; this is also considered to be a 'deficit' model, viewed from a biological perspective. It is considered mechanistic, in that the body is described as a machine that fails from time to time. Therefore, any dysfunction of the mind is an ailment that results from a disease process such as a chemical imbalance or physical changes in the brain. The medical model gives names to groups of symptoms and calls them a disease, and this gives rise to the notion that people become labelled through the process of diagnosis. Cure rests in the hands of the medical profession who are the knowledge experts and who hold the reins of power in health interactions.

Unwell or disabled people are viewed as deviant or in some way inferior; that their disability places restrictions on their ability to participate in economic activity and so they are burdens on the state.

Arguments against the medical model suggest the model is inflexible and fails to recognise its fallibility. Illich (1976) was a vocal protagonist in criticism of the model, citing iatrogenic causes such as clinical injury, cultural iatrogenesis (the disregard of cultural [lay] health practices) and the medicalisation of normal human conditions such as sadness, loneliness and bereavement. Psychiatric iatrogenesis includes misdiagnosis, the side effects of psychotropic medication and the medicalisation of adolescent disaffection.

THE SOCIAL MODEL

The social model offers explanations that are related to the experience of those suffering poor health. It recognises that notions of health are socially created, and that society has a mediating role through such things as the environment, education and housing. It regards an individual's environment and their health as being intrinsically linked, especially in terms of the conditions in which we live and work, the food that we eat and the products that we use. Lang (2001: 8) considers that 'disabled people are subject to oppression and negative social attitudes, that inevitably undermine their personhood and their status as full citizens'. Foucault (1973) suggested that modern medicine is part of a process of regulating and disciplining both individual bodies and the social body.

The breakdown of traditional community, loss of support by geographic mobility away from family and low socioeconomic status are all implicated. This does not exclude the wealthy and well educated from the model, but makes the point that society needs to adapt and to adopt more inclusive ways of being.

Arguments against the social model include its inability to find cures or develop successful treatments to alleviate the symptoms of disease and that the medical model is scrutinised, transparent and objective (Goldacre, 2008). Table 13.2 describes Charli's ailments and Figure 13.1 shows how they are explained using the two models.

THE PSYCHODYNAMIC AND COGNITIVE MODELS

The psychodynamic model is premised on the work of Sigmund Freud and the notion that childhood experiences are crucial in shaping adult personality (McWilliams, 2009). Whilst much of Freud's work is still contested, there is good evidence that unconscious processes influence our behaviour

Table 13.2 Charli's ailments

Charli is suffering from myalgia encephalomyelitis (ME), this is episodic, and Charli has good days and bad days
Charli also suffers from depression and poor self-efficacy; on bad days, Charli needs a carer to support the activities of daily living
On good days, Charli feels well enough to go to work but does not have a job that allows this flexibility

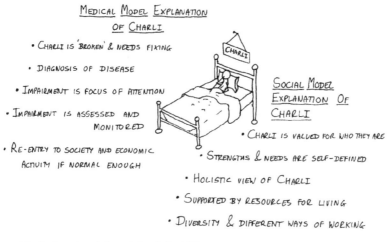

Figure 13.1   Medical and social models of disability

(Robinson and Gordon, 2011). Freud's model of the mind has withstood the test of time (Id, Ego and Super Ego) and psychodynamic analysts focus on Ego defence mechanisms when working with clients suffering anxiety. The cognitive model is premised on the notion that dysfunctional thinking can lead to poor mental health. It has strong links with the work of Jean Piaget and Edward Tolman, and this approach is considered analogous to the working of a computer's central processing systems (Atkinson and Shiffrin, 1968). Cognitive behavioural therapy (CBT) is one of the practical applications of this theory to mitigate established patterns of thinking habits such as negative self-censure or harsh self-criticism.

THE SPIRITUAL MODEL

The spiritual model (Figure 13.2) considers how belief in 'something greater than ourselves' can support people with poor mental health. For a long time, holding a religious belief was considered to be a symptom of mental illness (religious mania, voice hearing); certainly, Freud linked religion with neurosis. However, Turbott (1996) stated that a rapprochement between religion and psychiatry was essential for psychiatric practice to be effective. Whilst spirituality is a global phenomenon, it does not need to be anchored in any particular religious belief or tradition, whereas religious belief is in many ways 'institutionalised' spirituality with a specific set of rituals. Non-religious people often experience a spiritual void in their lives and seek answers to give hope and peace in their mind. Religious places provide a calm space and spiritual advisors who can give positive support; often they will offer this to both believers and non-believers alike.

Encouraging people to explore what is important to them spiritually can be a valuable self-help strategy and give meaning and direction to someone who feels lost.

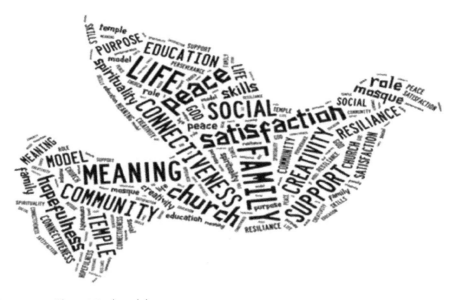

Figure 13.2   The spiritual model

THE BIOPSYCHOSOCIAL MODEL

Devised by cardiologists George Engel and John Romano in 1977, as a result of their awareness that cardiovascular disease is the result of not just biology but sociocultural and psychological influences too, this model incorporates features of the medical, social and psychological models. It is considered both scientific and humanistic. Engel (1977: 131) stated that 'no single illness or person is reduced to any one aspect'. The psychodynamic and medical models assert that the quality of our social relationships has a major impact on our physiological systems, especially in terms of our ability to cope with stress and the end states of depression and anxiety. Evidence has been found which shows that the chronically stressed may be vulnerable to subtle forms of brain damage (Sapolsky, 1996), resulting in memory loss and compromised immune functioning.

Healthcare workers should consider the biological, psychological and social domains (see Figure 13.3) in assessing the patient and in devising strategies to promote their health and to use participatory and empathetic interactions to cultivate a trusting relationship.

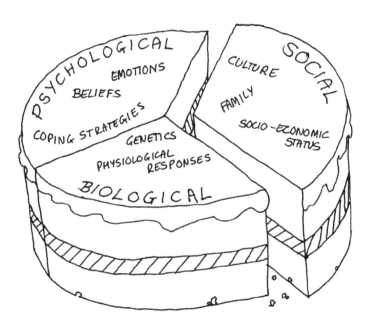

Figure 13.3   The biopsychosocial model

📋   Scenario 13.1

George is suffering from anxiety; he also has high blood pressure. When he talked to the nursing associate at his GP surgery well man clinic, he disclosed that he had a very stressful but lowly paid job: it paid just enough to cover his monthly bills. He said he ate a lot of junk food, high in salt, as he was too tired at the end of his day to cook properly. He also said that he didn't get out much and had few friends.
    Put George's disclosures into the model boxes below.

Biological	Psychological	Social

PSYCHIATRY

Psychiatry is a modernist approach, one that can trace its origins to the cultural transformations of the European Enlightenment and its quest to replace religious revelation with human reason as the path to truth and progress. Sigmund Freud (1856–1939) is thought of as the founder of psychiatry, although his work is considered contentious as it did not follow any scientific principles.

The term was coined by Johann Christian Reil in 1808, from the Greek meaning 'treatment of the soul'. Qualified psychiatrists are trained as physicians who then undertake postgraduate training to become psychiatrists. Patients are treated by taking a case history and a physical examination to determine if there is a biological cause for the illness. Recent research using MRI scanners and new discoveries in genomics and neuroscience are finding biological markers that underpin disorders once understood as failures in brain circuit processing. Health workers undertake mental health assessments which assess things such as the patient's speech, mood, phobias and obsessions, and abnormal experiences and beliefs as a way of aiding diagnosis and treatment.

Psychiatric treatment consists of drug therapy and psychological interventions, very occasionally surgical intervention (tumours, epilepsy) or electroconvulsive therapy.

Psychiatry has a mixed press, mainly due to its relationship with mental health legislation and the ability to 'section' people. Sectioning is the use of the various sections of the Mental Health Act 1983 (updated 2007) to place sufferers in secure accommodation and the enforcement of pharmacological treatment regimens (Community Treatment Orders). In the same way that physicians can confuse patients with use of diagnostic professional language, so can psychiatrists and psychiatric assessments, using language that is difficult to understand and that exploits the power differential between the doctor and patient (Figure 13.4).

Jerome Frank (1961) surveyed the world of psychotherapy. He came to the conclusion that all forms of therapy, even those with very different theoretical frameworks, worked on the basis of a common set of essential elements. These were:

- A helping relationship with a thoughtful and concerned listener
- A clearly defined space in which healing could take place
- The use of some 'ritual' which served to strengthen the relationship between therapist and client

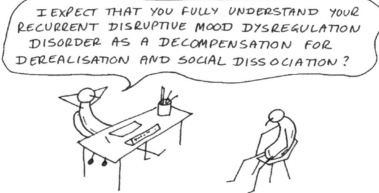

Figure 13.4   Power differential in psychotherapy

 Case Study 13.1   Student voice

This case study has been given by assistant practitioner Gillian, who is currently a trainee nursing associate.

Betty was admitted to hospital due to acute psychotic depression. When Betty arrived on the ward, she was disorientated and unaware of where she was. Due to ongoing risks of self-injurious behaviours, the multi-disciplinary team (MDT) placed Betty on a two person within arm's length observation criteria. This was to prevent her from causing more injuries. Observation levels were gradually reduced as she gained more insight into her mental health and her harmful behaviour stopped.

Prior to admission she had engaged in self-harming behaviours, extracting several teeth, and pulling her hair out. Betty refused to eat and drink, which led to a significant weight loss and her blood tests revealed that her body was lacking in specific vitamins due to lack of sufficient nutritional intake. Regular blood samples were obtained and analysed, this allowed the team to be aware of low counts regarding, plasma electrolytes, sodium, potassium, phosphate and magnesium.

Following an initial assessment from the MDT, it was decided the appropriate treatment would involve a 12-week course of electroconvulsive treatment (ECT).

Question

How would you approach supporting Betty with her treatment? Jot down some notes, then read the rest of Gillian's case study at the end of the chapter.

MENTAL HEALTH AND STIGMA

As explained earlier, whether a behaviour is considered normal or abnormal depends on the context and culture surrounding it. Archaeologists have found 7000-year-old skulls with holes drilled into them; no one really knows why but the current explanation is either to relieve headaches or to let demons out (possibly epilepsy). The ancient Greeks blamed the uterus (in women) and called it hysteria. In early medieval times, possession by the devil was the prevailing view and women were blamed and burned as witches. By the sixteenth century, asylums were established to contain the mentally ill and quite often these were seen as a source of entertainment. People went to places such as St Mary of Bethlehem in London (which gave us the name Bedlam) to watch the crazy people.

Asylums were generally overcrowded and custodial in nature. The rise of the age of Enlightenment in the early eighteenth century led to a different explanation, that of the medical model and the disease process, although many still felt that mental ailments were the products of moral defects in the character. In 1883, the German psychiatrist Emil Kräpelin (1856–1926) developed a naming system of psychological disorders that consisted of a grouping of symptoms. Kräpelin described what he called 'dementia praecox', which is now better understood as schizophrenia.

People throughout history have been stigmatised for being mentally ill and this is still true today. Social stigma considers that people are uncomfortable with people who are mentally unwell. They are viewed as 'abnormal'; in fact we still study 'abnormal' psychology. Such people are different, and they may be dangerous, they may behave in unexpected ways or be violent, therefore they are not to be trusted and should be treated with caution. The perpetuation of this view, especially through the media, can lead to self-stigmatisation. When the sufferer internalises stigma, this can significantly affect feelings of shame and lead to poorer treatment outcomes and increased social exclusion. Research by Livingstone and Boyd (2010) found that 'internalised stigma was positively associated with psychiatric symptom severity and negatively associated with treatment adherence'; this was especially true when researchers examined self-stigma in schizophrenia (Kung et al., 2008).

LABELLING THEORY

Society determines which behaviours are non-deviant and deviant; behaviours that do not fit with social expectations are labelled deviant. The consequences of being labelled as deviant can be far-reaching and have an impact on the labelled person's self-belief systems. Some choose deviancy (criminals), adolescents quite often go through a deviant phase (delinquency: Matza, 1964; Sykes and Mazda, 1957) and some have deviancy thrust upon them. People suffering poor mental health fall into the last description. Sociologists would explain that deviancy definitions are framed by the powerful and wealthy (judges, politicians, medical professionals) generally against the poor or marginalised and that they make the rules that define the context of deviant behaviour. An examination of prison populations showed that more than 70% of prisoners have two or more mental health disorders. Male prisoners are 14 times more likely to have two or more disorders than men in general, and female prisoners 35 times more likely than women in general (Social Exclusion Unit, 2004). Lord Bradley's (2009: 17) review of mental health and learning disabilities within the criminal justice system said that 'there are now more people with mental health problems in prison than ever before. While public protection remains the priority … custody can exacerbate mental ill health, heighten vulnerability and increase the risk of self-harm and suicide.'

Both Becker (1963) and Lemart (1967) examined notions of deviancy and they discussed the reaction of others in the explanation of deviance and considered that 'secondary deviancy' impacts on those labelled deviants. It is in response to this labelling that the person changes their behaviour in accordance with the label, so the label becomes a 'self-fulfilling prophecy'. Diagnosis by a medical professional can offer a person an explanation of the symptoms they are experiencing but the person's behaviour may reflect their internal understanding of what the diagnosis might mean. Goffman (1968) suggested that the label (diagnosis) can 'spoil the sufferer's identity'. Goffman called the social reaction to the diagnosis 'an enacted stigma' and the person's internal reaction 'felt stigma' (now called self-stigma). Diagnosis is not value neutral; some diagnoses such as depression or anxiety carry less stigma, whereas schizophrenia is value laden.

Link and Phelan (2001) describe five components of stigma: labelling, stereotyping, separation, status loss and discrimination within the context of a power differential. They consider that status loss and discrimination occur when the stigma interferes with a person's ability to participate fully in the social and economic life of her/his community, although Goffman considers that the discrimination can ripple out beyond the sufferer to their family and friendship networks (he called this courtesy stigma) and that these networks are tainted by association. This can further impact on the sufferer's self-belief by adding guilt to the mix. This is shown in the pool of social expectation in Figure 13.5.

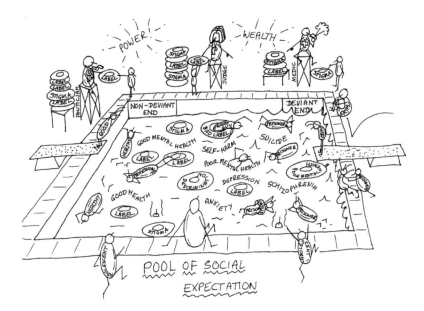

Figure 13.5   Pool of social expectation

The Mind/Time to Change Alliance carried out annual surveys on attitudes to mental health, which show that people are becoming more tolerant and understanding of people with mental health issues, but the last survey (2015) shows that people still feel unable to discuss poor mental health or mental health ailments with their employer as they fear repercussions for their career. Also striking was the number of people surveyed who considered those with poor mental health as 'likely to be violent', whereas the reality is that mentally ill people are more likely to be themselves victims of violence. Rethink's (2017) survey showed that people still think schizophrenics are violent and have a 'split personality'.

INTERSECTIONALITY IN MENTAL HEALTH

This discourse considers the effects of oppression on those with intersecting social, cultural and disabled identities. In the 1980s, Crenshaw and bell hooks opened a debate on black feminism and went on to develop a theoretical framework which brought together feminism and race. This was to remove the notion that feminism is a white enterprise, and to state that racial inequality and gender inequality are sides of the same coin. The debate has now widened to include all those who are marginalised by society for reasons such as gender, race, class, ability, sexual orientation, religion, caste, age and nationality. Intersectionality considers how such things can impact and interact on multiple levels, and the intersection perspective looks at the different types of discrimination (such as ageism, gender phobia, racism and bigotry) that an individual can suffer. Johnella Butler (2014) considers it is not just a quest for equality but a fight against injustice.

Seng et al. (2012) researched health disparities in post-traumatic stress syndrome and discovered that those with higher numbers of marginalised identities suffered from frequent discrimination leading to poor mental health. The social determinants of health play a major role in health and can compound health outcomes; those with multiple disparities can fall through health support networks and this has cumulative effects on health.

TREATMENTS AND INTERVENTIONS

The medical model supports pharmacological interventions, but this has led to accusations that this is the only available option (the 'one trick pony' theory), and some consider the relationship between the medical model and the pharmacological industry corrupt. There is a belief that the pharmacological industry is engaged in 'disease mongering' or constructing novel diseases to create new markets for commercially available drug treatments. This debate is typified by accusations that high cholesterol, which was once an indicator of disease, has now become a disease in itself. This debate was at its most vociferous during the creation of DSM 5, when it was revealed that two-thirds of the psychiatrists compiling the manual had a financial relationship with drug companies (Cosgrove and Krimsky, 2012).

THE PHARMACOLOGIC REVOLUTION

The first recognisable drugs to be used in mental health treatment were sedative, hypnotic and anticonvulsive – potassium bromide, chloral hydrate (1830) and paraldehyde (1880). The first barbiturate was Veronal (1903). The first major psychotropic drugs were the neuroleptic (antipsychotics) group, phenothiazines (tranquillisers), which became available in the early 1950s. This was considered the beginning of the 'pharmacologic revolution'.

Quite a few of the drugs prescribed for complex mental health conditions have off-target and unpleasant side effects, which is problematic for patients who have to balance using the drugs to control the ailment and living with the side effects. Many drugs can be given as a depot injection for those whose lives are too chaotic to take tablets or as a means of ensuring that medication is taken as part of a Community Treatment Order.

Schizophrenics are sometimes prescribed the drug Depixol (flupentixol), which in some people can lead to unwanted physical movements and facial tics, the so-called 'Depixol dance'. Depixol is also addictive and needs careful management.

Quite a few antipsychotics can be toxic when taken with alcohol and some patients prefer to self-medicate using alcohol and street drugs. This leads to accusations of non-compliance and the use of legally enforced medication.

INTERVENTIONS

Surgical intervention for psychiatric disorders is legal under the Mental Health (Treatment and Care) Act 1994 Section 70(1). Psychiatric neurosurgery includes frontal lobotomy and ablation of the basal ganglia. The pathways involved in psychiatric illness are poorly defined and surgical results are variable, therefore the practice of psychiatric neurosurgery has often been surrounded by controversy. Current practice tends to focus on the relief of symptoms, such as in epilepsy and Parkinson's disease, and it should be pointed out that fewer than 50 such surgical operations take place each year (in the USA and UK). Electroconvulsive therapy has had a mixed press, although evidence suggests that it can help with severe depression. Case study 13.1 has examined this.

The social model supports the various 'talking therapies', which include psychotherapy, psychoanalysis, counselling, cognitive behavioural therapy (CBT), acceptance and commitment therapy (ACT), neurolinguistic programming, dance and movement therapy, eye movement and desensitisation and reprocessing therapy (EMDR), assisted animal therapy, hypnotherapy and latterly nutrition therapy. There are many complementary therapies, which include (but are not limited to) aromatherapy, anthroposophy, Ayurvedic medicine, Bach Flower remedies, healing and touch therapies, homeopathy, hypnotherapy, massage, naturopathy, nutritional therapy, reflexology, traditional Chinese herbal medicine, Western herbal medicine, transcendental meditation and yoga. Government initiatives such as 'Improving Access to Psychological Therapies' (IAPT) (NHS, 2018) have promoted training for workplace staff to support employees at risk of losing employment due to depression and anxiety; as this is a stepped care model, NHS intervention is offered where needed. Treatment begins with support from a psychological wellbeing practitioner and can be escalated to specialised clinicians.

The recovery model of mental health acknowledges that some people have chronic long-term conditions and are never going to fully achieve their previous good mental health. Therefore, it focuses on supporting patients to make the best of their situation by emphasising resilience and control over problems and to live a meaningful life. As Goffman asserted, labelling spoils the identity of the sufferer, and so mentally unwell patients will need support to establish their identity based on who they are rather than what their diagnosis is. The caring nursing associate will know what is available in the community and can signpost patients to non-medical support groups such as Men in Sheds, Mind, Alzheimer's Society and Rethink local groups. During the Covid-19 pandemic lockdowns, concern was raised about the impact of isolation on mental health. Many reported being anxious, people under socioeconomic inequalities have been more likely to experience anxiety, panic, hopelessness, loneliness, and many said they were not coping well with the stress of the pandemic. The Covid-19 pandemic has exacerbated existing poor mental health as access to mental health provision has deteriorated due to demand and staff absence because of Covid-19. The Mental Health Foundation use the analogy 'we are all in the same storm, but we are all in different boats' and the divergence of experience has a socioeconomic context (Mental Health Foundation, 2021). Marmot et al.'s work (2021) on 'Build Back Fairer' cited the UK Household Longitudinal Study, which found that levels of psychological distress worsened during the Covid-19 lockdown. Respondents declared they suffered from a lack of concentration and/or sleep, and experienced feelings of unhappiness and loss of purpose. Women especially reported psychological distress, and it is not hard to imagine why. As soon as lockdown was lifted, many fled to the countryside or seaside to enhance their wellbeing.

Mental health support organisations offer such things as 'art for health' and 'walking for health'. Public Health England published a report (2016) which evidenced the benefits of art and exercise on health, and recent research by Frühauf et al. (2016) evidenced that exercise in the fresh air, even a short walk, had a measurable benefit for someone suffering depression. Interestingly, the game Pokémon Go! is encouraging people to walk and sufferers from poor mental health have stated that playing the game is getting them out and meeting people.

EVIDENCE-BASED PRACTICE

How do we know when we plan an intervention that it will work? Generally speaking, drug therapy has been through a rigorous process of testing before the drug comes to the market. Testing drugs for toxicity is a long process before it even gets to trials in human test subjects and costs run into several million pounds.

A key resource for evidence-based practice is the Cochrane Library, which offers high quality, independent evidence to inform healthcare decisions. It holds six databases of research documents, and the library is used to conduct meta-analyses of research reviews. Cochrane Reviews are systematic reviews of research in healthcare and the database (known as the CDSR) offers five types of review: intervention assessment, diagnostic test reliability, methodology reviews, qualitative reviews and prognosis reviews. The information generated can be used to influence practice; however, quite often best practice initiatives depend on healthcare professionals maintaining their CPD (continuing professional development), and searching out the best available evidence and finding means to implement initiatives into one's practice is not always an easy task, especially if funding is required.

MENTAL HEALTH IN A MULTICULTURAL SOCIETY

The cultural narrative explanation of mental health as formulated and categorised in the DSM reflects the normative values of American/Western Europe; however, this is not the whole world and different cultures have other explanations. Many early civilisations and societies were not literate and oral traditions were handed down by professional 'historians' or storytellers. The diaspora due to slavery or the genocide of Indigenous peoples by colonial invaders and settlers destroyed this repository of knowledge and forced a new Cartesian explanation of madness onto societies that had a spiritual explanation.

Box 13.1   The separation of mind and body

René Descartes (1596–1650) is considered 'the father' of modern Western philosophy. In his *Discourse on the Method and Principles of Philosophy* (1644) he states that he can prove his existence because he can think: *'cogito ergo sum'* – I think, therefore, I am.

In *The Description of the Human Body* (1648) he considered that the mind is separate from the body, suggesting that the body is a kind of machine, and this notion forms the basis of the biomedical paradigm because you can remove significant portions of the body, but the mind remains intact. This idea of the two separate entities (Cartesian dualism) is central to modern Western medicine.

Societies that explain ailments in a whole-body format (as opposed to dualistic) are now called 'holistic' and this is termed a 'metaphor', meaning a thing that is regarded as symbolic of something else. The term 'holistic' is applied to therapies such as counselling or massage, which is not its true meaning at all. Holistic medicine examines the individual in terms of their place in time and space and how they interrelate with their environment. This often includes their spirituality and the ways this is expressed, performing rituals and their place in relationship with their relevant gods or spirits. Holistic therapies look for 'soul health', the restoration of spiritual and moral wellbeing as the means to holistic health. Religious people take great comfort from their beliefs and perform rituals to enhance their relationship with their god. Whatever your own beliefs are, you need to respect other people's beliefs and support them to access their ministers when they need to.

CULTURAL IMPERIALISM AND MENTAL HEALTH

At the end of the nineteenth century, within British colonies in Asia, a part of the colonial medical officer's duties was to set up and run asylums. It was noticed that inmates who were judged mad smoked cannabis, and the British, being unaware that smoking cannabis was a normal social activity, determined that smoking cannabis made people insane (Mills, 2000).

At that time, very few non-Western countries used incarceration as a therapeutic intervention. In many rural areas, ritual, chants, herbal remedies, exorcisms and prayer were (and to some extents, still are) the normal healing practice. Some tribes welcomed those who heard voices, as they had clearly been chosen by the gods to become a shaman, the voice hearer, and their family were esteemed by the tribe. The Yoruba tribe in western Nigeria still practise traditional healing and pass on to trainees their knowledge verbally. Interestingly, the knowledge that they pass on is what works, and so it is continually updated through practical experience – an example of good evidence-based practice (Fernando, 2014).

MENTAL HEALTH FIRST AID

This programme was developed in Australia in 2000 by Betty Kitchener and Anthony Jorm and exported globally. It was adopted and launched in the UK by the Department of Health in 2007, and various organisations run training programmes for different sectors, organisations and communities, including the armed forces and youth leaders, in how to spot the signs of developing poor mental health and how to support someone evidencing the signs. It educates on suicide prevention, depression, anxiety, and psychosis.

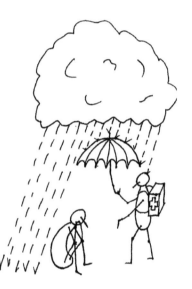

Figure 13.6   Mental health first aid

Would you know how to recognise the symptoms of someone becoming unwell?

- An unusually sad or irritable mood that does not go away
- Loss of enjoyment and interest in activities that used to be enjoyable
- Lack of energy and tiredness
- Feeling worthless or feeling guilty when the person is not at fault
- Thinking about death a lot or wishing they were dead
- Difficulty concentrating or making decisions
- Moving more slowly or, sometimes, becoming agitated and unable to settle
- Having sleeping difficulties or, sometimes, sleeping too much
- Loss of interest in food or, sometimes, eating too much; changes in eating habits may lead to either loss of weight or putting on weight

These are the classic symptoms of clinical depression (Mental Health First Aid, 2008).

MENTAL WELLBEING AND RESILIENCE FOR YOURSELF AND THE PEOPLE YOU CARE FOR

Research suggests that there are a number of variables that make a far greater contribution to happiness than external and superficial factors, such as wealth and possessions. Biology has an important role in developing depression.

THE ROLE OF NEUROTRANSMITTERS AND MENTAL HEALTH

Biologists would say only two things make you happy: dopamine (low amounts can produce anxiety and it has a relationship with schizophrenia) and serotonin (too little leads to depression, problems with anger control, obsessive-compulsive disorder, and suicidal ideation). These are neurotransmitters and they are the chemicals that allow the transmission of signals from one neuron to the next across synapses (see Chapter 6, Bioscience, for greater detail on the nervous system). Other neurotransmitters are norepinephrine and glutamate, which are important to the formation of memory, and which are reduced by the stress hormones (which is why stressed students have difficulty in remembering stuff). Endorphins are involved in pain reduction and pleasure, these slow down heart rate and respiration, and GABA (gamma-aminobutyric acid) acts like a brake on adrenaline but too little leads to anxiety.

PHYSICAL AND MENTAL HEALTH

It is a sad but true fact that patients with poor mental health have poorer outcomes for somatic ailments. Especially patients with non-affective psychotic disorders such as schizophrenia or psychotic episodes are at higher risk of somatic ailments and shorter life expectancy (–8 years); however, they often experience lower quality of somatic healthcare, underdiagnosis and undertreatment. Patients with severe mental illness also report more difficulties in accessing care than the general population (Küey, 2008). Coghlan and Lawrence (2002) researching in Western Australia found alarmingly high rates of physical illness in people with mental illness and evidenced that people with mental illness and serious physical illness were not hospitalised as often in comparison with somatic only disorders. Björkman et al. (2008) researched healthcare professionals' attitudes in Sweden and found that nurses treating somatic ailments reported negative attitudes to people with schizophrenia and considered them as being dangerous and unpredictable. At the same time, research in India by Poreddi et al. (2017) found that psychiatric ward attendants had more positive attitudes than general attendants towards psychiatric illnesses.

In the UK, Gateshill et al. (2011) compared attitudes towards mental disorders in medical and health professionals working in mental health and professionals working in different areas of medicine. Their research revealed that whilst both groups showed similar levels of empathy towards patients with poor mental health, those working in different areas reflected national attitudes described by 'Time to Change' respondents: 'When asked about how to describe someone who has a mental illness, nearly 40% agreed that they are prone to violence' (www.time-to-change.org.uk/home/about-us/our-impact, 2015). Both groups were also negative about substance misusers (alcohol and drugs), suggesting their use was a cause of poor mental health (rather than self-medication).

All this indicates that there is a near global perception by somatic nurses that mentally ill patients with somatic disorders are difficult to nurse, and that somatic nurses need training in understanding mental health disorders as there is a vacuum of practical guidance.

DIAGNOSTIC OVERSHADOWING (CHECK YOUR BIAS)

Diagnostic overshadowing has been usefully defined by Emerson and Baines (2010) as 'Symptoms of physical ill health are mistakenly attributed to either a mental health/behavioural problem or as being inherent in the person's learning disabilities'. People with poor mental health do not generally die from this, they die from preventable disorders which may have been treated but symptoms have been wrongly ascribed to their mental health condition. This is pertinent for people with a learning disability (LD): somatic nurses have a limited understanding of LD and comorbidity, such as the relationship between Down syndrome and cleft palate and cardiac abnormalities. Blair (2016) explains that 'Gastrointestinal cancers are approximately twice as prevalent in people with a learning disability, and coronary heart disease is the second highest cause of death for people with a learning disability.' Diagnostic overshadowing occurs when a healthcare worker observes someone with LD patting or rubbing their abdomen and assumes it is an LD behaviour rather than wondering if they are in pain; whereas paying close attention to nonverbal communication can save a life.

🗨 Case Study 13.2   Student voice

This case study is provided by trainee nursing associate Susan.

Whilst running my clinic in a GP surgery, a lady attended routinely for herself; during her appointment she expressed concern about her son Greg. He is a 33-year-old who has a learning disability and needed his Covid vaccination.

She told me that she had booked an appointment via the booking system. Both she and Greg attended the appointment, however when Greg saw the queue, he felt panicked and left without speaking to anyone. His mum then spoke to her GP who prescribed a mild sedative for him to take prior to attending his appointment, and some numbing cream for the site on his arm where the vaccine would be administered. She went on to make another appointment and attended again as planned, this time he managed to get into clinic room but then again panicked and left un-vaccinated.

Questions

What would you do in this situation? Make some notes then read Susan's thoughts at the end of the chapter, and compare them to your own.

Go Further 13.1

Look at the NHS RightCare Toolkit: Physical Ill-health and CVD Prevention in People with Severe Mental Illness found at: www.england.nhs.uk/rightcare/wp-content/uploads/sites/40/2019/03/nhs-rightcare-toolkit-cvd-prevention.pdf

---

The 'Track and Trigger' method (NEWS2) for physiological disorders, in order to identify any deterioration in patients, is in recent use in acute psychiatric hospitals and has been adapted to identify psychiatric patients who are experiencing mental health crisis.

The NHS Five Year Forward View for Mental Health plan (FYFVMH) promotes new models of care by using an integrated approach to care delivery. With a more integrated approach to mental health, it places an emphasis on combined mental health and physical health outcomes. Multispeciality Community Providers (MCPs) work together with Primary and Acute Care systems (PACs) to offer an integrated service so that people with complex and ongoing care needs have access to facilities staffed with teams who have MH expertise. James (2021) reviewed the targets of the FYFVMH and suggested some improvement in child and maternal mental health, but noted that failures such as NHS psychiatrist recruitment and reducing Out of Area Placements (OAPs) remain to be addressed. The impact of Covid-19 on service demand has increased waiting times, and provision is fragile in some areas. The government is funding a Covid-19 mental health and wellbeing recovery action plan, although it is not clear if funding is new money or reallocated money, taken from another part of the NHS.

The purpose of the new models of care is in recovery and relapse prevention in the community. In order to achieve these goals, staff training is core, in order to offer support for complex and comorbid physical and mental health conditions. Care teams are not just multi-disciplinary, they are also multi-sectoral, with the NHS working with both the private and the social enterprise sectors.

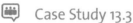

Case Study 13.3

Katie is a 23-year-old woman who received serious injuries in a car accident; her partner was killed in the accident. Katie has ongoing mobility issues due to injury to her pelvis and right hip; she is in constant distracting pain which has an impact on her ability to work. She suffers from depression and anxiety due to physical and emotional pain; she also has panic attacks if she gets into a car. She has financial worries and has returned to her parents' house to live as her landlord would not agree to her living in his flat while she is waiting for state benefits.

Katie's GP practice has integrated community-based physical and mental health services. Katie attends pain management and physiotherapy at her local clinic to support her physical recovery. She was signposted to grief counselling given by a local charity and recommended for CBT, offered by a local social enterprise company. She was also signposted to a welfare advisor from a national disability advisory service to support her application for benefits. This collaboration presents Katie with a holistic approach to her recovery.

COMMUNICATING WITH SOMEONE WHO IS MENTALLY UNWELL

Many people, including health workers, struggle to know what to say to someone with poor mental health; they don't know which questions to ask or how the person will respond. A genuine enquiry of 'how are you' and being prepared to listen is a recommended therapeutic intervention, allowing time and space for the patient to talk, tell their story and, equally importantly, feel like they are being heard; it is also a good de-escalation strategy. You cannot and should not try to 'fix' the person. Ask the patient who they would normally contact when they are mentally unwell, offer to ring them (on an office or ward phone, *never* your own mobile phone) and let them talk. If this is not possible, ask them what they would like to happen: this will allow the patient to be solutions focused, help them to break big problems into small manageable ones; ask them to identify which is the most important problem that needs attention and signpost them to get the help they want.

PERSONAL SAFETY

Whilst most people with poor mental health are not violent, sometimes they can be aggressive, and this can be frightening; always ensure your personal safety and never put yourself into danger. If you are in a small room, sit near the door, do not have furniture between you and an exit route. Be professional, be kind and listen to the person but be aware of your personal safety. If you feel threatened, offer to make tea/coffee, and find a colleague to support you or escalate to a senior.

Go Further 13.2

Active listening means leaning in, looking interested, and responding appropriately; this will help the patient to feel respected, accepted and cared about. If the patient can feel these things, they are likely to feel less isolated and establish trust in the care staff. This will give you the opportunity to understand the patient and their experience, read Chapter 9, Essential Skills for Care, for further detail on improving your interpersonal communication.

You could also read Nurse Kimberley Hodgson's article in the *Nursing Standard* on attitudes to people who self-harm when presenting to A&E. This can be found at: https://journals.rcni.com/doi/abs/10.7748/ns.30.31.38.s44

RESILIENCE

When working for health, it is important to take care not just of the patients and clients in your care, but to take care of yourself. Working for health is a stressful undertaking; many things can impact on your own mental health, such as worries, tiredness, workload, and financial problems can drag you down too. Many staff have suffered severe anxiety during the time of Covid-19. They have feared for themselves, their families and their patients; long-term stress can lead to distress and depression. Lack of appreciation by the government and intense pressure from managers have led many to consider leaving nursing altogether. Read the next few paragraphs on resilience and relate them to your own life and think about coping strategies that you can adopt to support yourself, so you do not become overwhelmed.

Seligman (2002) said that what distinguishes happy people from the unhappy is attitude, and that our attitude to our lives is determined by our character and genetics. He devised an equation to determine happiness:

H = Happiness

S = Set range (genetics)

C = Circumstances

V = Voluntary control (past, present, future)

- Past: Seligman says that when thinking about the past, people who are happy focus on good times rather than ruminating on the bad ones.
- Present: Seligman considers happy people take pleasure in their surroundings and their relationships and look for the good in each day.
- Future: Seligman says happy people are flexibly optimistic, they have a plan but are realistic in their goals and are not defeated if the plan doesn't pan out.

He also runs a website – www.authentichappiness.org – where you can take 'happiness' tests.

Dr Timothy Sharp and colleagues (2013) have shown that identifying your personal strengths and qualities can lead to higher levels of happiness. However, they say that often people take the opposite course of identifying and then mending their weaknesses. Sharp et al.'s research suggests that focusing on strengths develops resilience.

Resilience is the capacity to cope with stress and adversity. Developing healthy coping mechanisms results in individuals bouncing back to a previous state of happiness or using the experience of adversity to produce a hardening effect. Resilience is best understood as a process that promotes wellbeing or protects against being overwhelmed when in misfortune.

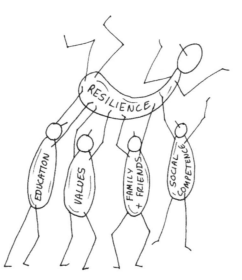

Figure 13.7   Resilience

Studies (Werner and Smith, 1992; Werner, 1970) show that the primary factor in resilience is having caring and supportive relationships within and outside the family – relationships that create love and trust, provide role models, and offer encouragement and reassurance help bolster a person's resilience (Figure 13.7). Table 13.3 shows you what other factors can add to resilience.

Prepare for feeling overwhelmed and stressed by developing strategies that can reduce these feelings. Stress produces a somatic response as your body thinks you are under attack or in a frightening situation (fight, flight or freeze). The stress hormones cortisol and adrenaline need to be worked off and the best way to do this is to work with natural processes by taking exercise. Walking is free and you don't need any special training or clothing to do it; singing aloud to uplifting music and dancing will have the same effect.

Table 13.3   Additional factors associated with resilience

The ability to make realistic plans and carry them out
A positive self-view and self-confidence
Communication and problem-solving skills
The ability to manage strong emotions

CHAPTER SUMMARY

- This chapter has discussed notions of mental health. You have considered the various models of mental health and how mental health is categorised.
- The system of nomenclature of groups of symptoms by reference to the DSM and ICD has been explained, and this has shown that interpretations of which groups of symptoms make up a disease are flexible and change over time.
- In order to help someone who is suffering poor mental health, you need to understand what can indicate that someone is becoming unwell. Understanding the way someone's behaviour is changing can help you to help them. Working for other people's health can tax your own, so developing personal resilience can support you in your role.

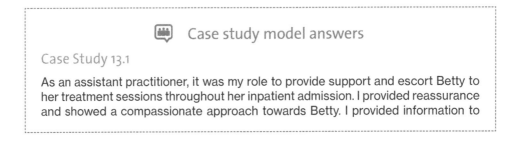

📖   Case study model answers

Case Study 13.1

As an assistant practitioner, it was my role to provide support and escort Betty to her treatment sessions throughout her inpatient admission. I provided reassurance and showed a compassionate approach towards Betty. I provided information to

Betty to help her understand what she could expect and the benefits of the treatment she would be receiving.

Post treatment, I would complete physical observations. This monitoring was an essential part of the recovery process. In the initial 6 hours following ECT I had to complete physical observations such as blood pressure, temperature, pulse, heart rate and oxygen levels. I documented Betty's vital observations on the online physical heath form.

With therapeutic engagement I was able to engage with Betty and offer support around the challenging behaviours she was displaying. Over time a positive relationship was formed, and Betty was extremely receptive of my approach and at times she asked for me personally.

I encouraged Betty to eat and drink and monitored both oral intake and urinary output. By encouraging and allowing her time her nutritional intake improved and she slowly started to gain weight.

After eight ECT appointments Betty was beginning to show insight into her condition; engagement became more structured as she was recovering from her psychotic depression. I have gained a lot of valuable skills to enable me to support people with psychotic depression

I cannot stress enough the importance of positive engagement when a service user is unwell. It took 6 months for Betty to become well again. She was then transferred to a rehabilitation ward to support her with her activities of daily living skills.

Assistant practitioner & nurse associate: Gillian

Case Study 13.2

As a trainee nursing associate, it was clear to me that the clinic setting was not the appropriate place for Greg to attend, as it was too overwhelming for him. I allocated time in my clinic to be able to give Greg enough time to chat, feel calm and advised mum to speak to the GP again to see if a sedative would be required.

Both Greg and his mum attended his appointment as planned. I approached Greg in a calm way and on his level asking about his hobbies, etc. I then went on to ask if he understood why he was here. He had a good knowledge of Covid, and the vaccine so had capacity for consent.

We got right up to the point of administering the vaccine, talking all the time of what I was doing, but he started to panic and flinched away which then posed a danger for me also with the needle. I advised mum that although she was asking if 'I could just give it' I refused as he was expressing his wishes and although I understood the predicament, it was not in my remit of care as a TNA to do this and I cannot forcibly give vaccine against his will.

I explained to mum that although Greg would be un-vaccinated, as are many people in community, there are still good ways of keeping safe by using mask/hand hygiene and avoiding large groups of people.

We agreed to have another attempt. One more appointment was booked, but this failed as a communication error with reception meant she missed the appointment. I phoned her and she understood that both she and the clinic had reached a bit of an impasse in trying to get this done. She would continue to speak to Greg and given time he may feel more confident. I assured her I would do all I could to help. I liaised with our learning disability service which assured me we had done all we could to help.

An issue during the pandemic that we have found within the vaccination programme is that although LD facilities are well catered for by community teams going to places of residential units, there is no facility in place for LD people who are being cared for in their own homes by parents.

Trainee nursing associate: Susan

FURTHER READING

WEBSITES

- Mind, the mental health charity: www.mind.org.uk
- Rethink Mental Illness: www.rethink.org
- Alzheimer's Society: www.alzheimers.org.uk
- Search on the NHS website for mental health: www.nhs.uk

BOOKS AND ARTICLES

All of these texts can support you in developing your understanding of mental health. You can read journal articles online and watch YouTube videos to deepen your knowledge:

- Frank, J. (1991) *Persuasion and Healing: A Comparative Study of Psychotherapy.* Baltimore: Johns Hopkins University Press.
- Gabe, J., Bury, M. and Elston, M. (2006) *Key Concepts in Medical Sociology.* London: Sage.
- Goffman, E. (1968) *Stigma: Notes on the Management of Spoiled Identity.* Englewood Cliffs, NJ: Prentice-Hall.
- Link, B. and Phelan, J. (2001) Conceptualizing stigma. *Annual Review of Sociology*, 27: 363–85.
- Seligman, M. (2002) *Authentic Happiness: Using the New Positive Psychology to Realise Your Potential for Lasting Fulfilment.* London: Simon & Schuster.

VIDEOS

- BBC Mental: A History of the Madhouse: www.youtube.com/watch?v=oswUssXzFlY
- The Role of Medication in Mental Health: www.youtube.com/watch?v=ZXOPsO-W6Cw
- NHS Frontline: Mental Health Rehabilitation: www.youtube.com/watch?v=Rg9RsIQRzL8
- Discrimination Firsthand – Experiences of Mental Health-related Stigma and Discrimination: www.youtube.com/watch?v=rWuKtrgT160

REFERENCES

Allderidge, P. (1979) Hospitals, madhouses and asylums: cycles in the care of the insane. *British Journal of Psychiatry*, *134*: 321–34.

Atkinson, R.C. and Shiffrin, R.M. (1968) Human memory: a proposed system and its control processes. In K.W. Spence, and J.T. Spence (eds), *The Psychology of Learning and Motivation* (Vol. 2). New York: Academic Press. pp. 89–195.

Becker, H. (1963) *Outsiders*. New York: Simon & Schuster.

Björkman, T., Angelman, T. and Jönsson, M. (2008) Attitudes towards people with mental illness: a cross-sectional study among nursing staff in psychiatric and somatic care. *Scandinavian Journal of Caring Sciences, 22*(2): 170–7.

Blair, J. (2016) Diagnostic overshadowing: see beyond the diagnosis. *British Journal of Family Medicine*, March/April: 37–41.

Bradley Report (2009) *Lord Bradley's Review of People with Mental Health Problems or Learning Disabilities in the Criminal Justice System*. Executive Summary. London: Department of Health.

Butler, J. (2014) *Leveraging Intersectionality: Seeing and Not Seeing*. Phoenix, AZ: Richer Press.

Coghlan, R. and Lawrence, D. (2002) Health inequalities and the health needs of people with mental illness. *NSW Public Health Bulletin, 13*(7): 155–8.

Cosgrove, L. and Krimsky, S. (2012) A comparison of *DSM*-IV and *DSM*-5 panel members' financial associations with industry: a pernicious problem persists. *PLoS Medicone, 9*(3): e1001190.

Crenshaw, K. (1989) Demarginalizing the intersection of race and sex: a black feminist critique of antidiscrimination doctrine, feminist theory and antiracist politics. Available at: https://chicagounbound.uchicago.edu/cgi/viewcontent.cgi?article=1052&context=uclf

Emerson, E. and Baines, S. (2010) Improving health and lives: Learning Disability Observatory. Available at: https://digital.nhs.uk/services/general-practice-gp-collections/service-information/learning-disabilities-observatory

Engel, G. (1977) The need for a new medical model: a challenge for biomedicine. *Science, 196*: 129–36.

Fernando, S. (2014) *Mental Health Worldwide Culture, Globalization and Development*. Basingstoke: Palgrave Macmillan.

Foucault, M. (1973) *The Birth of the Clinic*. London: Taylor and Francis.

Frank, J. (1961) *Persuasion and Healing: A Comparative Study of Psychotherapy*. Baltimore: Johns Hopkins University Press.

Frühauf, A., Niedermeier, M., Elliott, L., Ledochowski, L., Marksteiner, J. and Kopp, M. (2016) Acute effects of outdoor physical activity on affect and psychological well-being in depressed patients: a preliminary study. *Mental Health and Physical Activity*. Available at: www.sciencedirect.com/science/journal/17552966

Gabe, J., Bury, M. and Elston, M. (2006) *Key Concepts in Medical Sociology*. London: Sage.

Gateshill, G., Kucharska-Pietura, K. and Wattis, J. (2011) Attitudes towards mental disorders and emotional empathy. *The Psychiatrist, 35*: 101–5.

Goffman, E. (1968) *Stigma: Notes on the Management of Spoiled Identity*. Englewood Cliffs, NJ: Prentice-Hall.

Goldacre, B. (2008) *Bad Science*. London: HarperCollins.

hooks, b. (2014) [1984]) *Feminist Theory: From Margin to Center* (3rd edn). New York: Routledge.

Illich, I. (1976) *Limits to Medicine: Medical Nemesis – The Expropriation of Health*. London: Boyers Publishing.

James, A. (2021) The end of the Five Year Forward View – what is next for mental health? Available at: https://blogs.bmj.com/bmj/2021/04/15/adrian-james-the-end-of-the-five-year-forward-view-what-is-next-for-mental-health/

Küey, L. (2008) The impact of stigma on somatic treatment and care for people with comorbid mental and somatic disorders. *Current Opinion in Psychiatry, 21*(4): 403–11.

Kung, K., Tsang, H. and Corrigan, P. (2008) Self-stigma of people with schizophrenia as predictor of their adherence to psychosocial treatment. *Journal of Psychiatric Rehabilitation, 32*(2): 95–104.

Lang, R. (2001) *The Development and Critique of the Social Model of Disability*. Paper given to the University of East Anglia. Available at: www.ucl.ac.uk/epidemiology-health-care/sites/epidemiology-health-care/files/wp-3.pdf

Lemart, E. (1967) *Human Deviance, Social Problems, and Social Control*. London: Prentice-Hall.

Link, B. and Phelan, J. (2001) Conceptualizing stigma. *Annual Review of Sociology, 27*: 363–85.

Livingstone, J. and Boyd, J. (2010) Correlates and consequences of internalized stigma for people living with mental illness: a systematic review and meta-analysis. *Journal of Social Science Medicine, 71*(12): 2150–61.

Marmot, M., Allen, J., Goldblatt, P., Herd, E. and Morrison, J. (2021) *Build Back Fairer: The COVID-19 Marmot Review*. Available at: www.instituteofhealthequity.org/resources-reports/build-back-fairer-the-covid-19-marmot-review

Matza, D. (1964) *Delinquency and Drift*. New York: Wiley.

McWilliams, N. (2009) Psychoanalysis. In I. Marini and M.A. Stebnicki (eds), *Professional Counsellor Desk Reference*. New York: Springer. pp. 289–300.

Mental Health First Aid (2008) Depression guidelines. Available at: https://mhfa.com.au/resources/mental-health-first-aid-guidelines#mhfaesc

Mental Health Foundation (2017) What is mental health? Available at: www.mentalhealth.org.uk/your-mental-health/about-mental-health/what-mental- health

Mental Health Foundation (2021) Coronavirus: The divergence of mental health experiences during the pandemic. Available at: www.mentalhealth.org.uk/coronavirus/divergence-mental-health-experiences-during-pandemic

Mills, T.L. (2000) Depression, mental health, and psychological well-being among older African Americans: a selective review of the literature. *Perspectives, 7*: 93–104.

Mind and Time to Change (2015) Latest survey shows public are less likely to discriminate against people with mental health problems. Available at: www.mind.org.uk/news-campaigns/news/latest-survey-shows-public-are-less-likely-to-discriminate-against-people-with-mental-health-problems/

NHS (2018) Adult Improving Access to Psychological Therapies programme. Available at: www.england.nhs.uk/mental-health/adults/iapt/

Parsons, T. (1951) *The Social System*. London: Routledge & Kegan Paul.

Poreddi, V., Rohini, T. and Suresh, B. (2017) Medical and nursing students' attitudes toward mental illness: an Indian perspective. Available at: www.scielo.org.co/pdf/iee/v35n1/2216-0280-iee-35-01-00086.pdf

Public Health England (2016) *Arts for Health and Wellbeing: An Evaluation Framework*. Available at: www.gov.uk/government/uploads/system/uploads/attachment_data/file/496230/PHE_Arts_and_Health_Evaluation_FINAL.pdf

Rethink (2017) Available at: www.rethink.org/news-and-stories/news/

Robinson, M.D. and Gordon, K.H. (2011) Personality dynamics: insights from the personality social cognitive literature. *Journal of Personality Assessment, 93*(2): 161–76.

Sapolsky, R. (1996) Why stress is bad for your brain. *Journal of Science, 273*(5276): 749–50.

Seligman, M. (2002) *Authentic Happiness: Using the New Positive Psychology to Realise Your Potential for Lasting Fulfilment.* London: Simon & Schuster.

Seng, J.S., Lopez, W.D., Sperlich, M., Hamama, L. and Meldrum, C.D.R. (2012) Marginalized identities, discrimination burden, and mental health: empirical exploration of an interpersonal-level approach to modelling intersectionality. *Journal of Social Science and Medicine, 75*(12): 2437–45.

Sharp, T., Moran, E., Kuhn, I. and Barclay, S. (2013) Do the elderly have a voice? Advance care planning discussions with frail and older individuals: a systematic literature review and narrative synthesis. *British Journal of General Practice, 63*(615): e657–e668.

Social Exclusion Unit (2004) Mental health and social exclusion. Available at: www.centreformentalhealth.org.uk/sites/default/files/mental_health_and_social_exclusion.pdf

Sykes, G. and Mazda, S. (1957) Neutralization and drift theory. *American Sociological Review, 22*: 664–70.

Szasz, T. (1961) *The Myth of Mental Illness.* New York: HarperCollins.

Turbott, J. (1996) Religion, spirituality and psychiatry: conceptual, cultural and personal challenges. *Australian Journal of Psychiatry, 30*(6): 720–30.

Wakefield, J. and Horwitz, A. (2006) The epidemic in mental illness: clinical fact or survey artifact? Contexts, 5: 19–23. https://journals.sagepub.com/doi/pdf/10.1525/ctx.2006.5.1.19

Werner, E.E. and Smith, R.S. (1992) *Overcoming the Odds: High-risk Children from Birth to Adulthood.* Ithaca, NY: Cornell University Press.

Werner, J.A. (1970) To nursing practice. *Perspectives in Psychiatric Care, 8*: 248–61.

World Health Organization (2014) Mental health. Available at: www.who.int/features/factfiles/mental_health/en/

Zola, I.K. (1973) Pathways to the doctor – from person to patient. *Journal of Social Science Medicine, 7*(9): 677–89.

14

PROTECTING CHILDREN AND VULNERABLE ADULTS

JANETTE BARNES AND JADE CARTER-BENNETT

STANDARDS OF PROFICIENCY FOR NURSING ASSOCIATES (2018)

Relevant Platforms include:

Platform 1:1.4 Demonstrate an understanding of, and the ability to challenge or report discriminatory behaviour.

Platform 2:2.5 Understand the importance of early years and childhood experiences and the possible impact on life choices, mental, physical and behavioural wellbeing.

Platform 3:3.21 Recognise how a person's capacity affects their ability to make decisions about their own care and to give or withhold consent.

Platform 3:3.22 Recognise when capacity has changed and understand where and how to seek guidance and support from others to ensure the best interests of those receiving care are upheld.

Platform 3:3.24 Take personal responsibility to ensure that relevant information is shared according to local policy and appropriate immediate action is taken to provide adequate safeguarding and that concerns are escalated.

Platform 5:5.6 Understand and act in line with local and national organisational frameworks, legislation, and regulations to report risks, and implement actions as instructed, following up and escalating as required.

Annex B Recognise and escalate signs of all forms of abuse 1:1.6.

For most parents, our children are everything to us: our hopes, our ambitions, our future. Our children are cherished and loved. But sadly, some children are not so fortunate. Some children's lives are different. Dreadfully different. Instead of the joy, warmth and security of normal family life, these children's lives are filled with risk, fear, and danger: and from what most of us would regard as the worst possible source – from the people closest to them.

Tony Blair (2003) Foreword to *Every Child Matters*

This chapter has been co-written by a social worker who has worked predominantly with children and by an adult transitions social worker in order to give a holistic appreciation of the role of safeguarding across the life span. Janette discusses the assessment process involved in safeguarding children using the Every Child Matters/Helping Children Achieve (ECM/HCA) framework, while Jade discusses the *No Secrets* policy in adult social services and the Care Act, which replaced it in 2014; she also discusses the use of advocates and the Mental Capacity Act 2005, and makes reference to the temporary use of the Coronavirus Act 2020 during the Covid-19 pandemic.

Glossary

* **Abuse** A form of maltreatment either by commission or omission
* **Advocacy** Someone who supports the client to ensure their rights are protected and asserted
* **Assessment** This could be of a developmental nature or a needs-led survey
* **Child in need** Under Section 17 (10) of the Children Act 1989, a child who is unlikely to achieve or develop without the support of the local authority
* **Child protection** Supporting a child suffering, or likely to suffer, significant harm
* **Common Assessment Framework (CAF)** A standardised approach to conducting an assessment
* **Single Assessment Process** This is replacing the CAF, but the information collected is similar

INTRODUCTION

The quotation that opens this chapter comes at the beginning of the government's initial consultation document entitled *Every Child Matters*, which was published in 2003 as a response to the findings of the Laming Report that same year after the death of Victoria Climbié. It lays out the nature of child protection. However, sadly, despite all best efforts to date, we still have children who are in dire need of help, support and protection. In March 2020, the number of children who were 'looked after' was 80,080, a 2% increase from the previous year (Gov.uk, 2020).

Alongside these concerning statistics for children, there have also been many cases of severe harm resulting in the death of vulnerable adults despite the *No Secrets* White Paper (Department of Health, 2000). Following the murder of Steven Hoskin, a man with a learning disability who lived alone and was tortured before his death in 2006, a serious case review in 2007 found that agencies including health, social care and police had missed signs that should have initiated adult protection procedures. In 2014, the Care Act set out a legal framework which details safeguarding duties for local authorities and introduced core principles to protect vulnerable adults and prevent abuse and neglect from occurring.

In this chapter, we hope to give you an insight into the five essential building blocks for children to develop and grow into well-balanced happy young adults. We will also look at different aspects covered in the assessment process used by local authorities' social services departments, and how these form a holistic mechanism to allow you and other practitioners to make reasoned judgements about safety and needs once in possession of the relevant information. We will also aim to give an insight into how this is relevant within adult social services because it supports the identification of eligible social care needs in terms of ensuring every opportunity for support to parents is offered. This is explained later in the text, with reference to the Care Act 2014. Also, we describe how local authorities can use toolkits such as the Signs of Safety model, originally created for 'keeping children safe', which has been adapted to identify and manage risks to vulnerable adults.

We will look at the importance of attachment; how this combined with structure and boundaries, and in addition to basic needs for care and love, fosters resilience, growth and development throughout childhood. You will note that we have focused most closely on the needs of the children; however, we will also look at the needs of parents in terms of support and guidance to ensure their children are safe and well looked after and how such support can impact their ability to effectively parent their children and keep them safe.

Go Further 14.1

Read the Children Act 1989/2004 (or see Working with Kids, 2017, for a good practical explanation) and other guidance and legislation, such as the Signs of Safety model. Your knowledge and understanding of these will support your practice. The Children and Social Work Act 2017 introduces 'Corporate Parenting Principles' and states that a Personal Advisor should be offered to all children leaving care up to age 25 (regulations determined April 2018). It also highlights the necessity to look at educational support needs for children previously looked after, in addition to those currently being looked after. Legislation includes an amendment to the Children Act 2004 to incorporate the Child Safeguarding Practice Review Panel (to strengthen the serious case review guidance) and which renamed the Local Safeguarding Board as 'Safeguarding Partners' – namely the local authority, clinical commissioning group and the chief officer of police.

EVERY CHILD MATTERS/HELPING CHILDREN ACHIEVE

Every Child Matters (ECM) and its subsequent incarnation as *Helping Children Achieve* (HCA) sets out five aspects that should be addressed for all children so that they can have a safe and happy childhood wherever possible with their birth family. It covers all the things that a child needs to ensure their safety, development and happiness as they grow, and the aspects can be remembered with the acronym SHEEP.

Staying safe: Protecting children from harm, neglect, or abuse while they are growing up; and equipping them with the skills for independence. There is lots of guidance and information around safeguarding children, but you need to know where to look. Activity 14.1 offers you some help.

⚙ Activity 14.1

What protocols does your own organisation follow and how will you contribute to this for the children and families you meet through your work?

Reflect on your current knowledge. Imagine a child discloses something untoward to you that will impact on their safety:

- What do you do?
- What are your organisation's procedures; do you know where this information is?
- Who can you talk to? And what is your moral obligation to the child?
- What are your observations – for example, home conditions, child's presentation, parent's actions/inactions? Consider how Bronfenbrenner's Systems Theory (1979) helps to explain how a child's development is affected by their environment
- Is it putting the child at risk/significant risk?
- What can you do (this may depend on your role and moral obligations)?
- Who else can help (other professionals, family, school, police)?

Doing nothing, if you have concerns, **is not an option**.

Staying healthy: Ensuring children have good physical, emotional and mental health by ensuring they have a healthy lifestyle. How will you know this?

When you are with a child, observe them for the following factors:

- Child's presentation – physically and mentally: are their appearance and reactions as you might expect? For example, injuries, stature, cleanliness, confidence, eye contact.
- How does the child interact/react with parent/s or primary caregiver?
- How does the child interact with others? Confident, quiet, withdrawn, fearful?

Doing nothing, if you have concerns, **is not an option**.

Enjoying and achieving: As is their right, all children should be enabled to enjoy their lives and get the best out of it while achieving their potential for living independently. What can you do to help?

- Do parents help the child/ren to develop skills for future life?
- Are there opportunities for the child to socialise and learn from others?
- Is disability and support looked at positively?
- Do parents need support to help their children?

Doing nothing, if you have concerns, **is not an option**.

Economic wellbeing/overcoming poverty: Overcoming children's socioeconomic disadvantages to achieve their full potential in life.

- Do parents have knowledge of and access to universal and targeted benefits for the child?
- Housing – does this meet needs? If not, how can this be addressed?
- Do parents keep the child safe, and give them a secure social structure in which to live and thrive?
- Is the child loved by family and friends, do they have continuity of love and support from principal caregivers – positive attachment and ultimately the basis for resilience? And does the child have self-esteem, confidence? Is the child able to achieve in life, education, social scenarios?

Yes, you guessed it – doing nothing **is not an option!**

Go Further 14.2

Maslow, A. (2014 [1962]) *Towards a Psychology of Being* (3rd edn). Bensenville, IL: Lushena Books. Read Essays 13 and 14 to deepen your knowledge.

Positive contribution: Enabling children to make a positive contribution to their community and society, and not engaging in antisocial or offending behaviour.

In what way does Maslow's pyramid (Figure 14.1) relate to children's needs, consider the lower two tiers and consider what opportunities might a child need to self-actualise.

What opportunities does the child have?

- Are disability or socioeconomic issues a barrier? If so, how can this be overcome?

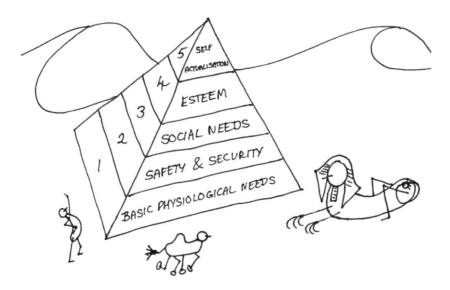

Figure 14.1   Maslow's pyramid of needs

- What are the significant issues in the child's life preventing achievement?
- Does this relate to Maslow? Where is the gap in meeting lower-level needs which inhibit self-actualisation?
- What can you do to help break barriers/enable needs to be met?

We will be taking a closer look at how these areas are assessed when a child and their family are facing difficulties. The failure of one or more of these areas to be addressed may lead to difficulties in other areas, for example, un-addressed bullying of a child at school may lead to poor educational achievement and/or attendance, and increased friction at home, perhaps an escalation in unacceptable behaviours at home or in social settings. It is not always the case that the child is willing or able to articulate their fears or concerns and it is up to others – family, friends, school, GPs and others – including you – to help them by spotting the signs and symptoms, and ensure the right support is sought and put in place for them.

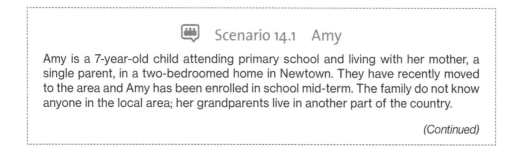

Scenario 14.1   Amy

Amy is a 7-year-old child attending primary school and living with her mother, a single parent, in a two-bedroomed home in Newtown. They have recently moved to the area and Amy has been enrolled in school mid-term. The family do not know anyone in the local area; her grandparents live in another part of the country.

(Continued)

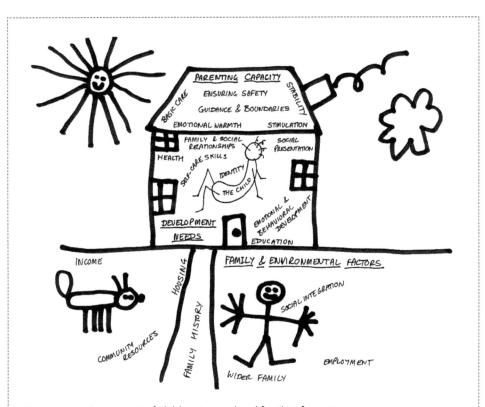
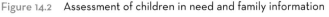

Figure 14.2   Assessment of children in need and family information

Source: © Alan Davidson, The Scottish Government, Better Life Chances Unit

For the past week Amy has been late to school on several occasions. She has been dressed in appropriate clothing, but the clothing is dirty, and she appears to have had only a minimal wash. She has been noted to be hungry, swooping on food at lunch break and taking crisps and biscuits from the children who bring packed lunches. When challenged about this she says she is hungry because she did not eat her breakfast. She appears wary and does not make eye contact with her teacher, shunning other children who taunt her, calling her names, 'Smelly' and 'Piggy'.

Today, Amy arrives at school late, subdued and remains quiet all morning. Just before lunch she is excused to go to the toilet and when she returns to class just as the children are lining up to go to lunch, it becomes obvious that she has had an 'accident'. The classroom assistant takes Amy to one side, then to the school nurse, as it is apparent that the child is both embarrassed and in some discomfort. When the school nurse attempts to assist Amy, not only is it evident that she has soiled, but she also has some red and purple blotches on her upper thighs which were noticeable when she lifted her dress.

What happens next ...?

Think about your organisation's protocols and relevant legislation or if you are not working in a child environment think about what you would do if a friend was telling you this scenario, what advice would you give her/him?

> Think about the children and young people you know in your professional or private life. How might you notice the signs of need, or a child who needs protection? How might you play your part in dealing with this, or helping to ensure the need is met? Using the signposts from the Assessment of children in need and family information (Figure 14.2), how would you help Amy?

NO SECRETS/THE CARE ACT (2014): SAFEGUARDING VULNERABLE ADULTS

No Secrets (DoH, 2000) guides the development and implementation of policies and procedures to protect vulnerable adults from harm and abuse. Although superseded by the Care Act 2014, the guidance includes the broad definition of a 'vulnerable adult' as a person 'who is or may be in need of community care services by reason of mental or other disability, age or illness; and who is or may be unable to take care of him or herself, or unable to protect him or herself against significant harm or exploitation'. The *No Secrets* guidance details the different forms of abuse as physical, sexual, psychological, financial, neglect, discriminatory and organisational, however the Care Act 2014 recognises those listed and introduces additional forms of abuse to the *No Secrets* guidance (repealed in 2015), including domestic violence/abuse, self-neglect and modern slavery. Table 14.1 offers guidance. The Care Act replaces *No Secrets* with a statutory duty placed upon professionals to protect vulnerable adults.

Where a safeguarding concern has been raised, the local authority holds a duty to investigate and determine further action; however, safeguarding is everyone's concern and key partners include health, social care, the Care Quality Commission (CQC) and the police, who all have a duty to support. Neglect and self-neglect fall within this duty due to risks to and wellbeing of the person. More information on risk and capacity in relation to self-neglect can be found in the Care Act 2014 statutory guidance. A link is given under Further reading.

Following the Covid-19 pandemic came the implementation of the Coronavirus Act 2020. This included temporary but substantial powers for local authorities and across services, including the temporary registration of nurses, nursing associates and midwives. While changes were made in the way assessments were carried out, the safeguarding of vulnerable adults duties and responsibilities remained. You can find out more about the Coronavirus Act 2020 and its changes to legislation on the Gov.uk website. A link is provided in the Further reading section.

Go Further 14.3

This document gives detail of general and specific duties. It can be found at: https://assets.publishing.service.gov.uk/government/uploads/system/uploads/attachment_data/file/315993/Care-Act-Guidance.pdf

---

Table 14.1   Remember: abuse can take place anywhere

1. What do you do if you suspect abuse is occurring? As described previously, this may depend on your role. However, doing nothing is not an option.
2. Are you familiar with your organisation's adult safeguarding policy? You need to ensure you know what process to follow.
3. Who can help? Consider your line manager, police, CQC, the Adult Safeguarding department of your local authority, or if you are on placement and at college, your college safeguarding team can signpost you.
4. Consider mental capacity in accordance with the Mental Capacity Act 2005. This is particularly relevant as informed consent may inform your intervention. Advocacy is also important – this is mentioned in more detail later in this chapter.

Think about adults you have met both professionally and personally. Would you recognise the different forms of abuse as detailed in the Care Act 2014? What would you do next? What evidence is there to inform your intervention? Read the case study in Scenario 14.2 and consider how you would react. We all have a part to play in ensuring the safety and prevention of harm to adults. Safeguarding adults includes the responsibility of supporting people to make informed choices and having control of their lives. In health and social care, there are principles set out that are agreed within the Care Act 2014 that help us to understand how to safeguard adults, particularly those who are considered vulnerable. These are:

1. Empowerment: Ensuring people have all the information available to them in order to make their own decisions.
2. Prevention: Taking preventative measures before harm can occur.
3. Proportionality: The least restrictive or intrusive intervention to risk presented.
4. Protection: Support, advocacy and representation.
5. Partnership: Solutions through the exploration of services within the community.
6. Accountability: Transparency and accountability within the practice of safeguarding.

Scenario 14.2   Mary

Mary is a 25-year-old woman with a learning disability. Mary lives with her mother and two siblings, who are also adults but do not have learning disabilities. Mary is currently pregnant with her first child. The relationship between her siblings and Mary is volatile, often resulting in verbal arguments.

Mary told her midwife that she currently sleeps on her mother's sofa due to her sibling moving into her bedroom and Children's Services are involved due to concerns around Mary's capacity to parent her child effectively and safely without support because of her own learning needs.

During a meeting, Mary presented as wearing weather-inappropriate clothing and stated that she did not have enough money to buy a coat. Mary went on to say that this was because she had given her mother money for the rent, and she had needed to pay for the household weekly shop as her mother could not afford it.

1.   What types of abuse may be occurring here?

2.   What would you do next in supporting Mary to remain safe?

PROFESSIONAL STANDARDS: ETHICS, CONDUCT AND PERFORMANCE

Social workers, occupational therapists, teachers, doctors, nurses and nursing associates, to name but a few, are accountable to a code of conduct, performance and ethical standards for practice. Many health professions are regulated by the Health Care and Professionals Council (HCPC), however social workers moved to a new regulatory body in 2019 with the introduction of Social Work England. Nurses and nursing associates are required to register with the Nursing and Midwifery Council (NMC) before they are able to legally practise. While Social Work England and the HCPC set out different standards for practice, under their guidelines, all registered professionals have a duty to be committed to promoting and protecting the interests of service users and carers. To communicate appropriately and effectively, 'respect confidentiality and adhere to the General Data Protection Regulation 2018, and to report concerns about safety'. Similarly, The NMC Code gives guidance around ensuring nurses and nursing associates prioritise people, practise effectively, preserve safety and promote professionalism and trust (NMC, 2015, updated 2018 to reflect the regulation of nursing associates).

The evolution of policies, legislation and guidance has meant that professional development is at the forefront of social work, ensuring the continuous updating of knowledge so that standards can be consistently adhered to, and there is accountability for those professionals who do not. Perhaps the most common of these knowledge frameworks is the Professional Capabilities Framework, developed by the Social Work Reform Board. This standards framework sets out the expectations of social workers at each career stage

Many employer organisations also have their own professional development systems, which promote and support the performance of the professionals within it. For more information about ethical codes, read Chapter 4, Practising Values and Ethics in Health and Care Settings.

ASSESSMENT, SUPPORT AND ADVOCACY

ASSESSMENT OF NEEDS: CHILDREN

When concerns are raised about a child to the local authority, either by an individual or an organisation, the local authority has a duty to make enquiries, and take whatever action to consider whether the child is a child in need or a child at risk, as described in the Children Act 1989/2004 and Working Together to Safeguard Children 2018.

You will always have someone in your organisation that you can share concerns with and seek guidance from, and there is likely to be a delegated person who will ensure the local authority is informed. One of the most important things you should do is to ensure you make an accurate record of your concerns, of anything that a child discloses to you, and then take it to the appropriate person. This will enable social services to make their enquiries and assess needs if this is necessary.

The Children Act 1989/2004 provides a two-tiered assessment process with Child in Need (S17), and Child Protection (S47), each setting out a legal duty of meeting the needs of the child.

While local authorities will have different formats for collecting the information necessary to assess a child's needs, this is usually initiated by a single point of referral which is then triaged to determine what action and assessment, if any, is required. This is called an Early Help Assessment (EHA), which replaced the Common Assessment Framework (CAF). The 'My World Triangle' details child-centred factors for consideration when writing an assessment (see Figure 14.3).

Despite the change in name and perhaps format, the Early Help Assessment continues to maintain the principles that were enshrined in the Common Assessment Framework: that is, the holistic assessment of the child and family to determine needs and the systems/theories and strategies needed to protect and enhance children's lives. Wherever possible, this would be achieved with a child remaining in the care of their birth parent(s), when this can be done safely and in the child's best interests. It is a national approach to assessing any unmet needs that a child may have.

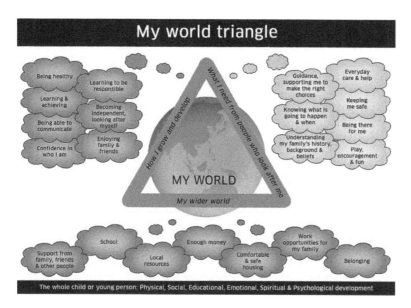

Figure 14.3   My World Triangle

Source: ©Scottish Government, Better Life Chances Unit. Reproduced with permission, under the terms of the Open Government Licence

The Children Act 1989 states in Section 20 (or s.31, depending on which section of the Act you are applying) that where possible, required action should be taken without recourse to the courts. All assessments should have the child at its centre and should ensure that the child's voice is heard. It must, in addition to the needs of the child, assess the ability of the parents or main caregivers to parent the child successfully. In effect, the same areas as the CAF addressed should still be covered:

- The child's development needs
- Parenting capacity
- Environmental factors

There is, rightly, great emphasis on the assessment allowing the child's voice to be heard throughout. The child's needs, and the risks they are or may be exposed to, must be assessed and analysed together with the child's own strengths, including their quality of attachment to parents. This is alongside their parents' strengths and resilience and the support they can call on from the wider family network. Equally, the protective factors need to be assessed – many families and parents would struggle without the help of others, be they extended family and friends, or professional support from schools, health and other professionals in the social care or health-care system.

The EHA forms the initial part of that process and allows for essential help to be put in place as quickly as possible.

Here are the areas that may be covered.

For the child:

1. Health and the actions to ensure this is maintained – diet, exercise, physical and social stimulation
2. Learning and achieving – educational support and attainment, extra-curricular activities and interests
3. Sense of self-confidence in who they are
4. A sense of their belonging and place within the family, extended family and their world
5. The child's social skills within the family and beyond
6. Self-care skills, and the child's level of independence
7. The support the child gets from family, friends, and other significant people in their lives

This assessment relies heavily on the skills of the assessor in engaging the child and establishing their feelings and wishes. It is important for all professionals working with the child to be honest and open with them. Many children lack the confidence and trust to talk to others about how they feel, and this may mean that the process of getting to know the child and the causes of their problems might be slow. This also might mean that the information you have, along with any evidence, including any disclosures made to you, is important to those carrying out an assessment.

It is important to ensure that your communication and actions support this process rather than inhibit it. Ensure you speak to children in a place that they feel comfortable, use language that they will understand and ensure they feel safe. Listening to the child is very important, as is clarifying information without leading the child's responses. It is very important not to ask any leading questions. Leading, which some might see as encouraging, might just get you what you want to hear and not necessarily what the child really wants to say/tell.

While there are occasions where children are removed from parents either immediately or after a period of time, there are many more children and parents who receive help and support from other sources in order to ensure their needs are met and they are deemed safe.

ASSESSMENT OF NEEDS: ADULTS

'Excellent social work is about emphasising the use of professional engagement and judgement, as opposed to procedural approaches. With a focus on the individual, taking a holistic and co-productive approach to keeping the person at the centre of all decisions. A move to outcome and needs based assessment would put the individual and their views, needs and wishes at the centre of the work, as the setting of outcomes is both a personal and subjective process.' (Romeo, 2017) Though cited by Chief Social Worker Lyn Romeo back in 2017, person-centred practice and strengths-based approaches remain at the heart of social work. The Department of Health and Social Care published a Practice Framework for strengths-based practice in 2019 which stated: 'Factors such as organisational context, structure and mandate, access to resources, legislation, theoretical cultures and professional knowledge influence and have the potential to shape professional practice for social workers working with vulnerable adults, families and communities' (Connolly, 2007: 830).

Every adult who appears to require care and support has a right to an assessment of their needs, regardless of their likely eligibility to receive state-funded care and support. The duties of the local authority in relation to assessing need are set out in the Care Act 2014, with a focus on how a person's needs can impact upon their wellbeing as well as what outcomes they wish to achieve. The Act set out to put people in control of their care and support; it also introduced an assessment of needs for carers. Eligibility decision making has consideration for three criteria:

1. The adult's needs arise from a physical or mental impairment or illness
2. As a result of their impairment, the adult is not able to achieve two or more outcomes
3. There is, or is likely to be, a significant impact on the adult's wellbeing

The assessment outcomes for adults are:

1. Managing and maintaining nutrition
2. Maintaining personal hygiene
3. Managing toilet needs
4. Being appropriately clothed
5. Being able to make use of the home safely
6. Maintaining a habitable home environment
7. Developing and maintaining family and personal relationships
8. Accessing and engaging in work, training, education or volunteering
9. Making use of necessary facilities or services in the community
10. Carrying out the caring responsibilities the adult has for a child

Assessing the needs of an adult will differ in the process and eligibility of service to that of a child. However, safeguarding is paramount to social care across the life span and it is important to know what to do when concerns arise.

A key part of the assessment process is the consideration of mental capacity and ensuring that the person has been given every opportunity to communicate their wishes. The person should be supported to make decisions about their own life whether capacity is determined or not. It is important that the person is supported to ensure their views are central to the assessment process.

ADVOCACY AND MENTAL CAPACITY

Advocacy is very important within adult social care because it shapes the intervention, ensuring the service user's views remain central. Professionals must ensure that every person receiving an assessment is offered advocacy to assist them in the decision-making process. Quite often, a person will have an informal carer, friend or relative who may be able to take on an advocacy role. Independent Mental Capacity Advocates (IMCAs) are required when someone is assessed as lacking the mental capacity to make a specific decision. This was introduced by the Mental Capacity Act 2005, which provides the legislation for safeguarding people who lack capacity. This includes decisions about where someone lives and about receiving medical treatment.

The Mental Capacity Act 2005 provides a legal framework that ensures everyone is given every opportunity to communicate their wishes whether capacity is determined or not. It is important that the person is supported to ensure their views are central.

The Act aims to protect and empower those who lack capacity to make decisions and applies to every person aged 16 and above. Its code of practice provides guidance which it is the duty of all professionals to comply with and is underpinned by five statutory principles, which are set out in Table 14.2.

There is also a duty for independent advocacy under the Care Act 2014, which means that local authorities have a duty to ensure people are involved in decisions about their care and support. Advocacy is required to support people in expressing their wishes and making decisions where appropriate. More information can be found about advocacy within the Care Act 2014.

Table 14.2   Core principles of capacity

1. The presumption of capacity
2. Individuals being supported to make their own decisions
3. The right to make unwise decisions
4. Best interests
5. The least restrictive option

SUPPORT FOR MEETING ADULTS' NEEDS

Looking at the Care Act compliant needs assessment, and identifying the social care needs, the next stage is looking at how these needs can be met – whether with a Personal Assistant (PA) or a care agency, within a day care opportunity or with respite.

Support is usually provided via a direct payment or a commissioned service, however it is important to consider if there are community resources which may be of benefit, or whether reablement is appropriate.

It is worth noting that adult social services are not free – once 18, a young person will undergo a financial assessment to assess if they are required to contribute towards their care. This can range from zero to the full cost.

Often, a person will have both social care and health needs that are unmet, and so multi-agency working is imperative in ensuring the most appropriate support for someone. This may include a learning disability service, mental health services and education.

SUPPORT FOR CHILDREN AND FAMILIES

There is support for both children and their parents/primary carers. For example, there are a range of parenting programmes available for parents to support and enhance their parenting skills and resilience. This alone may be sufficient for the quality of parenting to be deemed 'good enough' after a period of monitoring. Support workers may be assigned to the family to help parents to establish routines and boundaries, help parents to build skills in communicating with their children, providing suitable stimulation, ensuring their health and safety, putting the child's needs at the centre of what they do. Equally they may need more specific support to help cope with issues such as disability or mental health needs (either the parent's or the child's). Health and social care professionals will work together to provide appropriate support.

Consider the models of multi-agency working, including the link into adult assessment for parents, support from mental health professionals and Education and Health Care Plans (EHCPs), which are reviewed annually and can run until a person is 25 years old and so cross the transition between children's and adult services.

Support for adults is not limited to parents however, with the implementation of personal independence budgets and direct payments for adults with eligible social care needs. This means that adults are now given the opportunity to choose and manage their own support should they wish and have the mental capacity to do so. Support is often to promote the safety of an individual and, while meeting assessed unmet needs, encourages independence wherever possible. Much like children's services, a multi-agency approach may be needed to ensure effective outcomes when it comes to support. Examine the scenario below and think about the multi-agency response needed to protect and support this family.

> ### 🗔 Scenario 14.3
>
> A referral is received by social services from an anonymous source about a family of four living near Newtown. The information is that the house is plagued by mice and there is rotting rubbish in both front and back gardens as well as pieces of rotting furniture, including bed frames. The children, who range from age 2 to 12, are often in the garden unsupervised and look dirty, dishevelled and undernourished. Sometimes the youngest child is even to be found playing in the street, which, although not a main road, does have above-average through-flow of cars as it is used as a shortcut to bypass the town.
>
> Initial enquiries reveal that the children are often dirty and hungry at school, and often off sick, with the youngest two children having continence problems. Although there are no serious health concerns recorded by the family doctor, it is discovered that the mother is supporting her children alone, is dependent on benefits, and has in the past had problems with anxiety and depression.
>
> The referral was made because a known drug dealer has been seen going into the house several times recently and the referrer said they believed he was living there some of the time.
>
> 1. Consider the family circumstances and list the different types of help they may need.
>
> 2. Where do you think that help will come from?
>
> 3. What action do you think is required?
>
> 4. Who will deal with this?
>
> 5. Support for both adults and children – how might this differ?

TRANSITION FROM CHILDHOOD TO ADULTHOOD

Regardless of whether or not a child receives services from the local authority, if they are likely to have needs following their 18th birthday, the Care Act 2014 states that the local authority must carry out an assessment. This includes transition assessments for children, young carers and those detained in the youth justice system, and young people receiving mental health services. The Care Act 2014 as well as the Children and Families Act 2014 provides legal guidance for young people with support needs who are preparing for adulthood. This process involves collaborative working across agencies. A pivotal point within this process is that while the child's needs and wishes should be at the forefront of any intervention, once an adult they have a legal right to make their own decisions around their care and support. The Mental Capacity Act 2005 applies to individuals aged 16 and over and is therefore a vital piece of legislation in the promotion of strengths-based practice during this transition process.

Currently, included within the Act is the process of Deprivation of Liberty Safeguards. This part of the legislation is prescribed when it is necessary to deprive someone who lacks the mental capacity to consent to restrictions within their care and support. In May 2019, the Mental Capacity (Amendment) Bill was passed as law and will replace the current Deprivation of Liberty Safeguards with a scheme called Liberty Protection Safeguards in April 2022. The updated process will mean people from the age of 16 will have their liberty safeguarded, evolving the duty of care from the previous minimum age of 18.

A key point to remember when someone is approaching adulthood is the notion of independence vs protection. Parental responsibility refers to the 'rights, duties, powers, responsibilities and authority which by law a parent has in relation to a child' (Children Act 1989) and lasts until the person is 18. However, the Mental Capacity Act defines a child as under the age of 16. The MHA Code of Practice (36.10) provides guidance that two points should be considered when determining whether a decision comes within the zone of parental control:

- Is the decision one that a parent would be expected to make?
- Are there any indications that the parent might not act in the young person's best interests?

Transition to adulthood can be fraught with complexities, and it is important to understand the legislation that promotes the safeguarding of young people as well as adults.

ATTACHMENT THEORY

Attachment theory (Bowlby, 1951) considers that a strong emotional and physical attachment to at least one primary caregiver is critical to a child's personal development. (Further detail about attachment theory can be found in Chapter 5, Applied Health Sciences.)

We know from Bowlby's research that attachment develops from very early on in a child's life and that different types of attachments are formed (Ainsworth, 1973), while attachment shapes and affects a child's sense of self, and their relationship with others. The lack of secure attachment in early childhood, when left unaddressed, will set the pattern of action and reaction to caregivers in later life, and may inhibit the developing child from forming positive attachments to others, sometimes for the rest of their lives.

A good understanding of attachment theory and the behaviours that might ensue from different types of attachment is essential when working with children and families. Not only will there be issues for the child who does not have a secure attachment, but the inability to support that secure attachment may stem from the parent's inability to form secure and lasting attachments themselves. Their own childhood and development may have been shaped by a lack of secure attachment.

Attachment types:

1. **Secure:** The positive attachment to a primary caregiver who is there for the child and supports them to grow and develop healthily, developing self-confidence in life. Children who have a secure attachment are likely to be more resilient and able to make positive attachments to others and use their positive experiences in childhood when they become parents themselves.

2. **Avoidant:** A child demonstrating this type of attachment may be very compliant with a parent's requests and instructions in order to avoid being rejected. These children don't want to appear needy or wanting attention as this leads to the parent being angry or resentful. They become self-reliant and independent, showing little reaction when separated from the parent. The parent is likely only to show a positive response when the child is well behaved and not in need of attention, being hostile and rejecting at other times.

3. **Ambivalent:** Arises where the caregiver is inconsistent in caring for their child and is neglectful through being unable to empathise with the child and their needs. The parent is likely to be responsive to the child more to meet their own need and not the child's. Children subject to this will both seek and reject parental attention and support, leaving them confused and with low self-esteem.

4. **Disorganised:** This results from the parent or caregiver being angry, rejecting, or displaying behaviour that frightens the child. There is no emotional attachment or commitment, and this is often linked to parental dependence on drugs, alcohol or other substances. Their own needs are of greater importance than the child's. The resultant anxious child may seek solace from the parent who has also been the initial cause of their anxiety. Children with disorganised attachment are often very disturbed, unable to form positive social relationships, and often display aggression that is difficult to address.

Many children in the care system will display evidence of insecure attachment of some kind. Hopefully with patience, support and therapeutic interventions, practised consistently, the child may be able to learn to form positive attachments with alternative caregivers and gain resilience and the ability to cope better with future life and its changes.

ATTACHMENT THEORY, FROM CHILDHOOD TO ADULTHOOD

Numerous studies suggest that it is infant attachment that is paramount in the shaping of personality and relationships. There may be many challenges in adulthood as a result of an insecure attachment and it is argued that our primary caregivers can have a significant effect on this.

While this does not suggest that a child with poor attachment will be unable to create or maintain meaningful relationships or lead a fulfilling life, many studies have found that there are some developmental patterns typical of insecurely attached children. Bowlby's monotropic theory proposed the idea that a child's attachment type may be reflected in later relationships throughout their life. These challenges may include emotional detachment, fear of trusting relationships and confusing self-image as well as a lack of ability to manage complex and aggressive behaviours. By looking at the different attachment styles, we can hypothesise how this may impact a child as they approach and enter adulthood (see Table 14.3).

There is no clear 'treatment' for an adult who has experienced an insecure attachment as a child; however, it has been suggested that professional intervention may support and encourage an adult to learn to change behaviours over time, thus promoting meaningful and fulfilling relationships throughout their life. If this intervention, be it through mental health, social or counselling services, is to be at its most effective, it is suggested that support is given at an earlier stage of an adult's life.

Table 14.3   Attachment in later life

Secure	An adult may be empathetic and be able to create and maintain meaningful relationships. A child who experiences a secure attachment may have more confidence in relationship building and creating boundaries.
Avoidant	As a result of a rejecting attachment or indeed an unavailable one, once an adult, the child may themselves be avoidant in close relationships, possibly intolerant and critical of others in the relationship. The child may learn to behave in such a way as to not appear to want attention and this may continue into later life.
Ambivalent	Due to the unpredictability of this attachment style, in that a parent is inconsistent in their caring role, this may lead to an adult being insecure and unpredictable in their relationships. Without having been given an opportunity to learn about meaningful relationships, future relationships may create anxiety and possible controlling behaviour.
Disorganised	Abusive relationships may result from a disorganised attachment and the child who experiences this type of attachment may become insensitive in later relationships during adulthood. This type of attachment can create fear in a child, which may lead to behaviours where it is felt acceptable by the adult to mimic the behaviours they experienced. Where a child who experiences this type of attachment may seek comfort from the caregiver who installs this fear, this may be a trait that is transferred into adulthood, meaning that the now adult may be at higher risk of abuse and/or neglect than an adult who had a secure attachment during childhood.

In addition to previously mentioned relationship behaviours, it is important to understand that this is not an exhaustive list of risks during adulthood and its transition, but rather an insight into how attachment theory may explain how relationships with others can be impacted upon. Studies show that children who do not experience a secure attachment are at higher risk of depression and substance misuse, however there have also been studies that suggest these behaviours can be attributed to many other factors and may or may not put an adult at further risk of abuse or neglect. Preventative measures are key in reducing these risks.

CHAPTER SUMMARY

- We hope that you now understand the critical thinking and structure around identifying the holistic and specific needs of children, families and vulnerable adults.
- Children must have their basic needs met to a level where they can develop and enjoy life and reach their full potential, ensuring safety and promotion of independence.
- You will understand the importance of listening to the child and ensuring their views are heard alongside assessing the skills and abilities of the primary caregivers, and how this is mirrored in adult services through the use of advocacy.
- You will also have an understanding of why mental capacity is so important and the legislation that underpins this.
- In addition to an understanding of your role and responsibilities around safeguarding children and adults in your care, you will have an appreciation of the many facets of the assessment process and your role in this, if any. You have looked at underlying theories, primarily attachment theory, and the importance of this to a child's development from conception onwards as well as the approaches within adult social care and how these often intertwine.
- This chapter would need to be a book on its own to give you all the answers and information available, but we hope it will give you food for thought and invite you to engage in further reading and research.

📖 FURTHER READING

RELEVANT LEGISLATION AND GUIDANCE

All of these can be found at: www.legislation.gov.uk

- Working Together to Safeguard Children 2018
- Children and Social Work Act 2017

- Children Act 1989 and 2004
- Children and Families Act 2014
- Care Act 2014
- Mental Capacity Act 2005
- The Coronavirus Act 2020
- No Secrets: Guidance on Protecting Vulnerable Adults in Care (2000)
- Framework for the Assessment of Children in Need and their Families (2000)
- Working Together to Safeguard Children (reviewed in 2017, updated in 2018)

WEBSITES

- Pocket guide to adult safeguarding: www.england.nhs.uk/wp-content/uploads/2017/02/adult-pocket-guide.pdf
- NSPCC safeguarding guide. Safeguarding children and child protection: https://learning.nspcc.org.uk/safeguarding-child-protection

BOOKS

These key texts will support your knowledge development and understanding of issues in working with children and families:

- DfE (Department for Education) (2013) *Working Together to Safeguard Children: A Guide to Inter-Agency Working to Safeguard and Promote the Welfare of Children (Safeguarding Children in Education)*. London: Shurville Publishing. Available at: www.gov.uk/government/publications/working-together-to-safeguard-children--2
- Fowler, J. (2002) *A Practitioner's Tool for Child Protection and the Assessment of Parents*. London: Jessica Kingsley.
- Howe, D. (2011) *Attachment Across the Lifecourse: A Brief Introduction*. Basingstoke: Palgrave.
- Linden, J. and Webb, J. (2016) *Safeguarding and Child Protection: Linking Theory and Practice* (5th edn). London: Hodder Education.
- Maslow, A. (2014 [1962]) *Towards a Psychology of Being* (3rd edn). Bensenville, IL: Lushena Books.
- Northway, R. and Jenkins, R. (2017) *Safeguarding Adults in Nursing Practice* (2nd edn) (Transforming Nursing Practice Series). London: Sage.
- Pitcher, D. (2014) *Inside Kinship Care: Understanding Family Dynamics and Providing Effective Support*. London: Jessica Kingsley.

VIDEOS

- NHS Safeguarding: www.youtube.com/watch?v=HYJWtv7CEHU
- Child Protection and Safeguarding: www.youtube.com/watch?v=gkxu5KjrW8U
- Safeguarding: Disclosure: www.youtube.com/watch?v=a0WAMExLq70
- Enfield Safeguarding Adults – www.youtube.com/watch?v=YMcP2C34DZw

REFERENCES

Ainsworth, M.D.S. (1973) The development of infant–mother attachment. *Review of Child Development Research, 3*: 1–94.

Blair, T. (2003) Foreword to *Every Child Matters*. Green Paper. Cm 5860. London: The Stationery Office.

Bowlby, J. (1951) *Maternal Care and Mental Health*. Geneva: World Health Organization Monograph.

Bronfenbrenner, U. (1979) *The Ecology of Human Development: Experiments by Nature and Design*. Boston: Harvard College Press.

Connolly, M. (2007) Practice frameworks: conceptual maps to guide interventions in child welfare. *The British Journal of Social Work, 37*(5): 825–37.

Department of Health (2017) *Strengths-based Social Work Practice with Adults*. Foreword. Available at: https://assets.publishing.service.gov.uk/government/uploads/system/uploads/attachment_data/file/652773/Strengths-based_social_work_practice_with_adults.pdf

Department of Health (2000) *No Secrets: Guidance on Developing and Implementing Multi-agency Policies and Procedures to Protect Vulnerable Adults from Abuse*. London: DoH.

Gov.uk (2020) Children looked after in England including adoptions. Available at: https://explore-education-statistics.service.gov.uk/find-statistics/children-looked-after-in-england-including-adoptions/2020

Laming Report (2003) *The Victoria Climbié Inquiry: Report by Lord Laming*. Cm 5730. London: The Stationery Office.

NMC (Nursing and Midwifery Council) (2018) *The Code*. Available at: www.nmc.org.uk/standards/code/

Romeo, L. (2017) Chief social worker for adults' annual report: 2017 to 2018. Available at: www.gov.uk/government/publications/chief-social-worker-for-adults-annual-report-2017-to-2018

Social Work England (2020) *Professional Standards*. Available at: www.socialworkengland.org.uk/standards/professional-standards/

Working with Kids (2017) Children Act 2004. Available at: www.workingwithkids.co.uk/childrens-act.html

15

ADDITIONAL NEEDS AND CHALLENGING BEHAVIOURS IN ADULTS AND CHILDREN

KEVIN GRAHAM AND GILLIAN ROWE

STANDARDS OF PROFICIENCY FOR NURSING ASSOCIATES (2018)

Relevant Platforms include:

Platform 1:1.4 Demonstrate an understanding of, and the ability to challenge or report discriminatory behaviour.

Platform 1:1.9 Communicate effectively with a range of skills and strategies with colleagues and people at all stages of life and with a range of mental, physical and cognitive and behavioural health challenges.

Platform 1:1.10 Demonstrate the skills and abilities required to develop, manage, and maintain appropriate relationships with people, carers and colleagues.

Platform 1:1.11 Provide, promote, and where appropriate, advocate for non-discriminatory, person-centred and sensitive care at all times. Reflect on people's values and beliefs, diverse backgrounds, cultural characteristics, language requirements, needs and preferences, taking into account any need for adjustment.

Platform 1:1.12 Recognise and report any factors that may adversely impact safe and effective care provision.

Platform 2:2.5 Understand the importance of early years and childhood experiences and the possible impact on life choices, mental, physical and behavioural health and wellbeing.

(Continued)

> Platform 3:3.4 Demonstrate the knowledge, communication and relationship management skills required to provide people, families and carers with accurate information that meets their needs before, during and after a range of interventions.
>
> Platform 3:3.20 Understand and apply the principles and processes for making reasonable adjustments.
>
> Platform 6:6.5 Identify when people need help to facilitate equitable access to care, support and escalate concerns appropriately.
>
> Annex A 2.4–2.9, 3.1, 3.2, 4.1–4.5.

Remember, no-one can make you feel inferior without your consent.

Eleanor Roosevelt

This chapter introduces you to theories that explain additional needs and challenging behaviours. It will consider what these terms mean and how they are used in settings to describe and explain various cognitive disabilities and how such disabilities can result in challenging behaviour. Children with a learning disability and cognitively and physically disabled people suffer from not just their disability but the prejudice that society expresses, and this chapter will help you to understand how stereotyping can impact on people's self-esteem. You will also consider the legal and ethical frameworks in which your practice takes place.

Glossary

- **Additional needs** A need for additional support
- **ADHD** Attention deficit hyperactivity disorder
- **Behavioural, emotional and social difficulties (BESD) and social, emotional and mental health (SEMH)** Someone with an adjustment disorder such as obsessive-compulsive disorder (OCD) or who exhibits disruptive, antisocial and aggressive behaviour
- **Challenging behaviour** Culturally abnormal behaviour
- **Dementia** A cluster of symptoms relating to memory loss
- **Disability** A substantial long-term physical or mental impairment
- **Dyslexia** Difficulty in learning to read or interpret words or other symbols; does not affect general intelligence
- **Learning disability/difficulty** Reduced intellectual ability
- **SEN** Special Educational Needs

INTRODUCTION

As caregivers, we need to gain an understanding of how our responses to additional needs and challenging behaviours are informed by a combination of theoretical and practical models. It is also important for any aspiring practitioner to develop their own understanding of inclusion in work-based settings. This chapter will help you to understand a range of approaches, linked to best practice, and develop your recognition of the causes of challenging behaviours.

Scenario 15.1

David is a 14-year-old boy. Although short and obese, he has a usually friendly nature. He suffers from Prader–Willi syndrome and has autistic tendencies. He is sensitive to noise and picks his skin when anxious. David is assessed as SEN and has a higher-level teaching assistant to support him. David is frequently teased as he is cross-eyed; this leads to anger outbursts, which if not mediated quickly, can deteriorate into violence towards his tormenter.

1. Can you think how David can be supported and what strategies could be used to prevent his anger outbursts?

2. Write down your ideas and then revisit your writing after you have read the chapter.

ADDITIONAL NEEDS

How do we consider a service user to have what we would describe as an 'additional need'? We would start by acknowledging that a service user could be identified as falling within what is termed 'atypical development'. This means development does not follow the recognised pattern seen in most people and therefore would result in the individual needing some form of support to ensure they are able to access the same opportunities as everyone else.

Please note: the term *additional needs* is often used interchangeably with the commonly used *special needs*, which would mean an individual or service user ordinarily requires support to enable them to partake in day-to-day activities. Section 20 of the Children and Families Act 2014 defines a child as having Special Educational Needs (SEN) if he or she 'has a learning difficulty or disability which calls for special education provision to be made for him or her'. So the use of the term Special Educational Needs (SEN) denotes that a learner has significantly greater difficulty in learning than most children of their age.

Provision to support someone with SEN is generally defined relative to the provision that is normally available. However, for adult service users, and client groups in a healthcare perspective, the term 'additional needs'

not only encompasses the area of impairment to learning, but also of physical disabilities or difficulties and conditions that can often result in challenging behaviours.

As nursing associates, you may sometimes find the actions of an individual service user particularly difficult or hard to cope with. Whilst we appreciate that this is part of the job, you do need to develop an approach that is not only appropriately responsive but underpinned by your own professional sense of ethical practice and inclusive working. As a TNA, you are preparing to work in a sector where you will be in daily contact with individuals who will need support with activities of daily living. Such work takes resilience matched with a knowledgeable appreciation of the difficulties that can present themselves in a number of different, yet commonly recognisable areas.

DISABILITIES

The Equality Act 2010 defines a disabled person as someone who has 'a physical or mental impairment which has a substantial and long-term adverse effect on his or her ability to carry out normal day-to-day activities'. It is the effect on their ability to carry out normal day-to-day activities that should be considered. To be defined as a disability, the effect must be long term and substantial. A common misperception is that only disabled people are protected in law; however, the Equality Act enshrines nine protected characteristics (see Table 15.1) for a vast range of individuals belonging to groups who have traditionally been subjected to discriminatory behaviour. Do you know them?

Table 15.1   The protected characteristics

Age
Disability
Gender reassignment
Marriage and civil partnership
Pregnancy and maternity
Race
Religion or belief
Sex
Sexual orientation

SEN AND DISABILITY

An individual who has an impairment in learning is not by default considered to be disabled. The definition of SEN includes many, but not necessarily all, disabled children:

- A disabled child has SEN if they have a disability and need special educational provision to be made for them to be able to access the education that is available locally.
- The largest group of pupils who may be disabled but do not have SEN are likely to be those with a range of medical conditions – for example, those with severe asthma, arthritis or diabetes may not have SEN but may have rights under the Equality Act.

Similarly, not all children with SEN will be defined as having a disability under the Equality Act:

- Many of the pupils who have SEN or who are in School Action Plus will not count as disabled.
- Some children whose emotional and behavioural difficulties have their origins in social or domestic circumstances are identified as having SEN but may fall outside the definition of disability in the Equality Act.

However, those with a mental health condition are likely to be included where their impairment has a substantial and long-term adverse effect on their ability to carry out normal day-to-day activities.

Ailments considered as likely to require special educational support include:

- Attention deficit (hyperactivity) disorder (ADHD/ADD)
- Autism, including Asperger's syndrome
- Communication difficulties
- Emotional and behavioural difficulties (EBD)
- Epilepsy and cerebral palsy
- Obsessive-compulsive disorder
- Specific learning difficulties such as dyslexia

DISABILITY AND THE MEDICAL MODEL VS THE SOCIAL MODEL

The discussion around how best to support someone with additional needs has centred traditionally on the conflict between the medical and social model approaches. The medical model views the individual's disability as the root problem, which does not concern anyone other than the individual affected. For example, if a wheelchair user cannot get into a building because of some steps, this model would suggest that this is because of the wheelchair, rather than the steps. However, the social model of disability would see the steps as a barrier, drawing on the idea that it is society that disables people, through designing everything to meet the needs of people who are not disabled. The social model argues that there is a great deal that society can do to reduce and remove disabling barriers, and this is the responsibility of society, rather than the person with the disability.

GENETIC RESEARCH

There are currently two main methodologies for genetic research into psychological functioning: quantitative genetics and molecular genetics.

Quantitative genetics is based on quantifying how genetic and non-genetic factors, such as the surrounding environment, determine the consistent occurrence of particular traits or disorders within groups of people. This approach mainly uses studies which focus closely on the relative influence of the aforementioned factors on human development. The general principle of this methodology is that variation in traits is caused by the cumulative, small effects of many genes, combined with environmental factors. Studies using quantitative genetics have found major interplay between the two factors, and as such, suggest that disorders cannot be exclusively attributed to either.

Molecular genetics looks at how genes transferred from generation to generation determine an individual's susceptibility to particular mental and physical ailments. For instance, the first autism twin study (Folstein and Rutter, 1977) found that autism is highly heritable. However, over 50 years of genetic study has failed to identify an 'autism gene' or indeed an established combination of genes. The largest study to date (Grove et al., 2019) involved 18,000 autistic and 27,000 non-autistic people; this research revealed 12 regions of the genome that hosted common variants but no smoking gun.

Many studies tried to locate a more definitive causal factor without success, it is considered that both genetics and environment likely play a role but this ill-defined notion has led to many misconceptions (bad parenting, vaccines) that do not hold up under research.

Benard's (1991) book *Fostering Resiliency in Kids* (available as a pdf download, it's old but still useful) found that half to two-thirds of children growing up with environmental contributors to behavioural, emotional and social difficulties (BESD) were eventually able to adapt to normal behaviour. Her data sample included populations of:

- Children with mentally ill, alcoholic, abusive or criminally involved parents
- Children growing up in war-torn or economically depressed regions

---

Go Further 15.1

You can read Benard's research as a free pdf at: https://kaching.socialwork.hku.hk/Workshop%20Notes/Resiliency/Foster%20Resiliency.pdf

---

AUTISM

Autism is a lifelong developmental disability that affects how a person communicates with, and relates to, other people. It also affects how they make sense of the world around them.

This condition is called a spectrum, as the symptoms are measured against levels of severity. Individuals on the autism spectrum experience difficulties in social interaction and communication and may have rigid and repetitive ways of thinking and behaving. These behaviours are thought to be underpinned by difficulties in both the flexible generation of ideas and the understanding of other people's thoughts and feelings. There is, however, much variation in the way that children and young people with autism show these different behaviours.

Autism is a developmental condition and the presentation in any individual will change with age, with some children experiencing periods of rapid improvement and others stasis or plateauing of development. Low self-esteem, failure at tasks, social isolation and irrational thoughts are common difficulties for people with autism and can contribute to the development of mental health disorders. Children on the autism spectrum may also have a reduced awareness of their own emotional states, meaning that they are less able to plan to avoid stress.

Classical symptoms include:

- Not responding to their name
- Avoiding eye contact
- Not smiling when you smile at them
- Becoming very upset if they do not like certain tastes, smells, colours or sounds
- Repetitive movements, such as flapping their hands, flicking their fingers or rocking their body
- Not talking as much as other children

Until recently, many children with autism were not diagnosed until 4 or 5 years of age, and even later for those with good language skills and of average or above-average ability (sometimes referred to as 'high functioning autism'). However, progress has been made in the earlier identification of autism, and many children, especially those with a more classic presentation of autism in combination with language delay, are now often identified before the age of 5. In 2013, Asperger's syndrome became part of one umbrella diagnosis of autism spectrum disorder (ASD) in the *Diagnostic and Statistical Manual of Mental Disorders 5* (DSM 5).

Other factors that research points to as a potential cause are as follows:

- Brain injury in the womb
- High levels of oestrogen in the womb
- Dietary aspects in infancy
- Low brain stimulation in first weeks
- Associated behaviours (copying that of siblings or parents, for instance)

Some of the distinguishing features of autism are outlined next to help you understand the different ways in which people with autism may behave and think.

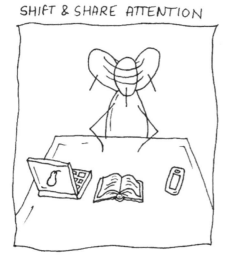 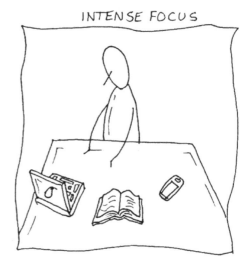

Figure 15.1   Polytropic and monotropic

MONOTROPISM VS POLYTROPISM

The terms 'monotropism' and 'polytropism' refer to the ability to shift and share attention, as seen in Figure 15.1. The polytropic mind can multitask and tends to put a moderate amount of attention into many areas of interest. People with autism are more likely to be monotropic. This means an intense focus on something of interest, and the reduced ability to switch quickly from one task to another.

THE THEORY OF MIND

Sometimes called 'mentalising' or 'mindreading', the theory of mind (often abbreviated to 'ToM') describes the social ability to understand the motives, intentions and beliefs of others, and to see something from another's point of view – even when that perspective is different from our own. Simon Baron-Cohen has been one of the leading researchers involved in ToM. He explains:

> In my early work, I explored the theory that children with autism spectrum conditions are delayed in developing a theory of mind (ToM): the ability to put oneself into someone else's shoes, to imagine their thoughts and feelings. ... We not only make sense of another person's behaviour (... Why did their eyes move left?), but we also imagine a whole set of mental states (they have seen something of interest, they know something or want something) and we can predict what they might do next. ... [This] theory proposes that children with autism and Asperger's syndrome are delayed in the development of ToM. (Baron-Cohen, 1997a: 113)

The Sally–Anne test is a psychological test used to measure social cognitive ability to attribute false beliefs to others (see Figure 15.2). The test involves two dolls, 'Sally' and 'Anne'. Sally has a basket. Anne has a box. Sally puts a ball in her basket and then leaves the scene. While Sally is away and cannot watch, Anne takes the ball out of Sally's basket and puts it into her box. Sally then returns, and the child is asked where she/he thinks Sally will look for her ball. Children are said to 'pass' the test if they understand that Sally will most likely look inside her basket before realising that her ball isn't there. Children under the age of 4, along with most autistic children (of older ages), will answer 'Anne's box', seemingly unaware that Sally does not know her ball has been moved.

CENTRAL COHERENCE THEORY

People on the autism spectrum tend to focus in on detail and may have difficulty understanding the 'bigger picture'. Children with developing minds will tend to seek out context, so have a strong central coherence often described as the ability to understand surrounding contexts or see 'the bigger picture' (Richardson et al., 2018). Baron-Cohen (1997b, 2008) captured the essence of this theory by suggesting that people on the autistic spectrum have problems in integrating information to make a coherent, global picture. Instead, they will often focus on the small, local details in a scene. The neurotypical mind, with strong central coherence, is more likely to attend to the gist, rather than the nitty-gritty.

Some theorists suggest that people with autism process faces and therefore emotions in unconventional ways. For example, some individuals with autism can easily recognise faces upside down – a task that neurotypical individuals find more difficult. This suggests that people with autism use individual features of the face to recognise people and emotions, rather than the whole face. These differences in facial processing may lead to difficulties in recognising emotions, and individuals may confuse the feelings

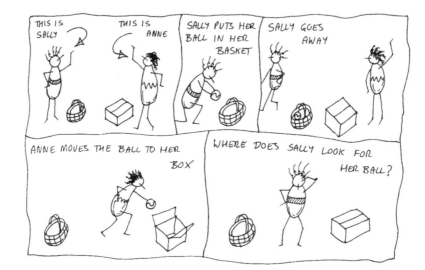

Figure 15.2   Sally and Anne (taken from a description by Baron-Cohen, 1997a)

of others. This confusion is not only limited to facial expression, and may apply to other forms of communication, such as body language.

THE EFFECT OF COLOUR

Colour can be an important factor in affecting the mood of a child with autism. Different colour schemes may have a calming, stimulating or even disturbing effect on those with autism. Studies have found that certain colour schemes are preferred, subdued or pastel colours mixed with grey, colours in blue or green hue and colours in solid, unpatterned blocks were preferential.

Noise reduction strategies can be useful for some individuals on the autism spectrum. Those oversensitive to noise could go to quiet areas or wear ear defenders. In terms of practice, alterations to the environment may go a long way to address challenging behaviours.

AUTISTIC ADULTS

Recent research undertaken by Cambridge University Autism Research Centre has shown that autistic adults are more likely to be gender diverse and are vulnerable to many types of negative life experience, including employment difficulties, financial hardship, domestic abuse and 'mate-crime' (Griffiths et al., 2019), leading to poor mental health conditions such as anxiety and depression, which are extremely common in autistic adults. Autistic adults often suffer from discrimination in the job market and discrimination in the workplace.

LEARNING DISABILITY

Over time, thinkers, researchers, psychologists and theorists have provided many reasons for poor achievement. The term 'learning disability' consequently evolved. There is also a lack of consensus as to what this term actually means. However, learning disability is defined by the Department of Health (2001) as a 'significant reduced ability to understand new or complex information, to learn new skills (impaired intelligence), with a reduced ability to cope independently (impaired social functioning), which started before adulthood'.

A learning disability affects the way a person understands information and how they communicate. Around 1.5 million people in the UK have a learning disability (MentalHealth.org, 2021). This means they can have problems with:

- Understanding new or complex information
- Learning new skills
- Coping independently

Box 15.1   Children with a learning disability in England 2018 (latest figures available)

- 28,241 children identified as having Moderate Learning Difficulties (MLD) – a reduction of 31% from 2010
- 29,492 children identified as having Severe Learning Difficulties (SLD) –
- an increase of 17% from 2010
- 10,032 children identified as having Profound Multiple Learning Difficulties (PMLD) – an increase of 16% from 2010

Public Health England (2021)

In the UK, the terms *profound, severe, moderate* and *mild* have been used to describe people with learning disability, but there are no clear dividing lines between the groups. Furthermore, there is no clear cut-off point between people with mild learning disability and the general population, and you may hear the term *borderline learning disability* being used. In the past, a diagnosis of a learning disability and understanding of a person's needs was based on IQ scores; today the importance of a holistic approach is recognised, and IQ testing forms only one small part of assessing someone's strengths and needs. Table 15.2 identifies each category in more detail.

Table 15.2   Categories of learning disability

Profound intellectual and multiple disabilities	This refers to people with a profound intellectual disability (an IQ of less than 20) and in addition they may have other disabilities such as visual, hearing or movement impairments, or they may have autism or epilepsy. People in this category have the highest levels of care needs in our communities.
Severe learning disability	This refers to people with an IQ of between 20 and 35. Many need a high level of support with everyday activities, but they may be able to look after some if not all their own personal care needs.
Moderate learning disability	This refers to people with an IQ of 35 to 50. They are likely to have some language skills, which means they can communicate about their day-to-day needs and wishes. Some people may need more support caring for themselves, but many will be able to carry out day-to-day tasks.
Mild learning disability	This refers to people with an IQ of 50 to 70. They are usually able to hold a conversation and communicate most of their needs and wishes. They may need some support to understand abstract or complex ideas. People are often independent in caring for themselves and doing many everyday tasks.

LEARNING DISABILITY AND THE MEDICAL MODEL VS THE SOCIAL MODEL

As discussed earlier, the social and medical models have had a profound influence on society's approaches to inclusion and care of the vulnerable. Here we will consider them in relation to learning difficulties more specifically.

The medical model asserts that an individual's level of ability is the main determining cause of low attainment. It looks at learning disability as an individual issue, so someone struggling to keep up with their peers may be deemed 'slow', without considering the wider context of their environment. In more general terms, this model places the onus on how a disability impairs an individual and makes them 'different' from the rest of society, rather than looking at surrounding factors that define this. It is the physical impairment (or in the case of identifying a learning disability) that makes the person disabled, rather than the limitations of the world in which they live. Bunbury (2019) explains that disability law is predicated on the medical model and considers this may strengthen some of the underlying factors that contribute to segregation and discrimination of disabled people.

By contrast, the social model focuses on the effects of the surrounding environment on an individual. When taking the perspective of this model, difficulties with learning, such as those experienced by children identified as having a form of mild learning disability, are due to shortcomings in support from the educational environment or at home. In contrast to the medical model, this viewpoint considers circumstances to be failing the child and as such emphasises the need for organisational change. In a wider context, it looks at how people's surrounding environments and society's negative attitudes, exclusions and barriers can exacerbate impairments and turn them into disabilities.

Practitioners must understand and be mindful of both approaches, taking account of all factors when evaluating anyone. How this is achieved in practice essentially comes down to the use of the practitioner's own reflective thinking and observations. Making reasonable adjustments to access and providing one-to-one support are all practical measures commonly pursued to ensure a basic but effective form of inclusion. Recall that the NMC Code states that you should keep to all relevant laws about mental capacity that apply in the country in which you are practising, and make sure that the rights and best interests of those who lack capacity are still at the centre of the decision-making process (4.3).

DYSLEXIA

Dyslexia is a language processing disorder that can hinder reading, writing, spelling and sometimes even speaking. Dyslexia is not a sign of poor intelligence or laziness. The Rose Report (Rose, 2009) said dyslexic difficulties 'are best thought of as existing on a continuum from mild to severe, rather than forming a discrete category'. While it stated there was no sharp dividing line between having or not having dyslexia, it defined three characteristic features:

1. Phonological awareness
   i. This is the ability to hear and analyse the sounds within words. It is understood to be the key skill required for learning phonics and acquiring the alphabetic principle.
2. Verbal memory
   ii. Verbal memory difficulties may give the impression that a child has not been paying attention, and include an inability to recall verbal instructions, failing to respond or responding slowly to questions. Issues with note taking, essay planning and self-organisation can be seriously troublesome for older students with greater than usual difficulties in verbal memory.
3. Verbal processing speed
   iii. This is the time it takes to process familiar verbal information, such as letters and digits. In your practice, this could involve the provision of additional time to assimilate information and complete tasks.

BEHAVIOURAL, EMOTIONAL AND SOCIAL DIFFICULTIES (BESD) AND SOCIAL, EMOTIONAL AND MENTAL HEALTH (SEMH) DIFFICULTIES

Challenging behaviour is that which does not follow a socially and culturally normative pattern and is both complex and challenging in many ways. Behavioural, emotional and social difficulties (BESD) and social, emotional and mental health difficulties (SEMH) are umbrella terms to describe a range of complex and chronic difficulties experienced by many individuals. Some commonly recognised traits include the following:

- Being withdrawn or isolated
- Displaying a disruptive and disturbing nature
- Being hyperactive and lacking concentration
- Having immature social skills
- Presenting challenging behaviours arising from other complex special needs

The frequency, intensity and duration of such behaviour is of a much higher level and the need for additional support in developing various emotional competencies is much more crucial to social and emotional development in an individual. For these reasons, behavioural disorders are judged to be more challenging for the practitioner to deal with. However, as you get to know your service user, you will gain a better understanding of their triggers to challenging behaviours and their particular preferences.

Current approaches recognise a complex relationship between environmental and genetic factors. In *Genes and Behaviour: Nature–Nurture Interplay Explained* (2006), Sir Michael Rutter argues that environmental factors will influence a genetic predisposition towards behavioural problems, either by increasing or decreasing its effects. In the 1960s, there was broad acceptance of the lasting and irreversible effects of early childhood experiences. There was also a consensus that social disadvantage was a major cause of BESD. During the 1980s, research found that the same or similar environmental factors could lead to a range of outcomes between various individual cases. As we moved away from this outlook, the nature of behavioural disorders was explored in much greater depth, and thus consideration was given to individual competence and how practice could support people's autonomy.

Goleman (2011), who expanded Meyer, Caruso and Saveloy's 1999 model, identified five emotional competencies, which are of arguable significance to the development of social and emotional skills:

1. Awareness of self and others. Essentially, this is an appreciation of the impact on each other's feelings as well as our own.
2. Mood management. The control of impulses and anger.
3. Self-motivation. Working towards specified goals, despite setbacks and occasional surmountable barriers.
4. Empathy. The ability to see things from other people's perspectives and to understand resultant associated emotions both cognitively and affectively.
5. Relationship management. The ability to cooperate with others when necessary and to form friendship, whilst resolving conflicts appropriately.

Therefore, support mechanisms must be created and put in place to facilitate the development of each competency, and these should address the barriers that result from challenging behaviour. The effectiveness of individual strategies that are used is therefore assessable against best practice measures and can be adjusted according to the circumstances at any given point. Given the shifting nature of attitudes towards behavioural disorders over time, it is important that we consider some of the more prominent disorders that fall into the BESD category to enhance our own professional understanding of the approaches used to enable support.

ATTENTION DEFICIT HYPERACTIVITY DISORDER (ADHD)

Attention deficit hyperactivity disorder (ADHD) describes the behaviours displayed by some children who are extremely restless and energetic. These children are often impatient and find it difficult to filter out other things going on around them. Typically, they will have an incredibly short attention span and find it difficult to concentrate on specific tasks. ADHD is the most common childhood-onset behavioural disorder, and it affects around 1:20 children in the UK (AA-DD UK, 2017). Recent research by Martin (2019) confirms Nøvik's (2006) work which suggests that it is approximately three times more common in boys than in girls, Martin suggests that girls express ADHD differently and symptoms may be missed. The symptoms of ADHD (NICE, 2019) are:

- Disorganisation and problems prioritising
- Excessive activity or restlessness
- Frequent mood swings
- Impulsiveness
- Lack of stress coping skills
- Low tolerance to frustration
- Poor planning ability
- Poor temper control
- Poor time management skills
- Problems focusing on a task and completing tasks
- Problems with multitasking

Methylphenidate (Ritalin) is widely prescribed to raise chronically low levels of dopamine activity in people with ADHD. In studies of its effects, 80% of children were able to improve their focus, attention span and impulse control.

However, some participants reported side effects, such as:

- Reduced appetite and weight loss
- Mild sleep disturbance
- Headaches

Professionals recommend that Ritalin is used only to treat children older than 6 years of age, and that treatment should be halted periodically to assess its impact. Adults with ADHD usually have at least one other poor mental health condition such as depression or anxiety (NICE, 2019).

MODEL OF ANGER

This model can help practitioners to raise awareness about the processes of anger with service users using social learning theory. Visual representations such as 'the match', 'the fuse' and 'the explosion' (Figure 15.3) help people to understand responses to anger by mapping an anger model to pictures. In this case, the match represents the anger trigger, the fuse represents escalation, and the explosion represents the crisis phase.

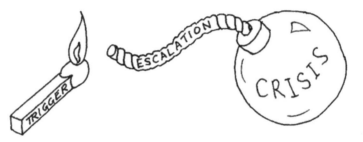

Figure 15.3   Model of anger

Go Further 15.2

Read the materials at www.advanced-training.org.uk/ to enhance your understanding of anger triggers and how to manage them. This is an excellent resource for those working with SEN children in schools and residential settings.

OPPOSITIONAL DEFIANT DISORDER (ODD)

Oppositional defiant disorder (ODD) is a psychiatric disorder. It is typically characterised by hostile behaviour towards figures of authority – and of a far more severe nature than what can usually be expected from normal childhood behaviour.

Typical behaviours will last over 6 months and will include:

- Swearing or use of obscene language
- Deliberately annoys other pupils or staff at school

- Child often angry and resentful
- Argumentative nature
- Child is often spiteful or vindictive
- Problems with losing temper
- Refusal to work or follow instructions
- Easy to offend or becomes oversensitive

The causes of oppositional defiant disorder are poorly understood but influence from parents is thought to be a contributing factor. Other factors may include:

- The environment in which a child is brought up, including lack of supervision, poor quality of housing or instability in the family
- A genetic predisposition may be present
- The nature of the child or adolescent such as 'touchiness' or spiteful-ness will increase the chances of developing ODD

Ensuring a comfortable environment and gaining a greater understanding of the traits that express themselves through ODD is crucial to accommodating it. An example would be to adjust your approach so that the service user feels less threatened and oppressed within your environment.

Pathological demand avoidance (PDA) describes children who will avoid everyday demands and expectations to an extreme extent and have an anxiety-driven need to be in control. PDA falls within the circle of Autistic Spectrum Disorders, whereas ODD does not.

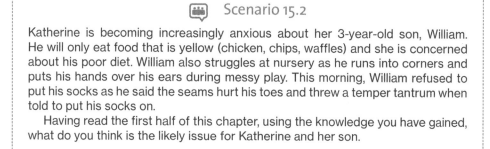

🗨 Scenario 15.2

Katherine is becoming increasingly anxious about her 3-year-old son, William. He will only eat food that is yellow (chicken, chips, waffles) and she is concerned about his poor diet. William also struggles at nursery as he runs into corners and puts his hands over his ears during messy play. This morning, William refused to put his socks as he said the seams hurt his toes and threw a temper tantrum when told to put his socks on.

Having read the first half of this chapter, using the knowledge you have gained, what do you think is the likely issue for Katherine and her son.

COMMUNICATION AND LEARNING DISABILITY

Communication is key to reducing challenging behaviours: people who are misunderstood or considered 'too difficult' to talk to, or who have their wishes and preferences ignored tend to get upset. When communicating always use accessible language, use body language and facial expression, where possible use diagrams or pictures or photographs when explaining something complex. Always reflect back to check for understanding before moving on. There are many communication resources available such as the 'Beyond Words' series. Digital resources include 'talking mats' (found at www.talkingmats.com/where-you-work/talking-mats-and-health/), widgits (found at www.widgit.com/sectors/health-emergency-justice/index.htm) and Makaton symbols for human body parts (found at https://makaton. org/TMC/Free_resources_)

Remember that the NMC Code requires you to:

7.1 use terms that people in your care, colleagues and the public can understand

7.2 take reasonable steps to meet people's language and communication needs, providing, wherever possible, assistance to those who need help to communicate their own or other people's needs

7.3 use a range of verbal and non-verbal communication methods, and consider cultural sensitivities, to better understand and respond to people's personal and health needs

7.4 check people's understanding from time to time to keep misunderstanding or mistakes to a minimum

NMC.org (2021)

PHYSICAL DIFFICULTIES

Physical disability pertains to total or partial loss of a person's bodily functions (e.g. walking, gross motor skills, bladder control) and total or partial loss of a part of the body (e.g. an amputation).

Examples of physical disability include:

- Cerebral palsy
- Muscular dystrophy
- Acquired brain injury
- Cerebrovascular event (stroke)
- Alzheimer's disease and vascular dementia

There are many kinds of disability and a wide variety of situations which people experience:

- The disability may exist from birth or be acquired later in life
- A person may have one disability or a number of disabilities or ailments (comorbidity)

- A person may be treated as having a disability when in fact they do not
- A person's disability may be apparent, such as loss of a limb; or hidden, such as epilepsy or deafness
- Disability may be more (or less) severe in its impact
- People with the same disability are as likely as anyone else to have different abilities
- Situations where a brain injury has occurred since birth

Historically, disabled people have been viewed with a variety of emotions including suspicion, ridicule and pity. Until recently, they have been excluded almost completely from all aspects of community life. Our culture is full of disablist language and imagery which has the effect of maintaining the traditional fears and prejudices which surround impairment. This has been noticeable during the time of Covid as clinically vulnerable disabled people were disproportionately reflected in the death statistics as they failed to receive the care support needed.

PHYSICAL DISABILITY AND THE MEDICAL MODEL VS THE SOCIAL MODEL

Many people think that disability is caused by an individual's health condition or impairment (the medical model). In this view, one might say that by fixing their body, disabled people will be able to participate in society just like everyone else. The social model of disability, on the other hand, suggests that disability is created by barriers in society itself, which generally fall into three categories:

- **The environment** – including inaccessible buildings and services
- **People's attitudes** – stereotyping, discrimination and prejudice
- **Organisations** – inflexible policies, practices and procedures

There are a variety of physical disabilities that impact on the approaches you will have to take in supporting those with impairments such as traumatic brain injury.

TRAUMATIC BRAIN INJURY

Traumatic brain injury is the result of things happening outside of the body – such as an accident to the head in a car or bike accident. Non-traumatic brain injury is the result of happenings inside the head, such as a tumour or stroke. Brain injuries, howsoever caused, can lead to impairments and challenging behaviours such as:

- Cognitive (the processes that go on in our head): Limited attention span, trouble remembering things, difficulties processing information

- Emotions and behaviour: Self-esteem, feelings of being behind, difficulties controlling emotions, distractedness, impatience, frustrations, trouble socialising
- Physical: Pain or discomfort, for children: lack of access to parts of the school, restrictions to getting involved in PE, and for children and adults: tiredness/fatigue, sleep disruption, seizures

DEMENTIA

Dementia is a cluster of symptoms based on memory loss. There are several different causes, the most common being Alzheimer's disease. Alzheimer's disease is currently thought to be the build-up of proteins in the brain which then form structures called 'plaques' and 'tangles' (Andrews, 2015). The loss of connections between nerve cells breaks the message-transmitting ability and leads to the death of nerve cells and loss of brain tissue. The next most prevalent cause is vascular dementia, which is due to brain cell death by lack of oxygen, which might be caused by a stroke or mini stroke (transient ischaemic attack or TIA). The blood vessels become blocked or clogged by cholesterol plaques or blood clots. Vascular dementia is characterised by a 'stepping down' of the sufferer's cognitive ability rather than the steady decline of Alzheimer's. The third main cause of dementia is Lewy bodies. Lewy body dementia (DLB) shares symptoms with Alzheimer's and with Parkinson's disease and is caused by Tau protein build-up within nerve cells. In the early stages of the disease the sufferer may experience visual or auditory hallucinations. They also have 'good' days and 'bad' days, which may in fact be good/bad weeks. DLB is progressive and the person slowly declines over time.

It is useful to understand that it is not just those of an older age who develop dementia. There is a small but increasing number of young people (early onset) who develop this; the Alzheimer's Society (2019) suggests 42,325 or 5% of those with dementia are younger than 65. People with Down syndrome may develop dementia in their 30s and people with learning disability in their 40s. The Alzheimer's Society considers early onset dementia likely to be hereditary (familial Alzheimer's) or, in some cases, caused through substance misuse (mainly alcohol). However, this may be reversed with abstinence and a good diet rich in thiamine.

CHALLENGING BEHAVIOUR AND DEMENTIA

Behaviour is a form of communication and body language is as eloquent as the spoken word. Behaviour is culturally mediated (see Chapter 13, Introduction to Mental Health and Wellbeing, for further detail) and each culture has different behavioural expectations. Common behaviour for sufferers of dementia is 'wandering' and 'rummaging'; clearly the person is engaged in some activity which is meaningful to them. It is unusual for dementia sufferers to be violent, unless they feel they are being threatened. It is important that health workers, care staff, family and friends explain clearly and in a language the person understands any activity they wish them to participate in, and that consent is obtained before any intervention takes place (see Chapter 9, Essential Skills for Care, for further details about consent).

The Mental Capacity (Amendment) Bill 2019 replaces the Deprivation of Liberty Safeguards (DoLS) with a scheme known as the Liberty Protection Safeguards. There are some concerns about this legislation as Liberty Protection Safeguards commence at age 16, not 18. Deprivation of liberty has to be authorised in advance by the 'responsible body'; this could be a hospital manager (NHS), a clinical commissioning group (GP) or for social care, the local authority. In order to authorise a deprivation of liberty, the person needs to be:

- Lacking the capacity to consent to the care arrangements
- Suffering from a mental disorder

These arrangements are necessary to prevent harm to the cared-for person and proportionate to the likelihood and seriousness of that harm. If the person objects to being deprived of their liberty, their case must be reviewed by an Approved Mental Capacity Professional (AMCP). The Act is effective from April 2022.

PROFESSIONAL APPROACHES TO ADDITIONAL NEEDS AND CHALLENGING BEHAVIOURS

Abrams (2010) defines prejudice as 'bias which devalues people because of their perceived membership of a social group'. Prejudice ultimately involves stereotyping and prejudging people. A stereotype is a highly simplified idea held about a group. When we create a stereotypical concept, we make shortcuts in our thinking which, in some situations, can be damaging. For patients and service users, their sense of identity can be affected if they are at the receiving end of negative attitudes towards them, and/or the group to which they belong. They may feel that certain options are not available or open to them.

So, is it possible to stop prejudicial views? Abrams (2010) found in research that the more contact there is with people from other groups and cultures and the more understanding there is, the more likely prejudice and discrimination will be reduced. There is an ongoing need for those working with the healthcare sector to be involved in training that is high quality and relevant to the sector. Training, however, is not enough on its own, as there are personal qualities and competencies that those working within the sector need. We should ultimately recognise that inclusion is about fostering the individual needs of each person and offering an equal opportunity to reach their potential. Inclusion and inclusive practice are requirements that support the individual needs of all disabled people and break down barriers to segregation and exclusion.

There are issues to be addressed before full inclusion becomes a reality and inclusion is the right of all individuals, and these issues need consideration by all practitioners. All staff should take a leadership role within their workplace to discuss and find measures to mitigate the following:

- Policies (both local and national) are often ineffective
- Training is not provided for all grades
- Pay amongst practitioners varies greatly depending on sector
- The profile of workers needs to be improved in many cases
- Access to resources needs to be widened
- More focus on 'needs-led' provision as opposed to 'budget-led' provision
- Funding issues need to be addressed

You can read more on leadership skills in Chapter 3, Leadership and Teamwork.

So, what then is good practice? In theory, it is the removal of barriers, the promotion of diversity, the creation of equal opportunities and the challenging of discrimination. We have a duty not to discriminate against people with disabilities and to make reasonable adjustments where required to support individuals with additional needs. These include accommodation and access, alongside other additional adjustments to enable access to health for all.

DISCRIMINATION

Discrimination is failing to take reasonable steps to ensure you do not place a disabled person at a 'substantial disadvantage'. Key to any student practitioner's understanding and appreciation of how to tackle discrimination is to understand that to treat someone differently as a result of their difference is not automatically a negative act.

Occasionally, a person will be discriminated against in favour of another, in which case we are deemed to be taking what is often referred to as 'positive discrimination' or in most cases, 'positive action'. The purpose of positive action is to allow disadvantaged people the same rights and opportunities as advantaged people.

Health and social care settings adhere to the stipulations laid down in the Equality Act 2010; translating this into practice, we are ever mindful, however, that our day-to-day work with vulnerable client groups necessitates the requirement to maintain awareness and understanding of how discrimination can manifest itself. Sometimes this is in the form of the most basic behaviours, which can carry substantial impacts with service users, no matter how harmless our approaches seem to us as practitioners.

SAFEGUARDING

The Care Act 2014 sets out the clear legal frameworks for each local authority and the need for multi-agency adult safeguarding boards (Local Safeguarding Partnerships). The board must review cases where abuse is suspected and there is concern that the local authority has not responded appropriately.

Abuse can be neglect, physical, mental, financial, sexual, domestic, discriminatory or organisational. It is incumbent upon you as a nursing associate to undertake safeguarding training, and to familiarise yourself with your organisation's policies and procedures in order to know where to turn if you witness or suspect abuse. Further information on safeguarding is found in Chapter 14, Protecting Children and Vulnerable Adults.

SAFEGUARDING STAFF

Patients (and family members) sometimes exhibit challenging behaviours that lead to violence towards staff. In 2018, the NHS Violence Reduction Strategy was announced to protect the NHS workforce against deliberate violence and aggression from patients and their families and members of the public. The Assaults on Emergency Workers (Offences) Act 2018 legislation was introduced to support the police, prison officers, custody officers, fire service personnel, search and rescue services and paramedics as well as community and district nurses. In 2018 over 17,000 attacks were committed against NHS staff, and this legislation will ensure that convicted perpetrators will serve a minimum of a year in prison.

A&E staff usually have access to an onsite trained response team when a patient becomes aggressive, Spector (2014) stated 'nurses in high-risk settings are working with people who are in pain, under stress, and often feel they have lost control of their lives'. Long waits in A&E can add to problems. As Professor C. Cooper (cited in Nelson, 2014) said, people are sick, injured, anxious, worried, intoxicated, and it is easy to see how the aggression builds up. Violence can be reduced by giving patients and families more information and by spending time addressing their concerns.

The majority of assaults occur in mental health or learning disability settings. Staff should receive training in anticipating triggers that can lead to aggressive behaviour, and how to defuse them using techniques for distraction and calming, and ways to encourage relaxation. Staff training should include skills to assess why behaviour is likely to become violent or aggressive, and should include personal, constitutional, mental, physical, environmental, social, communicational, functional and behavioural factors. Staff in acute psychiatric settings use assessment tools such as the Dynamic Appraisal of Situational Aggression (DASA-IV) to gauge the likelihood of a patient becoming aggressive, but this is usually not used in general health settings, and many are unaware this tool exists. Skills training should include breakaway techniques, which are physical skills to help separate or break away from an aggressor in a safe manner (NICE.org, 2018) to reduce the use of restraint or rapid tranquillisation.

Go Further 15.3

You can download the DASA-IV from here: www.rcpsych.ac.uk/docs/default-source/improving-care/nccmh/reducing-restrictive-practice/resources/dasa-information.pdf?sfvrsn=d779798b_2

LEARNING DISABILITY AND COVID

NICE have published guidelines to support health workers who work in both mental health and learning disability settings. Changes in routines and care can be particularly stressful for people with learning disabilities and/or autistic people, especially now that staff must wear a mask. This change needs to be explained carefully in order not to distress the client. The client needs to be encouraged to engage in enhanced infection control procedures and if possible, mask wearing themselves.

NICE suggest trying these things:

1. Try to explain in simple and familiar terms why things are changing, emphasising what will remain normal and how long change will likely last for.
2. Think about the things that can remain consistent, for example, whether it is possible to keep contact with the usual staff who provide support with certain tasks.
3. Consider where you can support the person you care for to continue doing what they enjoy and what calms them down.

Further advice and guidance can be found at the Challenging Behaviour Foundation: www.challengingbehaviour.org.uk/information-and-guidance/covid-19/covid-our-resources/

CHAPTER SUMMARY

- The number of conditions we have considered in this chapter is by no means an exhaustive list.
- We should not overlook the fact that the debate around causes and impacts of a variety of additional needs and challenging behaviours will continue to develop, creating an ever-changing perception of the barriers that people face, in turn fuelling changes in the way that we as practitioners conduct our duties.
- However, this chapter's aim has been to provide you with a starting point for your professional practice and to get you to think more deeply about how you can work with service users, patients and families in the best possible way and in line with their needs, regardless of their abilities and conditions.
- Your approaches in your healthcare practice will be shaped, morphed and informed further through ongoing reflective exercises, based upon the familiarity you will have with individual client groups during the course of your practice.
- Observing matters from the perspective of the service user remains key to addressing any barriers to opportunity and progress that you may encounter, as ultimately you are there to provide a service to support, enable and fulfil the needs of those who are less advantaged than ourselves.

FURTHER READING

You can deepen your knowledge and understanding of additional needs and challenging behaviours by visiting these websites and reading the recommended texts.

WEBSITES

- Alzheimer's Society: www.alzheimers.org.uk
- Advanced training materials for a range of learning and behavioural difficulties: www.advanced-training.org.uk
- The National Autistic Society: www.autism.org.uk
- The Challenging Behaviour Foundation: www.challengingbehaviour.org.uk/

TEXTS

- Andrews, J. (2015) *Dementia: The One-Stop Guide: Practical Advice for Families, Professionals, and People Living with Dementia and Alzheimer's Disease*. London: Profile.

- Baron-Cohen, S. (1997) *Mindblindness: An Essay on Autism and the Theory of Mind* (Learning, Development and Conceptual Change Series). Cambridge, MA: MIT Press.
- Baron-Cohen, S. (2008) *Autism and Asperger Syndrome (The Facts)*. Oxford: Oxford University Press.
- Daley, G. (2008) *Anger: A Solution Focussed Approach for Young People*. Bromley: Optimus Education.
- Kelly, N. and Norwich, B. (2004) *Moderate Learning Difficulties and the Future of Inclusion*. Abingdon: Routledge/Falmer.
- Northway, R. and Jenkins, R. (2017) *Safeguarding Adults in Nursing Practice* (2nd edn) (Transforming Nursing Practice Series). London: Sage.

VIDEOS

- Understanding Challenging Behaviour: www.youtube.com/watch?v=BUvEn8ejGm0
- The Lives of People with Learning Disability: www.youtube.com/watch?v=VhFUO-VshBg
- Positive Behavioural Support: It Happens for a Reason! www.youtube.com/watch?v=1l4Il65WyW8

REFERENCES

AA-DD UK (2017) *What is ADHD?* Available at: http://aadduk.org

Abrams, D. (2010) *Processes of Prejudice: Theory, Evidence and Intervention*. Available at: www.equalityhumanrights.com/en/publication-download/research-report-56-processes-prejudice-theory-evidence-and-intervention

Alzheimer's Society (2019) What is young-onset dementia? Available at: www.alzheimers.org.uk/about-us/policy-and-influencing/what-we-think/demography

Andrews, J. (2015) *Dementia: The One-Stop Guide. Practical Advice for Families, Professionals, and People Living with Dementia and Alzheimer's Disease*. London: Profile.

Baron-Cohen, S. (1997a) *Mindblindness: An Essay on Autism and the Theory of Mind* (Learning, Development and Conceptual Change Series). Cambridge, MA: MIT Press.

Baron-Cohen, S. (1997b) Theories of the autistic mind. Available at: www.neuroscience.cam.ac.uk/publications/download.php?id=40524

Baron-Cohen, S. (2008) *Autism and Asperger Syndrome (The Facts)*. Oxford: Oxford University Press.

Bernard, B. (1991) *Fostering Resiliency in Kids: Protective Factors in the Family, School, and Community*. San Francisco: WestEd Regional Educational Laboratory.

Bunbury, S. (2019) Unconscious bias and the medical model: How the social model may hold the key to transformative thinking about disability discrimination. *International Journal of Discrimination and the Law, 19*(1): 26–47.

Folstein, S. and Rutter, M. (1977) Infantile autism: a genetic study of 21 twin pairs. *The Journal of Child Psychology and Psychiatry, 18*: 297–321.

Goleman, D. (2011) *The Brain and Emotional Intelligence: New Insights.* Florence, MA: More Than Sound Publishing.

Gov.uk (2001) *Valuing People – A New Strategy for Learning Disability for the 21st Century.* Available at: https://assets.publishing.service.gov.uk/government/uploads/system/uploads/attachment_data/file/250877/5086.pdf

Griffiths, S., Allison, C., Kenny, R., Holt, R., Smith, P. and Baron-Cohen, S. (2019) The Vulnerability Experiences Quotient (VEQ): A study of vulnerability, mental health and life satisfaction in autistic adults. *Autism Research.* Available at: www.cam.ac.uk/research/news/autistic-adults-experience-high-rates-of-negative-life-events

Grove, J., Ripke, S., Als, T.D., et al. (2019) Identification of common genetic risk variants for autism spectrum disorder. *Nature Genetics, 51*, 431–44.

MentalHealth.org (2021) Learning disability statistics. Available at: www.mental-health.org.uk/learning-disabilities/help-information/learning-disability-statistics-

Mayer, J.D., Caruso, D.R. and Salovey, P (1999) Mayer-Salovey-Caruso emotional intelligence test. Available at: www.eiconsortium.org/measures/msceit.html

Nelson, R. (2014) Tackling violence against health-care workers. *The Lancet, 383*(9926): 1373–4.

NICE (National Institute for Health and Care Excellence) (2019) Attention deficit hyperactivity disorder: Diagnosis and management. *Clinical guideline (CG) 87.* Available at: www.nice.org.uk/guidance/NG87

NICE.org (2018) Violence and aggression management. Available at: www.nice.org.uk/guidance/ng10/resources/violence-and-aggression-shortterm-management-in-mental-health-health-and-community-settings-pdf-1837264712389

NMC (Nursing and Midwifery Council) (2018) The Code: Professional standards of practice and behaviour for nurses, midwives and nursing associates. Available at: www.nmc.org.uk/globalassets/sitedocuments/nmc-publications/nmc-code.pdf

Nøvik, T.S., Hervas, A., Ralston, S.J., Dalsgaard, S., Rodrigues Pereira, R. and Lorenzo, M.J. (2006) Influence of gender on attention-deficit/hyperactivity disorder in Europe. *European Child & Adolescence Psychiatry, 15*(Suppl. 1): I15–24.

Nursing and Midwifery Council (2018) *Code of Standards.* Available at: www.nmc.org.uk/standards/code/read-the-code-online/

Martin, J. (2019) Why is ADHD more common in boys than girls? Available at: https://theconversation.com/why-is-adhd-more-common-in-boys-than-girls-92151

Public Health England (2021) Summary of children with special educational needs. Available at: www.gov.uk/government/publications/people-with-learning-disabilities-in-england/chapter-1-education-and-childrens-social-care-updates

Richardson, H., Lisandrelli, G., Riobueno-Naylor, A., et al. (2018) Development of the social brain from age three to twelve years. *Nature Communications, 9*: 1027.

Rose, J. (2009) *Independent Review of the Primary Curriculum: Final Report.* Available at: www.educationengland.org.uk/documents/pdfs/2009-IRPC-final-report.pdf

Rutter, M. (2006) *Genes and Behaviour: Nature–Nurture Interplay Explained.* Oxford: Wiley Blackwell.

Spector, P. (2014) Nurse exposure to physical and nonphysical violence, bullying, and sexual harassment: A quantitative review. *International Journal of Nursing Studies, 51*(1): 72–84.

APPENDICES

APPENDIX PART 1: STANDARDS

	Knowledge, skills, behaviours
Duty 1 Be an accountable professional, acting in the best interests of people, putting them first and providing nursing care that is person-centred, safe and compassionate	K1 K2 K3 K4 K5 S1 S2 S3 S4 S5 S6 B1 B2 B3
Duty 2 Communicate effectively, recognising and working within the limits of competence and being responsible for their own actions	K6 K7 K8 S5 S7 S8 S9 S10 S11 S12 B1 B2 B3
Duty 3 Promote health and prevent ill health to improve and maintain the mental, physical, behavioural health and well-being of people, families, carers and communities	K9 K10 K11 K12 K13 K14 S13 S14 S15 S16 S17 B1 B2 B3
Duty 4 Contribute to the ongoing assessment of individuals' nursing care needs, recognising when it is appropriate to refer to others for reassessment	K15 K16 K17 K18 K19 S18 S19 S20 B1 B2 B3
Duty 5 Provide and monitor nursing care to individuals and groups, providing compassionate and safe nursing interventions	K20 K21 K22 K23 K24 K25 K26 K27 K28 K29 S5 S21 S22 S23 S24 S25 S26 S27 S28 S29 S30 S31 S32 B1 B2 B3
Duty 6 Improve safety of individuals by identifying risks to safety or experience of care and taking appropriate action, putting the best interests, needs and preferences of people first	K30 K32 K35 S33 S34 S35 S36 B1 B2 B3
Duty 7 Improve quality of care by contributing to the continuous monitoring of people's experience of care	K31 K33 K34 S37 B1 B2 B3

Duty 8 Contribute to the provision of complex nursing and integrated care needs of people at any stage of their lives, across a range of organisations and settings	K36 K37 K38 K39 K40 K41
	S38 S39 S40
	B1 B2 B3
Duty 9 Work in teams collaborating effectively with a range of colleagues	K42 K43
	S43 S44
	B1 B2 B3
Duty 10 Support and supervise others in the care team	K6 K42
	S38 S41 S42
	B1 B2 B3

Apprenticeship standards: Knowledge	Chapters they are found in
K1: Understand the Code: Professional standards of practice and behaviour for nurses, midwives and nursing associates (NMC, 2018), and how to fulfil all registration requirements	2,3,4,8,9,10
K2: Understand the demands of professional practice and demonstrate how to recognise signs of vulnerability in themselves or their colleagues and the action required to minimise risks to health	2,3,9,14,15
K3: Understand the professional responsibility to adopt a healthy lifestyle to maintain the level of personal fitness and well-being required to meet people's needs for mental and physical care	2,3,9,14,15
K4: Understand the principles of research and how research findings are used to inform evidence-based practice	1,2,3,4,8,11,14,15
K5: Understand the meaning of resilience and emotional intelligence, and their influence on an individual's ability to provide care	2,3,9,14,15
K6: Understand and apply relevant legal, regulatory and governance requirements, policies, and ethical frameworks, including any mandatory reporting duties, to all areas of practice	4,7,8,9,10,13,14,15
K7: Understand the importance of courage and transparency and apply the Duty of Candour	3,4,14
K8: Understand how discriminatory behaviour is exhibited	4,14,12,13,15
K9: Understand the aims and principles of health promotion, protection and improvement and the prevention of ill health when engaging with people	4,7,13,14,15
K10: Understand the principles of epidemiology, demography, and genomics and how these may influence health and well-being outcomes	6,7,10,11,12,14
K11: Understand the factors that may lead to inequalities in health outcomes	5,11,13

(Continued)

(Continued)

K12: Understand the importance of early years and childhood experiences and the possible impact on life choices, mental, physical and behavioural health and well-being	5,6,7,9,13,14,15
K13: Understand the contribution of social influences, health literacy, individual circumstances, behaviours and lifestyle choices to mental, physical and behavioural health outcomes	2,5,7,11,12, 14
K14: Understand the importance of health screening	5,9,11,12,13
K15: Understand human development from conception to death, to enable delivery of person-centred safe and effective care	5,6,7,8,14
K16: Understand body systems and homeostasis, human anatomy and physiology, biology, genomics, pharmacology, social and behavioural sciences as applied to delivery of care	5,6,7,9,10,13,14
K17: Understand commonly encountered mental, physical, behavioural and cognitive health conditions as applied to delivery of care	5,6,7,9,13,14
K18: Understand and apply the principles and processes for making reasonable adjustments	13,14,15
K19: Know how and when to escalate to the appropriate professional for expert help and advice	3,6,8,9,10,13,14,15
K20: Know how people's needs for safety, dignity, privacy, comfort and sleep can be met	4,9,13
K21: Understand co-morbidities and the demands of meeting people's holistic needs when prioritising care	6,7,9,10,15
K22: Know how to meet people's needs related to nutrition, hydration and bladder and bowel health	4,6,9
K23: Know how to meet people's needs related to mobility, hygiene, oral care, wound care and skin integrity	6,8,9,10,13
K24: Know how to support people with commonly encountered symptoms including anxiety, confusion, discomfort and pain	5,7,9,10,11
K25: Know how to deliver sensitive and compassionate end of life care to support people to plan for their end of life	4,5,6,7,8
K26: Understand where and how to seek guidance and support from others to ensure that the best interests of those receiving care are upheld	4,7,8,9,10,13,1,4,15
K27: Understand the principles of safe and effective administration and optimisation of medicines in accordance with local and national policies	7,9,10
K28: Understand the effects of medicines, allergies, drug sensitivity, side effects, contraindications and adverse reactions	7,9,10,13
K29: Understand the different ways by which medicines can be prescribed	9,10
K30: Understand the principles of health and safety legislation and regulations and maintain safe work and care environments	8,9,10
K31: Understand how inadequate staffing levels impact on the ability to provide safe care and escalate concerns appropriately	8,9,10,14,15

K32: Understand what constitutes a near miss, a serious adverse event, a critical incident and a major incident	8,9,10
K33: Understand when to seek appropriate advice to manage a risk and avoid compromising quality of care and health outcomes	3,4,9,10
K34: Know and understand strategies to develop resilience in self and know how to seek support to help deal with uncertain situations	2,3,9,12,13,14,15
K35: Understand own role and the roles of all other staff at different levels of experience and seniority in the event of a major incident	3,8,10,11
K36: Understand the roles of the different providers of health and care	2,3,13
K37: Understand the challenges of providing safe nursing care for people with complex co-morbidities and complex care needs	3,8,13,14,15
K38: Understand the complexities of providing mental, cognitive, behavioural and physical care needs across a wide range of integrated care settings	13,14,15
K39: Understand the principles and processes involved in supporting people and families with a range of care needs to maintain optimal independence and avoid unnecessary interventions and disruptions to their lives	3,4,13
K40: Understand own role and contribution when involved in the care of a person who is undergoing discharge or a transition of care between professionals, settings or services	2,9,14,15
K41: Know the roles, responsibilities and scope of practice of different members of the nursing and interdisciplinary team, and own role within it	2,9,11
K42: Understand and apply the principles of human factors and environmental factors when working in teams	8,9,10
K43: Understand the influence of policy and political drivers that impact health and care provision	2,11,12,13

Skills

S1: Act in accordance with the Code: Professional standards of practice and behaviour for nurses, midwives and nursing associates (NMC, 2018), and fulfil all registration requirements	All chapters
S2: Keep complete, clear, accurate and timely records	2,3,4,8,9,10
S3: Recognise and report any factors that may adversely impact safe and effective care provision	2,3,4,8,9,10
S4: Take responsibility for continuous self-reflection, seeking and responding to support and feedback to develop professional knowledge and skills	2,3,9
S5: Safely demonstrate evidence-based practice in all skills and procedures required for entry to the register: Standards of proficiency for nursing associates Annex A & B (NMC, 2018)	8,9,10,14,15

(Continued)

(Continued)

S6: Act as an ambassador for their profession and promote public confidence in health and care services	2,3,4
S7: Communicate effectively using a range of skills and strategies with colleagues and people at all stages of life and with a range of mental, physical, cognitive and behavioural health challenges	3-15
S8: Recognise signs of vulnerability in self or colleagues and the action required to minimise risks to health	8,9,10,13
S9: Develop, manage and maintain appropriate relationships with people, their families, carers and colleagues	3-15
S10: Provide, promote, and where appropriate advocate for, non-discriminatory, person-centred and sensitive care at all times, reflecting on people's values and beliefs, diverse backgrounds, cultural characteristics, language requirements, needs and preferences, taking account of any need for adjustments	All chapters
S11: Report any situations, behaviours or errors that could result in poor care outcomes	7,8,9,10,14
S12: Challenge or report discriminatory behaviour	8,9,13,14,15
S13: Apply the aims and principles of health promotion, protection and improvement and the prevention of ill health when engaging with people	8,12,13
S14: Promote preventive health behaviours and provide information to support people to make informed choices to improve their mental, physical, behavioural health and wellbeing	7,8,9,10,13
S15: Identify people who are eligible for health screening	8,11
S16: Promote health and prevent ill health by understanding the evidence base for immunisation, vaccination and herd immunity	11,12
S17: Protect health through understanding and applying the principles of infection prevention and control, including communicable disease surveillance and antimicrobial stewardship and resistance	8,9,10,11
S18: Apply knowledge, communication and relationship management skills required to provide people, families and carers with accurate information that meets their needs before, during and after a range of interventions	3,4,7,8,9,10
S19: Recognise when capacity has changed and how a person's capacity affects their ability to make decisions about their own care and to give or withhold consent	4,9,13,14,15
S20: Recognise people at risk of abuse, self-harm and/or suicidal ideation and the situations that may put them and others at risk	13,15
S21: Monitor the effectiveness of care in partnership with people, families and carers, documenting progress and reporting outcomes	4-15
S22: Take personal responsibility to ensure that relevant information is shared according to local policy and appropriate immediate action is taken to provide adequate safeguarding and that concerns are escalated	4,9,12,13,14,15
S23: Work in partnership with people, to encourage shared decision making, in order to support individuals, their families and carers to manage their own care when appropriate	3-15

S24: Perform a range of nursing procedures and manage devices, to meet people's need for safe, effective and person-centred care	4,7,8,9,10
S25: Meet people's needs for safety, dignity, privacy, comfort and sleep	7,9,10
S26: Meet people's needs related to nutrition, hydration and bladder and bowel health	7,9,10
S27: Meet people's needs related to mobility, hygiene, oral care, wound care and skin integrity	7,9,10
S28: Support people with commonly encountered symptoms including anxiety, confusion, discomfort and pain	7,9,10,13,14,15
S29: Give information and support to people who are dying, their families and the bereaved and provide care to the deceased	9
S30: Recognise when a person's condition has improved or deteriorated by undertaking health monitoring, interpreting, promptly responding, sharing findings and escalating as needed	7,9,10
S31: Act in line with any end of life decisions and orders, organ and tissue donation protocols, infection protocols, advanced planning decisions, living wills and lasting powers of attorney for health	9
S32: Work collaboratively and in partnership with professionals from different agencies in interdisciplinary teams	3,7,9,10,13,14,15
S33: Maintain safe work and care environments	8,9,10,15
S34: Act in line with local and national organisational frameworks, legislation and regulations to report risks, and implement actions as instructed, following up and escalating as required	3, 8,9,10,15
S35: Accurately undertake risk assessments, using contemporary assessment tools	8,9
S36: Respond to and escalate potential hazards that may affect the safety of people	8,9
S37: Participate in data collection to support audit activity, and contribute to the implementation of quality improvement strategies	3,8,9
S38: Prioritise and manage own workload, and recognise where elements of care can safely be delegated to other colleagues, carers and family members	3,9,13
S39: Recognise when people need help to facilitate equitable access to care, support and escalate concerns appropriately	3,8,9,10
S40: Support and motivate other members of the care team and interact confidently with them	3,9,10
S41: Monitor and review the quality of care delivered, providing challenge and constructive feedback when an aspect of care has been delegated to others	4,9,10
S42: Support, supervise and act as a role model to nursing associate students, health care support workers and those new to care roles, review the quality of the care they provide, promoting reflection and providing constructive feedback	3,9,10

(Continued)

(Continued)

S43: Contribute to team reflection activities to promote improvements in practice and services	2,3,9
S44: Access, input, and apply information and data using a range of methods including digital technologies, and share appropriately within interdisciplinary teams	7,9,10

Behaviours

B1: Treat people with dignity, respecting individual's diversity, beliefs, culture, needs, values, privacy, and preferences	4,7,8,9,10,12,13,14,15
B2: Show respect and empathy for those you work with, have the courage to challenge areas of concern and work to evidence based best practice	2,3,4,7,9,10,13,14,15
B3: Be adaptable, reliable, and consistent. Show discretion, resilience, and self-awareness	4,7,9,10,13

APPENDIX PART 2

Nursing Associate Domains and Where They Can Be Found in This Book	Chapter found in
Domain 1. Professional values and parameters of practice	
Standards and values	4,7,12,13,14,15
Professional knowledge	All chapters
Keeping up to date	2,3,4,9,10,11,12
Limits of competence/authority	3,4,6,7,9,10,13,14
How to seek support	3,4,6,7,9,10,13,14
Reflection on performance	3,4,7,8,9,10,13,14
Importance of personal integrity	2,3,4,9,10,14
Resilience and wellbeing	4,7,9,10,13
The role of occupational health	2,3,4,8,10
Personal strategies	1,2,3,4
Importance of adhering to legislation, standards, policies, protocols and values	3,4,5,7,8,9,10,13,14,15
The importance of implementing health, safety and security policies	3,4,8,9,14,15
Report any actions or decisions which are not in the best interests of any person in receipt of care	3,4,9,10,14
Promote evidence-based professional practice in person-centred care	1,2,3,4,9
Act as a role model	2,3,4,9
Promote and exemplify safe and effective working	2,3,4,6,7,8,9,10,11,12,13,14,15

Domain 2. Person-centred approaches to care

The fundamental principles of nursing practice	3,4,6,7,8,9
Describe the delivery of person-centred care	4,5,6,7,8,9,10,14
Describe the importance of gaining consent	4,8,9,10,12
Explain the importance of giving people choices	4, 8,9,10,12
Consider services from the family's point of view	4,7,9,10,12,13
Discuss concepts of choice, autonomy, empowerment, respect, holism, parity of esteem, empathy and compassion	2,3,4,6,7,8,9,10,11,12,13,14,15
Consider changing plan of care to meet changing needs	4,7,9,12,1,14
Support individuals to maintain their identity and self-esteem using person-centred values	4,5,9,10,13
Explain the impact of promoting effective health and wellbeing, empowering healthy lifestyles.	5,11,12,13

Domain 3. Delivering care

Describe the structure and functions of the human body	6,7
Health and ill health (physical and mental)	All chapters
Societal impact	4,5,7
Behaviour and lifestyle choices	5,7,13,14
Genetics and genomics	6,7
Disability	5,6,7,9
Stage of life	5,6,7,9
Socioeconomic factors and wider determinants of health	5,6,7,9,11
The impact of conditions on individuals, their families and/or carers	5,6,7,9,11,13,14,15
Reflect on how health behaviours impact on outcomes	5,7,9,11,13,14,15
Population health and public health priorities	3,7,9,11,12,13,14,15
Using physiological assessments and observations, in detecting and acting on early signs of deterioration	7,9,10
Describe the role and practice of infection prevention and control and the potential signs of infection	8,9
Individual's nutritional status and the ways this impacts on their overall health and condition	7,9
Explain drug pathways and how medicines act	7,10
Describe the impact of an individual's physiological state on drug responses and safety	7,10
Explain pharmacodynamics, the role of drugs and their mechanisms of action in the body	7,10
Discuss medication in terms of risks versus benefits	7,10,13
Describe the role and function of the bodies that regulate and ensure the safety and effectiveness of medicines	7,10
Describe and discuss the management of adverse drug events	10

(Continued)

(Continued)

Explain the importance of consent with regard to administering medicines	10,13
Describe individual legal responsibility, personal accountability and regulatory requirements	3,4,7,8,9,10,13
Explain statutory requirements in relation to mental health	13,14,15
Describe and explain legislation that underpins practice relating to medicines	10
Explain the importance of the safe handling of medicines	10
Health promotion through the life course approach	11,12,13
Describe the genetic and genomic contribution to health and common disease	6,7,13
Explain the need to manage and organise workloads and the role of prioritising the delivery of care	3,7,9
Explain behaviour change concepts and skills in relation to health, wellbeing and self-care	7,9,11,12,13
Monitor and record nutritional status and discuss progress or change	4,9
Administer medicines safely and in a timely manner	10
Communicate and act on any concerns about or errors in the administering of medicines	10
Work within legal and ethical frameworks that underpin safe medicines management	10
Correctly and safely receive, store and dispose of medications	10
Use up-to-date information on medicines management and work within local and national policy guidelines	7,10
Use sound numeracy skills for medicines management, assessment, measuring, monitoring and recording	9,10
Use sound literacy skills to record and document accurately interventions	4,7,8,9,10,13,14
Work safely and effectively	All chapters
Engage collaboratively with a range of people and agencies	2,3,4,7,8,9,10,11,12,13,14,15
Treat individuals with dignity, respecting their diversity, beliefs, culture, needs, values, privacy and preferences	All chapters
Have the courage to challenge areas of concern	3,4, 8,9,10,14
Be adaptable, reliable and consistent, show discretion, resilience and self-awareness and provide leadership	3,4, 8,9,10,12,14,15
Promote and demonstrate a positive health and safety culture	3,8,9,12,15
Domain 4. Communication and inter-personal skills	
Explain the importance of clear and effective communication for person-centred care	1,2,3,4,8,9,10,12,13,14,15
Duty of care, candour, equality and diversity	3,4,8,9,10,14
Promote clear and effective communication	1,2,3,4,8,9,10,12,13,14,15

Overcome barriers to clear and effective communication	All chapters
Impact of verbal and nonverbal communication	2,4,9
Communicate complex, sensitive information to a variety of health and care professionals	3,4,8,9,10,13,14
Respond appropriately to verbal and nonverbal communication	4,9,10
Promote and use appropriate digital and other technologies to support effective communication	4,9,10,14,15
Document nursing care in a comprehensive, timely, logical, accurate, clear and concise manner	4,9,10,13,14,15
Promote effective communication using a range of techniques and technologies	All chapters
Domain 5. Team-working and leadership	
Describe the personal qualities required to develop leadership competencies	2,3,4,8,14
Critically reflect on performance to identify one's own personal qualities	2,3,4,8,14
Explain the importance of working with others in teams and networks to deliver and improve services	2,3,4,8,11,14
Discuss models of leadership	2,3
Describe the role of technological innovations in improving health outcomes for individuals	9,10
Critically examine supervisory and leadership opportunities and roles	2,3,4,9,10,14
Explain the ways health and safety systems and policies can be developed, monitored and assessed	3,8,9,10
Take a lead with peers and others where appropriate	2,3,9,10
Critically reflect on personal performance	2,3,4,9
Work effectively with others in teams and/or networks to deliver and improve services, encouraging and valuing the contribution of all	2,3,4,9,10,12,13,14,15
Contribute to and support quality improvement and productivity initiatives within the workplace	3,4,9,10,14
Use clinical governance processes to maintain and improve nursing practice and standards of healthcare	3,8,9
Demonstrate team working and leadership skills in the provision of a healthy work environment	2,3,4,9,10
Actively encourage, and work within, a team environment, including multi-disciplinary teams	3,4,9,10,13,14,15
Engage in continuous service improvement for better health outcomes	2,3,4,9,10,13,14,15
Champion safe working practices and a culture that facilitates safety	3,8,9,10
Promote the contributions and co-production by individuals	2,3,4,9,10,13,14,15

(Continued)

(Continued)

Domain 6. Duty of care, candour, equality and diversity	
Take reasonable care to avoid acts or omissions which can reasonably be foreseen as likely to cause harm	3,8,9,10,14
Describe duty of candour and the ways this can be demonstrated in practice	3,8,9,10,14
Define harm and abuse and identify sources of support and guidance to inform appropriate action	3,8,9,10,13,14,15
Describe and critically discuss the importance of the basic rights and principles of dignity, equality, diversity, humanity and safeguarding	3,4,5,8,9,10,13,14,15
Describe the ways individuals can contribute to their own health and wellbeing	4,5,12,13
Duty of care, candour, cultural competence, equality and diversity	3,4,5,8,9,10,13,14,15
Challenge areas of concern using appropriate behaviours and communication methods	4,5,12,13,14
Recognise the signs of harm or abuse and act on this appropriately	9,14,15
Treat all individuals, carers and colleagues with dignity and respect for their diversity, beliefs, culture, needs, values, privacy	4,9,12,13,14,15
Safeguard and protect adults and children	9,14,15
Encourage and empower people to share in and shape decisions about their own treatment	7,9,10,13,14,15
Demonstrate respect, kindness, compassion and empathy for all individuals, carers and colleagues	3,7,9,10,13,14,15
Avoid making assumptions and recognise diversity and individual choice	3,5,7,9,10,13,14,15
Domain 7: Supporting learning and assessment in practice	
Explain and critically discuss core theories of learning	1,2
Describe the importance of feedback and the range of methods for giving and receiving feedback	1,2,3
Applying the skills of reflection to identify personal development needs	1,2,3,9,13
Acting as a self-motivated professional	1,2,3,9,13,14
Contributing to a culture that values CPD in recognising strengths	2,3
Act as a role model for ongoing learning and development of professional knowledge, skills and capabilities	2,3,4
Domain 8. Research, development and innovation	
Explain the importance of research, innovation and audit in improving the quality of patient safety	2,7,9,10
Governance and ethical frameworks	3,4
Evidence-based practice	1,2,3,9

The role of statutory and advisory regulatory bodies	3,4,9,10,13,14
Apply critical analytical skills in a research/audit/service improvement context	1,2,3
Demonstrate research awareness in evidence-based practice	1,2,3,7,8,9,

INDEX